Midwifery Practice: Critical Illness, Complications and Emergencies

Case Book

Case Book Series

This book is part of a new series of case books written for nursing and other allied health profession students. The books are designed to help students link theory and practice and provide an engaging and focused way to learn.

Titles published in this series:

Paramedics: From Street to Emergency Department Case Book
Sarah Fellows and Bob Fellows

Midwifery: Emergencies, Critical Illness and Incidents Case Book
Maureen Raynor, Jayne Marshall and Karen Jackson

Mental Health Nursing Case Book
Edited by Nick Wrycraft

Learning Disability Case Book
Edited by Bob Hallawell

Nursing the Acutely Ill Adult Case Book
Karen Page and Aiden McKinney

Perioperative Practice Case Book
Paula Strong and Suzanne Hughes

Visit www.openup.co.uk/casebooks for information and sample chapters from other books in the series.

Midwifery Practice: Critical Illness, Complications and Emergencies

Case Book

**Edited by
Maureen D. Raynor, Jayne E. Marshall
and Karen Jackson**

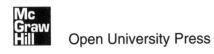

Open University Press

Open University Press
McGraw-Hill Education
McGraw-Hill House
Shoppenhangers Road
Maidenhead
Berkshire
England
SL6 2QL

email: enquiries@openup.co.uk
world wide web: www.openup.co.uk

and Two Penn Plaza, New York, NY 10121-2289, USA

First published 2012

A catalogue record of this book is available from the British Library

ISBN-13: 978-0-33-524273-3 (pb)
ISBN-10: 0-33-524273-1 (pb)
eISBN: 978-0-33-524274-0

Library of Congress Cataloging-in-Publication Data
CIP data applied for

Typesetting and e-book compilations by
RefineCatch Limited, Bungay, Suffolk
Printed and bound in the UK by Bell & Bain Ltd, Glasgow

Fictitious names of companies, products, people, characters and/or data that may be used herein (in case studies or in examples) are not intended to represent any real individual, company, product or event.

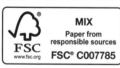
MIX
Paper from
responsible sources
FSC® C007785

The **McGraw·Hill** Companies

Parents are our role model to whom we would like to devote much praise. Maureen would like to thank her mother, Daphne, for being such a strength and for her words of encouragement during the evolution of *Midwifery Practice: Critical Illness, Complications and Emergencies Case Book*.

Jayne and Karen, on the other hand, wish to dedicate the book to their parents who have sadly died in recent years but who were the inspiration for them to pursue their academic careers in Midwifery Education and Practice. Without them all, such a project would never have come to fruition: to Colin and Mabel Marshall and Donald and Jean Jackson.

Contents

List of figures

List of tables

Contributors

ABOUT THE EDITORS

Maureen D. Raynor, MA, RMN, RN, RM, ADM, PGCEA, SOM, is employed by Nottingham University (City campus), Academic Division of Midwifery, where she works as a midwifery lecturer. She is also a supervisor of midwives, supporting both independent and NHS-based midwives. Maureen undertakes clinical practice on a weekly basis on the local Labour Suite and Maternity Assessment Suite, where she is link/liaison lecturer. This affords collaborative working opportunities with midwives and other disciplines. Her specialist interests including research are psychosocial issues, perinatal mental health/illness, intrapartum care, critical care, perineal care and developing/maintaining competence in new skills. She convenes the 'Best Practice' learning beyond registration module in perineal care offered at both Masters and first degree level, and is one of the named module leaders for the high dependency care course. Maureen is a member of Nottinghamshire Perinatal Mental Health Management Network Group, Partnership in Maternity Service (PIMS), i.e. the local Maternity Services Liaison Committee, United Kingdom and Northern Ireland Marcé Society (UKIMS), and a member of the local labour suite forum and management groups. Her publications have included journal articles, book chapters and popular midwifery text books which she has co-edited/co-authored, namely: *Decision Making in Midwifery Practice* and *Advancing Skills in Midwifery Practice* published by Elsevier, and *Psychology for Midwives* published by Open University Press. She also acts as a peer reviewer for *Midwifery* journal.

Jayne E. Marshall, PhD, MA, RN, RM, ADM, PGCEA, an experienced midwife and midwife lecturer, currently works at the University of Nottingham in the Academic Division of Midwifery, where she is Director of Learning Beyond Registration and Postgraduate Taught Courses (Midwifery) and Postgraduate Diploma/MSc in Midwifery. She has a particular interest in the complexities surrounding professional issues, law and ethics relating to midwifery practice and as well as facilitating modules at both undergraduate and postgraduate level, has written a number of publications in this area. She has co-edited the midwifery text books, *Decision Making in Midwifery Practice* and *Advancing Skills in Midwifery Practice* for Elsevier and has also contributed a number of chapters to the first edition of *Midwifery by Ten Teachers*, published by Hodder Arnold, adding to the established *Ten Teachers* series, popular among medical students. Jayne's first major piece of research involved evaluating the shared learning experiences of Pre-registration Diploma in Midwifery and Nursing students alongside the teachers of midwifery and nursing as part of her Masters degree at Loughborough University. In 2005, Jayne completed her PhD at the University of Nottingham by undertaking an ethnographic study examining informed consent during the intrapartum period through participant observation. Recently Jayne has completed a mixed methods study evaluating what effect the introduction of a work-based learning module, in a range of maternity settings, has had on the development of midwifery practice. Jayne is a member of the International Confederation of Midwives Research Standing Committee, the Research Advisory Network and the Education Advisory Network and as a member of the Royal College of Midwives since 1981, she also sits on the Ethics Advisory Committee. In addition, Jayne peer reviews for the ICM Congresses, the *Midwifery* journal and is an editorial board member of the new *International Journal of Childbirth* that was adopted by the ICM as its own journal at the 29th Congress in Durban.

Karen Jackson, MPhil, BSc (Hons), ADM, RM, RN, currently works at the University of Nottingham in the Academic Division of Midwifery, and is an experienced midwife and midwife lecturer. She has responsibility for pre-registration BMid (Hons) in Midwifery programmes and is module leader for Contraception and Sexual Health Modules for health care practitioners. She has a particular interest in all aspects of normal birth, including promoting normality and 'normalizing' more complicated cases, but is also a team member for the pre-registration 'complications and emergencies' modules, which enables a balanced approach to midwifery practice. Karen has written chapters in a number of textbooks including one on 'Sexuality' for the current *Mayes Midwifery* (Ballière Tindall). She has also had articles published widely on aspects of sexuality and childbirth, in various midwifery journals. Karen's first piece of research involved exploration of the role of the lecturer/practitioner in midwifery education and practice. In 2004, Karen completed her Master of Philosophy degree at the University of Nottingham by undertaking survey-based research on 'Aspects of sexuality and childbirth: Midwives' knowledge and attitudes'. Currently, Karen is studying for a doctorate by researching practices and decision-making in normal childbirth through a mixed methods approach. As part of her role as a midwife lecturer, Karen practises as a clinical midwife on the Queen's Medical Campus of Nottingham University Hospitals NHS Trust. Karen is a member of PIMS (Partnership in Maternity Service), i.e. the local Maternity Services Liaison Committee, and a member of the local labour suite forum and management groups. Karen is an active member of various research fora within the University of Nottingham. She is also a reviewer for the international peer-reviewed journal *Midwifery*.

ABOUT THE CONTRIBUTORS

Sam Bharmal, MB, BS, BMed Sci, FRCA, is a consultant anaesthetist and clinical lead for obstetric anaesthesia at the Queen's Medical Centre Campus of Nottingham University Hospitals NHS Trust. She has a number of specialist interests within education and training. These include maternity high dependency care, critical illness recognition and 'skills and drills' training of the multidisciplinary team. Sam has also contributed to a number of research initiatives such as the Comparative Obstetric Mobile Epidural Trial (COMET) Study Group UK that was published in *The Lancet* in 2001.

Susan Brydon, RN, RM, BSc (Hons), MSc, PGDipEd (Mid), Dip.Ap.Ssc, CertHp, Supervisor of Midwives (SOM), is employed by Nottingham University Hospitals NHS Trust. Susan is a senior midwife on the labour suite, and also works in the clinical education team, providing education to all grades of staff within the Family Health Division of the trust. Susan has a Diploma in Midwifery Education and contributes to undergraduate and postgraduate education. She also adds to the quality agenda by being an active member of the risk management committees and has been a Supervisor of Midwives since 1988. Her specialist interest is in developing and maintaining competence through education and training as well as the development of new skills. Susan has acted as an Expert Midwife in medico-legal cases for the past 18 years and has provided more than 500 reports for the Court.

Margaret M. Ramsay, MB, BChir, MA, MD, MRCP, FRCOG, is a consultant working in Fetomaternal Medicine at the Nottingham University Hospitals NHS Trust (Queen's Medical Centre campus). She has a particular interest in the care of women presenting with the complexities of medical conditions during pregnancy and has published widely in this area. Margaret is also passionate about the provision of obstetric high dependency care being effective among all members of the multidisciplinary team. She engages with the University of Nottingham, Academic Division of Midwifery in facilitating an annual module: *High Dependency Care of the Childbearing Woman*, to equip midwives for such an extended role.

Jane Rutherford, MBChB, DM, FRCOG, is a consultant obstetrician and subspecialist in Maternal Medicine at Nottingham University Hospitals NHS Trust. She runs a busy tertiary clinic for women with medical disorders in pregnancy and has particular interests in both medical disorders in pregnancy and in intrapartum care.

Andrew Simm, MD, MRCP, FRCOG, is a consultant obstetrician who practises at Nottingham University Hospitals NHS Trust (City campus). His special interests are maternal and fetal medicine, diabetes mellitus and intrapartum care. He co-chairs both the labour suite forum and the regular labour suite management meetings. He is also a member of the encephalopathy and clinical governance committees.

List of abbreviations

AAGBI	Association of Anaesthetists of Great Britain and Ireland
ABCDE	airway, breathing, circulation, disability, exposure/environment or secondary but more detailed examination
ACCP	American College of Chest Physicians
aCL	anticardiolipin antibodies
ACOG	American College of Obstetricians and Gynecologists
ADH	anti-diuretic hormone
AFE	amniotic fluid embolism
ALERT	acute life-threatening events recognition and treatment
ALT	alanine aminotransferase
APA	antiphospholipid antibodies
APEC	Action on Pre-Eclampsia
APH	antepartum haemorrhage
APS	antiphospholipid syndrome
APTT	activated partial thromboplastin time (see partial thromboplastin time [PTT])
ARDS	adult respiratory distress syndrome
ARM	artificial rupture of the membranes
ART	assisted reproductive therapy
AST	aspartate aminotransferase
AVPU	Alert, responds to Voice, responds to Pain or Unresponsive
BMI	body mass index
BP	blood pressure
BPM	beats per minute
BS	blood sugar
CAPS	catastrophic antiphospholipid syndrome
CEMACH	Confidential Enquiries into Maternal and Child Health (became CMACE in 2008)
CEO	Chief Executive Officer
CMACE	Centre for Maternal and Child Enquiries
CNST	Clinical Negligence Scheme for Trusts
COC	combined oral contraceptive
CPR	cardiopulmonary resuscitation
CQC	Care Quality Commission
CS	caesarean section
CT	computed tomography
CTG	cardiotocograph/cardiotocography

CVA	cerebral vascular accident (stroke)
CVP	central venous pressure
CVS	cardiovascular system
CXR	chest X-ray
DH	Department of Health
DIC	disseminated intravascular coagulation
DKA	diabetic ketoacidosis
DVT	deep vein thrombosis
EAACI	The European Academy of Allergology and Clinical Immunology
EBL	estimated blood loss
ECG	electrocardiogram
ED	Emergency Department
EFM	electronic fetal monitoring
EWS	early warning systems
FBC	full blood count
FDG	fibrin degradation products
FH/FHR	fetal heart/fetal heart rate
FHH	fetal heart heard
FSE	fetal scalp electrode
GAS	group A *Streptococcus*
GCS	Glasgow Coma Scale
GDG	Guideline Development Group (part of NICE)
GI	gastro-intestinal
GP	general practitioner.
Gp & S	group and save (serum)
Hb	haemoglobin
HCC	Health Care Commission (now replaced by CQC)
HELLP (syndrome)	haemolysis, elevated liver enzymes and low platelets
HFEA	Human Fertilisation and Embryology Authority
HIV	human immunodeficiency virus
HPL	human placental lactogen
HR	heart rate
IA	intermittent auscultation
ICM	International Confederation of Midwives
ICP	intrahepatic cholestasis of pregnancy
ICU	intensive care unit
IgE	immunoglobulin E
IM	intramuscular
INR	international normalized ratio
IOL	induction of labour
IPL/E	interprofessional learning/education
IUCD	intra-uterine contraceptive device
IUFD	intra-uterine fetal death
IUGR	intra-uterine growth restriction
IV/IVI	intravenous/intravenous infusion

IVIG	intravenous immunoglobulin
LA	lupus anticoagulant
LFTs	liver function tests
LMWH	low molecular weight heparin
LOA	left occipito anterior
LSCS	lower segment caesarean section
MAP	mean arterial pressure
MEOWS	Modified Early Obstetric Warning Score
MLU	midwifery-led unit
MODS	multiple organ dysfunction syndrome
MOET	managing obstetric emergencies and trauma
MRI	magnetic resonance imaging
NAD	nothing abnormal detected/no abnormalities detected
NCEPOD	National Confidential Enquiry into Patient Outcome and Death
NHS	National Health Service
NHSLA	National Health Service Litigation Authority
NICE	National Institute for Health and Clinical Excellence
NICU	neonatal intensive care unit
NMC	Nursing and Midwifery Council
NND	Neonatal Death
NPSA	National Patient Safety Agency
NRLS	National Reporting Learning System
NSAID	non-steroidal anti-inflammatory drug
NUH	Nottingham University Hospitals
OBPPI	obstetric brachial plexus palsy injury
OHSS	ovarian hyperstimulation syndrome
OSCE	objective structured clinical examination
P	pulse
PAPS	primary antiphospholipid syndrome
PCA	patient-controlled analgesia
PCT	Primary Care Trust
PE	pulmonary embolism
POP	progesterone only pill
PPH	postpartum haemorrhage
PPROM	pre-term pre-labour rupture of the membranes
PRECOG	pre-eclampsia community guideline
PTT	partial thromboplastin time
PV	per vaginam
RBC	red blood cells
RCA	Royal College of Anaesthetists
RCM	Royal College of Midwives
RCOG	Royal College of Obstetricians and Gynaecologists
RCPCH	Royal College of Paediatrics and Child Health
RCT	randomized controlled trial
RCUK	Resuscitation Council UK
ROA	right occiput anterior

ROL	right occipito lateral
ROSC	return of spontaneous circulation
RR	respiratory rate
SaFE	simulation and fire-drill evaluation
SANDS	Stillbirth and Neonatal Death Society
SAPS	secondary antiphospholipid syndrome
SBAR	Situation, Background, Assessment and Recommendation
SC	subcutaneous
SD	standard deviation
SIGN	Scottish Intercollegiate Guidelines Network
SIRS	systemic inflammatory response syndrome
SLE	systemic lupus erythematosus
SPD	symphysis pubis dysfunction
SPFH	symphysis pubis fundal height
SROM	spontaneous rupture of membranes
SSC	Surviving Sepsis Campaign
ST	Speciality trainee
SUI	serious untoward incident
T	temperature
TEDS	thromboembolic deterrent stockings
Temp	temperature
TPR	temperature, pulse, respiration
TVS	transvaginal scan
U & Es	urea and electrolytes
UDCA	ursodeoxycholic acid
UFH	unfractionated heparin
UK	United Kingdom
US/USS	ultrasound/ultrasound scan
UTI	urinary tract infection
VE	vaginal examination
VF	ventricular fibrillation
VKA	vitamin K antagonist
VTE	venous thromboembolism
WAO	World Allergy Organization
WBC	white blood cells
WCC	white cell count
XR	X-ray

Introduction
Maureen D. Raynor, Jayne E. Marshall and Karen Jackson

Globally the context of pregnancy and birth yields high morbidity and mortality figures. In the United Kingdom alone, 261 women lost their lives as a direct or indirect consequence of pregnancy, resulting in an overall maternal mortality rate of 11.39 per 100,000 maternities as reported by CMACE for the triennium 2006–2008 (CMACE 2011). Sepsis, pre-eclampsia and thromboembolic disorders are highlighted as the leading causes of maternal deaths in the UK. Tragically, it also brings to the fore the startling reality that in 70 per cent of direct deaths and 50 per cent of indirect deaths, care was substandard. A strong body of evidence points to the failure of staff to predict and recognize clinical deterioration. Coupled with this there is often delayed communication, not acting promptly or ignoring early warning signs and not informing/involving senior staff in a timely manner when an emergency or critical illness manifests (SIGN 2004; NCEPOD 2005; NPSA 2007; NICE 2007, 2008; DH 2009). These issues are also recurrent themes in the current and previous triennial reports (Lewis and Drife 2004; Lewis 2007; CMACE 2011).

Clearly, the key to preventing such devastating outcomes in pregnancy, labour and puerperium is the early recognition of critical illness in the childbearing woman in order to make a swift response, timely referral and achieve high quality care based on sound evidence. Care should be implemented by knowledgeable and skilled members of the multidisciplinary team, well rehearsed in the treatment of maternity emergencies and critical illness.

In pregnancy two lives are at stake – mother and baby. Hence the critically ill pregnant woman poses a unique set of challenges and complexity to midwives, obstetricians, anaesthetists and the wider interprofessional team. Pregnancy is deemed to be a state of altered health. The pregnant woman for the most part will still be in the flush of youth. Assessment of any deviation from normality during pregnancy must consider the physiological parameters. However, the physiological reserve and compensatory mechanisms of pregnancy make diagnosis difficult and conspire in preventing many of the classic signs and symptoms associated with the onset of critical illness from being recognized early and acted upon judiciously. This makes the pregnant woman vulnerable. Midwives and doctors should comprehend that the relative youthfulness of childbearing women and any ensuing morbidity culminating in maternal demise will be catastrophic. The ripple effect such devastation has is profound, not only for the immediate family but for all health care professionals involved in the woman's care.

The Northwick Park report by the former Health Care Commission (2006) and successive reports on the confidential enquiries into maternal deaths in the UK (Lewis and Drife 2004; Lewis 2007; CMACE 2011) have all emphasized the importance of effective team work in achieving optimal outcomes for mothers and babies.

ABOUT THIS BOOK

Midwifery Practice: Critical Illness, Complications and Emergencies Case Book is the result of a collaborative effort between midwifery lecturers, supervisors of midwives, obstetricians and anaesthetists, all grounded in practice and actively involved as key professionals in the management of maternity emergencies, critical illness and interdisciplinary skills and drills training relating to these issues. The book editors and chapter contributors therefore have the specialist knowledge, experience and enhanced skills to write authoritatively about each of the featured topics.

To the best of the editors' knowledge, the book is the first of its kind in midwifery that employs purely a case study approach as a platform in locating the exploration of the key issues relating to maternity emergencies and critical illness. A wide gamut of pathophysiology unique to pregnancy that may have grave sequelae are addressed. These include pre-eclampsia, eclampsia, thromboembolic disorder, H E L L P syndrome, disseminated intravascular coagulation, obstetric cholestasis, haemoglobinopathy crisis, haemorrhage, uterine rupture and inversion as well as anaphylaxis, sepsis, cardiac arrest and diabetic coma. The safety of mothers and babies in midwifery practice is the guiding principle of care. Risk assessment/management as part of a broader clinical governance strategy is of importance in health care. Risk assessment aids risk identification, early recognition of critical illness or complications likely to result in full-blown emergencies, which ultimately culminates in improved outcomes in practice. The education and training of midwives and doctors in the recognition and prompt response to emergencies and critical illness are paramount to stemming maternal morbidity and mortality. It is for these reasons that the decision was made to include a chapter on risk management and recognition of the critically ill woman.

Midwifery Practice: Critical Illness, Complications and Emergencies Case Book is essential reading for midwifery and medical students as well as midwives interested in high level care in order to build capacity and confidence at assessing, responding and evaluating acute conditions that may arise in practice. The book will assist with the honing of knowledge and skills in the recognition of critical illness, complications and generally women needing high dependency care. The book will also act as a valuable resource to paramedics as they are in the vanguard of care attending to emergency calls in the community setting.

Recognition of the critically ill woman has been included as a chapter rather than a case study as the content resonates with all the cases reflected in the book. It is suggested that this initial section and Case 2 are read first before exploring the rest of the cases presented in the book.

THE CASE STUDIES

With the exception of recognition of the critically ill woman, a standard approach to each case study is adopted, which includes pre-reading and self-assessment, allowing readers to test their knowledge on what they already know before engaging with the case studies. Summary boxes of key learning points are included as are text boxes, tables and figures to generate interest for the reader. However, due to the nature of some topics, a number of cases are combined and have two or three sections or additions to the case scenario to demonstrate how an initial complication can trigger a cascade of events, such as pre-eclampsia and

HELLP syndrome (Case 3). This will give the impression that some cases are more detailed in length than others, but the reader should bear in mind that this is done deliberately to illustrate the complexities of some conditions, ensure fluidity and to demonstrate that some factors are inextricably linked.

Where appropriate, copyright permission has been sought to reproduce evidence-based guidelines and algorithms to aid clarity and accessibility of salient points raised in the text.

Although the case studies are based loosely on clinical encounters and experience garnered over the years, the women in the case studies are given fictitious names and each of the case scenarios depicted has been altered to uphold the ethical considerations of confidentiality and anonymity.

For ease of reference throughout the book, the midwife is referred to by employing the feminine pronoun. However, it is acknowledged that there are also male midwives. Therefore, the male midwife is also inferred whenever the term midwife is used.

REFERENCES

CMACE (2011) *Saving Mothers' Lives: Reviewing Maternal Deaths to Make Motherhood Safer: 2006–2008. The Eighth Report of the Confidential Enquiries into Maternal Deaths in the United Kingdom.* Ed. G. Lewis. *BJOG: An International British Journal of Obstetrics and Gynaecology*, 118 (Suppl. 1): 1–203.

Department of Health (DH) (2009) *Competencies for Recognising and Responding to Acutely Ill Patients in Hospital.* Available at: http://www.dh.gov.uk/en/Publicationsandstatistics/Publications/PublicationsPolicyAndGuidance/DH_096989 (accessed 12 May 2011).

Health Care Commission (2006) *Investigation into 10 Maternal Deaths at, or Following Delivery at Northwick Park Hospital, Northwest London Hospitals NHS Trust between April 2002–April 2005.* Available at: http://www.cqc.org.uk. (accessed 10 May 2011).

Lewis, G. (ed.) (2007) *The Confidential Enquiry into Maternal and Child Health (CEMACH). Saving Mothers' Lives: Reviewing Maternal Deaths to Make Motherhood Safer, 2003–2005. The Seventh Report on Confidential Enquiries into Maternal Deaths in the United Kingdom.* London: CEMACH.

Lewis, G. and Drife, J. (eds) (2004) *Why Mothers Die: 2000–2002: The Sixth Report of the Confidential Enquiries into Maternal Deaths in the United Kingdom.* London: Royal College of Obstetricians and Gynaecologists.

National Confidential Enquiry into Patient Outcome and Death (2005) *An Acute Problem.* London: NCEPOD. Available at: http://www.ncepod.org.uk/2005aap.htm (accessed 10 May 2011).

National Institute for Health and Clinical Excellence (2007) *Acutely Ill Patients in Hospital: Recognition of and Response to Acute Illness in Adults in Hospital.* London: NICE. Available at: http://www.nice.org.uk/Guidance/CG50 (accessed 10 May 2011).

National Institute for Health and Clinical Excellence (2008) *Surgical Site Infection.* London: NICE. Available at: http://www.nice.org.uk/nicemedia/pdf/CG74FullGuideline.pdf (accessed 10 May 2011).

National Patient Safety Agency (2007) *Safer Care for the Acutely Ill Patient: Learning from Serious Incidents.* London: NPSA. Available at: http://www.npsa.nhs.uk/nrls/alerts-and-directives/directives-guidance/acutely-ill-patient/ (accessed 10 May 2011).

Scottish Intercollegiate Guidelines Network (SIGN) (2004) *Postoperative Management in Adults.* Edinburgh: SIGN. Available at: http://www.sign.ac.uk/pdf/sign77.pdf (accessed 10 May 2011).

ANNOTATED FURTHER READING

Maternal Critical Care Working Group (2011) *Providing Equity of Critical and Maternity Care for the Critically Ill Pregnant or Recently Pregnant Woman.* London: RCOA.

Provides useful background reading for the remainder of the book.

CASE STUDY 1
Recognition of the critically ill woman
Maureen D. Raynor

Pre-requisites for the chapter: the reader should have an understanding of:

- Normal physiological parameters of vital signs and haemodynamic monitoring in pregnancy.
- The physiological changes during pregnancy in all major bodily systems.
- Systematic assessment tools used to aid early recognition and mobilize rapid response to critical illness, namely ABCDE and AVPU methods.
- Basic and advanced cardiopulmonary resuscitation of mother and neonate.

Pre-reading self-assessment

Outline the adaptive changes that occur in the following maternal bodily systems to meet the increased metabolic demands of the mother/fetus and developing placenta:

1 respiratory
2 cardiovascular
3 gastrointestinal
4 renal/urinary.

Recommended prior reading

Billington, M. and Stevenson, M. (eds) (2007) *Critical Care in Childbearing for Midwives.* Oxford: Blackwell.
Maternal Critical Care Working Group (2011) *Providing Equity of Critical and Maternity Care for the Critically Ill Pregnant or Recently Pregnant Woman.* London: RCOA. Available at: http://www.oaa-anaes.ac.uk/assets/_managed/editor/File/RCoA/Prov_Eq_MatandCritCare.pdf
Mulyran, C. (2011) *Acute Illness Management.* London: Sage.
National Institute for Health and Clinical Excellence (NICE) (2007) *Acutely Ill Patients in Hospitals: Recognition of and Response to Acute Illness in Adults in Hospital.* CG50. London: NICE. Available at: http://www.nice.org.uk

BACKGROUND

Although midwives are the perceived guardians of and experts in normality, they are key public health professionals at the forefront of care charged with risk identification and timely referral to their medical colleagues of any deviation from normality (NMC 2004).

The Centre for Maternal and Child Enquiries (CMACE) (CMACE 2011) acknowledges that suboptimal care plays a significant part in a number of the maternal deaths reported in the UK, such as failure to recognize the onset of critical illness until it is too late. Yet, increasingly women with co-morbidities requiring specialist care choose to become pregnant, presenting the midwifery profession with a number of challenges. Critical care in midwifery practice is complex, requiring the midwife to gain additional skills to detect and assist with the care of women presenting with life-threatening conditions. Midwives have to be adequately prepared to rise to such a global challenge in being able to recognize critical illness. This is best realized via an interprofessional approach (Department of Health 2000, 2009; RCOG et al. 2007; RCOG 2008).

Against this background, a lack of critical care skills among student midwives, especially undergraduates from a non-nursing background, has been fiercely debated: a phenomenon not unique to midwifery. Similar criticism has been raised in nursing (Bench 2007; Kyriacos et al. 2011). The international definition of a midwife as identified by the ICM (2005) highlights the far-reaching responsibilities of the midwife. This includes prevention and detection of ensuing complications in mother/fetus/neonate coupled with timely referral for appropriate medical attention. The midwife is also required to undertake emergency measures when necessary.

In order to prepare student midwives to embrace their future autonomous, accountable role as practising midwives, the NMC (2009) sets the standards for the pre-registration midwifery programme that institutions of higher education must ensure students achieve. One such standard is to develop knowledge and skills in the recognition of critical illness and management of maternity emergencies.

A case scenario specific to this chapter has not been included as the issues raised are transferable to all the subsequent cases.

RECOGNITION OF ACUTE CRITICAL ILLNESS IN PREGNANCY

Acute critical illness in pregnancy covers a wide spectrum of disorders and fundamentally relates to any condition that seriously compromises the health and well-being of mother and baby that may ultimately result in death. Critically ill pregnant women vary considerably from non-pregnant adults who are gravely ill. Most illness encountered in everyday life is self-limiting in nature and poses minimal threat to the well-being of healthy individuals. However, if the cause of the illness is serious, it can disrupt physiological parameters leading to derangement of factors that would normally regulate homeostasis. In the pregnant woman such illnesses can escalate into a life-threatening or critical state that soon exhausts physiological reserves. Moreover, the physiological changes that occur in each system of the body during pregnancy may undermine the physiological responses needed to fight an acute illness, e.g. sepsis (Clutton-Brock 2011).

There are some conditions that are completely unique to pregnancy and bring their own set of complications for midwives and the wider interprofessional team. The complex physiological changes may not always be acknowledged as speedily as they should. A pregnant woman, for example, can quickly lose a litre of her circulating blood volume at term without showing any signs of compromise associated with hypovolaemia, as would be expected if the woman was not pregnant (Case 12) (Johanson et al. 2003; Grady et al. 2007). Early recognition of critical illness, timely referral and prompt response are therefore the cornerstones to safe-guarding the health and well-being of mother and baby.

Causes of acute critical illness in pregnancy

The reasons for women becoming acutely ill during pregnancy are manifold. These women, for simplicity's sake, can be categorized as those presenting with pregnancy-related complications and those who have pre-existing illness or co-morbidities. Examples of each category are outlined in Box 1.1.

Box 1.1 Some risk factors for critical illness in pregnancy

Women with pregnancy-related complications	Women with pre-existing co-morbidities
Antepartum/postpartum haemorrhage	Diabetes mellitus
Chorioamnionitis	Obesity
Acute fatty liver of pregnancy	Cardiomyopathy
Retained placenta	Renal disease
Puerperal sepsis	Haematological disorder
Pre-eclampsia/eclampsia and HELLP syndrome	Haemoglobinopathy
	Anaemia
Amniotic fluid embolism	Epilepsy
Venous thromboembolism	HIV infection

Women admitted to hospital presenting with marked physiological derangements affecting organ function, such as the cardiovascular, respiratory, neurological and renal systems, are likely to have been displaying clinical features of imminent life-threatening illness in the preceding hours (Stubbe 2006; Carrington and Down 2009; Jansen and Cuthbertson 2010). Women who are critically ill can be grouped as:

1 those with unstable conditions with the potential to progress to rapid deterioration, e.g. haemorrhage, pre-eclampsia and sepsis
2 those with marked physiological derangements leading to shock, cardiac or respiratory arrest (Cases 10–12).

Clinical features suggestive of critical illness

The clinical features of a critical illness are marked out by failing organ systems (Mitchell 2010). Therefore, the initial assessment performed by the midwife or doctor helps to identify the early warning signs of such an illness. Recognition of critical illness ensures intervention and escalation of care, which aims to significantly improve outcomes for mothers and babies. While emergencies and complications that may arise in midwifery practice may prove complex and perplexing to the novice midwife, effective care consists of having the ability and skills to employ very simple measures such as the ABCDE method of assessment. Box 1.2, adapted from Grady et al. (2007), highlights some of the features suggestive of clinical deterioration in the pregnant woman and the clinical features indicative of physiological compensation.

Box 1.2 Features suggestive of underlying critical illness and physiological compensation

Features suggestive of underlying critical illness	Features suggestive of physiological compensation
• Tachypnoea – RR > 20 breaths per min. • Restricted/obstructed airway. • Tachycardia P > 120 bpm. • ↓ Urine output < 0.5 mL/kg/hour consecutively. • Desaturation O_2 SATS < 95%. • Prolonged capillary refill time > 2 seconds. • Marked changes in systolic BP (< 90 or MAP < 65). • CVP reading > 10 or < 1.	Tachycardia – HR ↑ due to ↑ myocardial pump. Hb O_2 desaturation – O_2 is released more readily from the haem component of RBC. Oliguria – ↓ blood flow to kidneys → Na + H_2O retention. Cool and/or cyanosed peripheries – due to vasoconstriction. Circulatory volume maintained for a while as blood is diverted from the splenic capsule (see Case 12). Hyperglycaemia. Net result → metabolic acidosis.

Skills of assessment and monitoring

Recognition of critical illness, whatever the cause, starts with basic assessment and monitoring of vital signs or physiological observations. It is important to start initial assessment with careful history taking (Mitchell 2010).

A thorough systematic assessment of vital signs and level of consciousness will reveal changes in cardiovascular, neurological and respiratory function. The physiological parameters, as defined by NICE (2007), that should be considered in the event of a suspected critical illness and are a key component in any assessment plan are:

• heart rate
• respiratory rate
• systolic BP
• core body temperature.

Detailed history should consider common signs and symptoms of underlying life-threatening conditions such as haemorrhage, venous thromboembolism (VTE), shock or infection, as outlined in Figure 1.1.

Check for signs of organ dysfunction, especially if there is evidence of underlying infection as this could signify sepsis. A thorough examination of the woman is essential. Laboratory investigations such as those listed in Box 1.3 may be requested by the medical team.

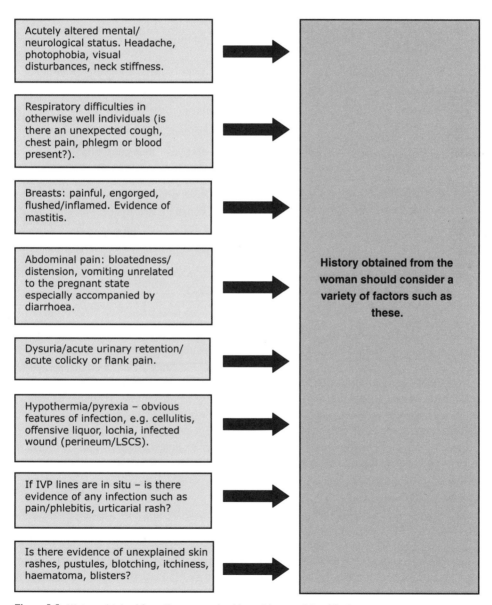

Figure 1.1 History obtained from the woman should consider a variety of factors

Box 1.3 Thorough examination required

- Need for O_2 therapy to maintain O_2 SATS > 90%
- INR > 1.5 or APTT > 60 seconds
- Lactate > 2 mmol/L
- Bilirubin > 4 mg/dL or 70 mmol/L
- Alkaline phosphatase level > 250 units per litre
- Platelets < 100 × 10^9/L

Changes in systolic BP and hourly urine measurements previously outlined.

Physiological and biochemical clinical signs of critical illness	
Biochemical features	Elevated or lowered WBC
	Reduced platelets
	Evidence of metabolic acidosis
	Elevated C-reactive protein concentration
	Elevated urea and creatinine levels
Physiological features	Systemic inflammation (see sepsis case study)
	Extremes of body temperature i.e. hyperthermia or hypothermia
	Tachypnoea
	Tachycardia

A systematic physiologically-based and effective approach to assessment and monitoring that aids the early recognition of the mother who is developing a critical illness is crucial. The ABCDE method of assessment, as outlined by Figure 1.2, highlighted by ALERT (2011), RCUK (2010) and Smith (2003) to respond to advanced cardiopulmonary life support and trauma, provides a simple tool for pattern recognition of critical illness. It should be ubiquitously employed by midwives and other members of the interprofessional team. The ABCDE approach underpins most of the case studies throughout this book. It is presented here as it forms the key to assessing women who display signs of illness. The ABCDE acronym is Airway, Breathing, Circulation, Disability, Exposure/Environment or secondary but more detailed Examination.

Airway

Any sudden maternal deterioration warrants the woman's airway being checked to detect signs of obstruction. If the woman is sitting up in bed and talking, this does not necessarily signify that all is well. A woman with early clinical features of sepsis, for example, may appear initially well.

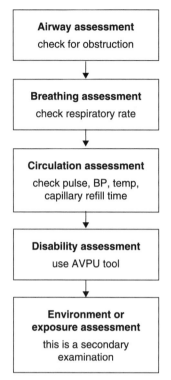

Figure 1.2 ABCDE systematic approach to assessment

Source: Adapted from ALERT (2011).

Check point

Adapted from Grady et al. (2007):

- Look, listen and feel for signs of obstruction.
- Use a head tilt or chin lift (see Case 12) where necessary to ensure adequate oxygenation.
- Pregnant women present a number of difficulties for airway management, e.g. the woman needs to be inclined laterally to secure airways, suction or remove foreign bodies.

Breathing

Respiratory rate is one of the most useful physiological parameters to be assessed as an increase in this most crucial measurement is telling of a developing or underlying critical illness (Grady et al. 2007); the woman's pattern of breathing will be influenced by a host of factors.

Think

Is the woman displaying any of the following conditions?

- asthmatic
- in pain
- anxious/frightened
- affected by opiate analgesia
- suffering from upper respiratory tract infection.

An increasing respiratory rate is an objective sign compared to shortness of breath, a more subjective symptom, as it may indicate pathogenesis in the cardiopulmonary system such as shock (Stubbe 2006). If the RR is > 20 breaths per minute, there should be cause for unease and the midwife should convey her concerns to the medical team. She should also try and determine the cause for the increase in respirations. RR > 24 breaths per min. should ring alarm bells and could prove life-threatening.

The rise and fall of the woman's chest movements should be observed and counted. The symmetry and depth of chest movements should be noted. Carrington and Down (2009) state that tachypnoea is a sensitive marker in the onset of critical illness. This, they state, may be the body's way of normalizing underlying metabolic acidosis associated with poor tissue perfusion. High concentration of oxygen therapy might be necessary. Pulse oximetry should be used to vigilantly monitor the woman's oxygen saturation levels.

Laboured respirations, air hunger/gasping for breath, sounds of grunting, wheezing or crackling should be promptly reported to the medical staff to enable timely implementation of remedial treatment. Emergency equipment such as an adult airway, suction apparatus, bag and mask, oxygen and appropriate drugs must be readily available.

Monitoring respiratory rate is particularly important as this is the first vital sign to be compromised in the development of any acute critical illness (SIGN 2004; NCEPOD 2005; NICE 2007; NPSA 2007). Notably, from experience, this is the area that midwives are most inconsistent in measuring. Care of the acutely ill pregnant woman will be premised on assessment, monitoring and ongoing evaluation of the effectiveness of each care intervention on maternal and fetal well-being implemented by the interprofessional team.

Check point

Due to the physiological changes in the respiratory system during pregnancy, the gravid uterus poses a number of difficulties (Grady et al. 2007):

Raised diaphragm + splayed ribs = restricted CPR.

Circulation

Assess circulation by checking:

- Is the woman shivery?
- Is she hot, cold, sweaty and clammy to touch?

Check the colour of her skin and extremities to detect any changes, e.g. pallor, ashen or cyanosed. Measure and record key vital signs, i.e. temperature, pulse, respirations (TPR) and blood pressure (BP). Tachycardia and changes to BP and temperature may signify a sympathetic response (Grady et al. 2007). If the BP is significantly lowered, the medical team may prescribe a fluid challenge and vasopressin.

Hypovolaemia may lead to hypoperfusion of vital organs and tissue hypoxaemia. This may manifest as hypotension, oliguria, cold and cyanosed peripheries as well as confusion or even coma (Carrington and Down 2009).

Check point

Due to the physiological changes in the cardiovascular system (CVS) during pregnancy, anticipate the following challenges (Grady et al. 2007):

- External cardiac massage is difficult to perform as left lateral tilt is needed to avoid aorto-caval compression (Case 12).
- Obesity might also be evident with significant breast hypertrophy.

Disability

It is important to assess for early signs of disability using the AVPU tool (Cases 10 and 11). Blood glucose measurement at the bedside using a glucometer is also important as outlined in Cases 10, 11 and 13.

Exposure–environment–examination

This is seen as a top-to-toe and front-to-back secondary assessment to aid decision making and planning (ALERT 2011). A detailed account of this aspect of the ABCDE tool is provided in Case 10.

Evaluate

Critical thinking and clinical judgement are paramount when using the ABCDE method of assessment. It is important not to progress from the initial stage of the assessment tool to the next step until the first one is adequately addressed. Evaluation of the thoroughness and effectiveness of each step of the assessment process should be done regularly. The woman may continue to deteriorate despite well-intended care intervention(s) or as a direct result of the treatment (Smith 2003). Call for help sooner rather than later whenever a critical illness is suspected.

Neurological status

Assess whether the woman is anxious or restless. Use the *AVPU* assessment tool (*Alert*, responds to *Voice*, responds to *Pain* or *Unresponsive*) outlined in Case 10 to determine if she has a lowered level of consciousness, is alert or confused. *P* and *U* values should be reported immediately to a senior doctor (see Case 12). Level of consciousness may necessitate additional monitoring, e.g. hourly urine output, pain assessment and biochemical analysis (blood glucose, lactate, base excess and arterial pH).

Resuscitation

The main goal of resuscitation is to restore normal organ function speedily, especially the vital centres such as the brain, heart, lungs, kidneys, gut and liver (Mitchell 2010). The main aims of this stage can be achieved through appropriate goal-directed therapy such as the *resuscitation* and *management* sepsis bundles identified in Case 11.

TRACK AND TRIGGER SYSTEMS OR EARLY WARNING SCORES

Because physiological deterioration or significant changes in vital signs often precede critical illness, use of a track and trigger system as recommended by NICE (2007), e.g. the MEOWS chart (see Case 2) helps in the timely recognition of potentially life-threatening conditions.

Successive reports on the Confidential Enquiries into Maternal Deaths in the UK (Lewis 2007; CMACE 2011) recommend use of the MEOWS tool to aid better recognition of early warning signs of impending maternal collapse and detection of life-threatening conditions such as amniotic fluid embolism (AFE), eclampsia and haemorrhage. The MEOWS system is adopted by many obstetric-led maternity units to aid in the early identification of the woman at risk of deterioration. As highlighted by NICE (2007) and SIGN (2004), detailed assessment should account for the following:

- Intelligent and consistent approach to monitoring and recording observations.
- Recognition of early signs of deterioration.
- Communicating with senior colleagues and accurate documentation of observations causing concern.
- Escalating concerns and making appropriate and rapid response to early signs of deterioration.

Early warning systems (EWS) or track and trigger systems are reported to have a high specificity but a low sensitivity and predictive value; hence their validity and reliability have been questioned (McGaughey et al. 2007; Jansen and Cuthbertson 2010; Kyriacos et al. 2011). Although there is no robust evidence base that identifies which of the EWS is the best fit for use in maternity care, CMACE (Lewis 2007; CMACE 2011) suggest that the MEOWS chart, purposefully adapted to meet the needs of childbearing women, adds value. A systematic approach to assessing and recording vital signs may trigger early response to deviations from normality (Case 2). Recording vital signs on the MEOWS chart means nothing without the midwife being able to exercise clinical judgement and responding appropriately to signs of physiological deterioration. Midwives work as part of the multiprofessional team and are the ones to alert doctors when a critical event such as an emergency or complication arises. Therefore, women's safety depends on the ability of the midwife to alert senior medical colleagues of abnormal clinical findings in order that immediate and appropriate response to care can be initiated.

INTERPROFESSIONAL COLLABORATION

As previously outlined, early recognition of critical illness in the pregnant woman can be a complex and challenging process. However, failure to do so is associated with adverse outcomes and remains a common criticism in key reports (Lewis and Drife 2001, 2004; Lewis 2007; HCC 2006; NICE 2007; NPSA 2007; CMACE 2011).

Effective teamwork between midwives and all relevant disciplines is particularly important in the management of critical situations when a clear chain of command, effective communication and a 'joined-up' approach to care are needed. Student midwives work alongside their mentors collaborating with other disciplines such as paramedics, obstetricians, anaesthetists, neonatologists, haematologists, theatre nurses, emergency department staff, gynaecology units and critical outreach teams in managing critical illness and emergency situations.

It is important to keep knowledge and skills regularly refreshed as critical illness and emergencies encountered during the childbearing continuum are rare. Findings from a number of randomized control trials (RCTs) have revealed that regular updates via the utilization of a skills-based 'fire-drill' approach is an effective way for midwives and doctors to practise managing critical illness and maternity emergencies (Black and Brocklehurst 2003; Crofts et al. 2007; Siassakos et al. 2009). Draycott et al. (2008) have developed a useful manual for the interprofessional team to manage such situations, which is successfully embedded, continuously audited and evaluated in Bristol, England.

Check point

- Effective care often involves very simple measures implemented well and skilfully by knowledgeable and competent midwives.
- General principles of critical care management when employed must be adjusted to take into consideration the pregnant woman's condition, e.g. the prevention of supine hypotension.

It is important to heed the findings and recommendations of key reports, namely CMACE (2011), Lewis (2007), Department of Health (2009), NCEPOD (2005), NPSA (2007) and SIGN (2004), which highlighted that much more could be done in relation to monitoring, recording and acting on vital signs. Key issues arising from these reports for midwifery practice are the importance of:

- assessing, monitoring, recording/reporting observations;
- recognizing early signs of deterioration;
- communicating observations causing concern, using the Situation, Background, Assessment and Recommendation (SBAR) tool (Case 2) to report and document information transferred by telephone to medical staff regarding concerns relating to women who are unwell;
- responding to the onset of critical illness appropriately and rapidly.

Summary of key points

- Recognition of critical illness in midwifery practice is vital.
- The onset of any critical illness signifies the need for urgency, vigilance and the escalation of care. Knowing how to recognize such an illness, what to do and how to do it can prevent full-blown emergencies and their sequelae.
- Outcomes for mothers and babies can be significantly improved with early and appropriate care interventions.
- The use of any track and trigger systems in the identification of the critically ill pregnant woman should demonstrate modification that considers the altered physiology of pregnancy, e.g. the MEOWS chart.
- The ABCDE system provides a systematic tool for assessing whether adequate oxygenation and stable cardiopulmonary function have been achieved.
- The AVPU tool is useful in assessing level of consciousness/neurological status.
- Interpretation of the result of haemodynamic monitoring in the critically ill pregnant woman requires a good working knowledge and understanding of the physiological parameters of pregnancy.

REFERENCES

ALERT (2011) *The ALERT System of Assessment.* Available at: http://www.alert-course.com (accessed 28 May 2011).

Bench, S. (2007) Recognition and management of critical illness by midwives: implications for service provision, *Journal of Nursing Management,* 15(3): 348–56.

Black, R.S. and Brocklehurst, P.A. (2003) Systematic review of training in acute obstetric emergencies, *British Journal of Obstetrics and Gynaecology,* 110:837–41.doi:10.1111/j.1471-0528.2003.02488.

Carrington, M. and Down, J. (2009) Recognition and assessment of critical illness, *Anaesthesia and Intensive Care Medicine,* 11(1): 6–8.

Clutton-Brock, T. (2011) Critical care, in CMACE *Saving Mothers' Lives: Reviewing Maternal Deaths to Make Motherhood Safer: 2006–2008: The Eighth Report on Confidential Enquiries into Maternal*

Deaths in the United Kingdom. Ed. G. Lewis. *BJOG: An International British Journal of Obstetrics and Gynaecology*, 118 (Suppl. 1): 173–80.

CMACE (2011) *Saving Mothers' Lives: Reviewing Maternal Deaths to Make Motherhood Safer: 2006–2008. The Eighth Report of the Confidential Enquiries into Maternal Deaths in the United Kingdom*. Ed. G. Lewis. *BJOG: An International British Journal of Obstetrics and Gynaecology*, 118 (Suppl. 1): 1–203.

Crofts, J.F., Ellis, D., Draycott, T.J., Winter, C., Hunt, L.P. and Akande, V.A. (2007) Change in knowledge of midwives and obstetricians following obstetric emergency training: a randomised controlled trial of local hospital, simulation centre and teamwork training, *British Journal of Obstetrics and Gynaecology*, 114: 1534–41. doi:10.1111/j.1471-0528.2007.01493.

Department of Health (2000) *Comprehensive Critical Care: A Review of Adult Critical Care Services*. London: DH. Available at: http://www.dh.gov.uk (accessed 11 May 2011).

Department of Health (2009) *Competencies for Recognizing and Responding to Acutely Ill Patients in Hospital*. Available at: http://www.dh.gov.uk/en/Publicationsandstatistics/Publications/Publications PolicyAndGuidance/DH_096989 (accessed 17 May 2011).

Draycott, T., Winter, C., Crofts, J. and Barnfield, S. (2008) *Practical Obstetric Multi-professional Training (PROMPT) Trainer's Manual*. London: RCOG.

Grady, K., Howell, C. and Cox, C. (eds) (2007) *Managing Obstetric Emergencies and Trauma: The MOET Course*, 2nd edn. London: RCOG.

Health Care Commission (2006) *Investigation into 10 Maternal Deaths at, or Following Delivery at Northwick Park Hospital, Northwest London Hospitals NHS Trust between April 2002–April 2005*. Available at: http://www.cqc.org.uk (accessed 10 May 2011).

International Confederation of Midwives (2005) *Definition of a Midwife*. Brisbane: ICM.

Jansen, J.O. and Cuthbertson, B.H. (2010) Detecting critical illness outside ICU: the role of track and trigger systems. *Current Opinion in Critical Care*, 16(3): 184–90.

Johanson, R., Cox, C., Grady, K. and Howell, C. (2003) *Managing Obstetric Emergencies and Trauma: The MOET Course Manual*. London: RCOG.

Kyriacos, N., Jelsma, J. and Jordan, S. (2011) Monitoring vital signs using early warning scoring systems: a review of the literature. *Journal of Nursing Management*, 19(3): 311–30.

Lewis, G. (ed.) (2007) *The Confidential Enquiry into Maternal and Child Health (CEMACH). Saving Mothers' Lives: Reviewing Maternal Deaths to Make Motherhood Safer: 2003–2005. The Seventh Report on Confidential Enquiries into Maternal Deaths in the United Kingdom*. London: CEMACH.

Lewis, G. and Drife, J. (eds) (2001) *Why Mothers Die, 1997–1999: The Fifth Report of the Confidential Enquiries into Maternal Deaths in the United Kingdom*. London: RCOG.

Lewis, G. and Drife, J. (eds) (2004) *Why Mothers Die 2000–2002: The Sixth Report of the Confidential Enquiries into Maternal Deaths in the United Kingdom*. London: RCOG.

McGaughey, J., Alderdice, F., Fowler, R., Kapila, A., Mayhew, A. and Moutray, M. (2007) Outreach and Early Warning Systems (EWS) for the prevention of Intensive Care admission and death of critically ill adult patients on general hospital wards, *Cochrane Database of Systematic Reviews*, Issue 3. Art. No. CD005529. doi: 10.1002/ 14651858. CD005529.pub2.

Mitchell, E. (2010) Specific features of critical care medicine: recognition of critical illness, in F.G. Smith and J. Yeung (eds) *Core Topics in Critical Care Medicine*. Cambridge: Cambridge University Press.

National Confidential Enquiry into Patient Outcome and Death (2005) *An Acute Problem*. London: NCEPOD. Available at: http://www.ncepod.org.uk/2005aap.htm (accessed 10 May 2011).

National Institute for Health and Clinical Excellence (2007) *Acutely Ill Patients in Hospital: Recognition of and Response to Acute Illness in Adults in Hospital*. London: NICE. Available at: http://www.nice.org.uk/Guidance/CG50 (accessed 10 May 2011).

National Patient Safety Agency (2007) *Safer Care for the Acutely Ill Patient: Learning from Serious Incidents*. London: NPSA. Available at: http://www.npsa.nhs.uk/nrls/alerts-and-directives/directives-guidance/acutely-ill-patient/

Nursing and Midwifery Council (2004) *Midwives Rules and Standards.* London: NMC.

Nursing and Midwifery Council (2009) *Standards for Pre-Registration Midwifery Education.* London: NMC. Available at: http://www.nmc-uk.org (accessed 12 February 2011).

Resuscitation Council (UK) (2010) *2010 Resuscitation Guidelines.* London: RCUK.

Royal College of Obstetricians and Gynaecologists (2008) *Standards for Maternity Care: Report of a Working Party.* London: RCOG.

Royal College of Obstetricians and Gynaecologists, Royal College of Anaesthetists, Royal College of Midwives, Royal College of Paediatrics and Child Health (2007) *Safer Childbirth: Minimum Standards for the Organisation and Delivery of Care in Labour.* London: RCOG.

Scottish Intercollegiate Guidelines Network (SIGN) (2004) *Postoperative Management in Adults.* Edinburgh: SIGN. Available at: http://www.sign.ac.uk/pdf/sign77.pdf (accessed 10 May 2011).

Sepsis Alliance (2010) *Surviving Sepsis Campaign.* Available at: http://www.sepsisalliance.org (accessed 12 June 2011).

Siassakos, D., Crofts, J., Winter, C. and Draycott, T., on behalf of the SaFE Study Group (2009) *Multiprofessional 'Fire-Drill' Training in the Labour Ward.* London: The Royal College of Obstetricians and Gynaecologists.11:1:55-60 DOI: 10.1576/toag.11.1.55.27469.

Smith, G. (2003) *ALERT: Acute Life-Threatening Events Recognition and Treatment,* 2nd edn. Portsmouth: University of Portsmouth.

Stubbe, C. (2006) Recognition and assessment of critical illness, *Anaesthesia and Intensive Care Medicine,* 8(1): 21–3.

ANNOTATED FURTHER READING

Intensive Care Society (2009) *Levels of Care for Adult Patients: Standards and Guidelines.* London: Intensive Care Society. Available at: http://www.ics.ac.uk/intensive_care_professional/standards_and_guidelines/levels_of_critical_care_for_adult_patients (accessed 10 May 2011).

Uses a classification system to identify the levels of critical care as recommended by CEMACH (Lewis and Drife 2004).

James, A., Endacott, R. and Stenhouse, E. (2011) Identifying women requiring maternity high dependency care, *Midwifery,* 27: 60–6. DOI: 10.1016/j.midw.2009.09.001.

Article explores the concept of critical care and levels of high dependency care.

Price, L.C., Germain, S., Wyncoll, D. and Nelson-Piercy, C. (2009) Management of the critically ill obstetric patient, *Obstetrics, Gynaecology and Reproductive Medicine,* 19(12): 350–8.

Addresses the physiological parameters of pregnancy alongside organ-specific aims of assessing and treating critical illness.

Obesity: risk management issues
Jayne E. Marshall and Susan Brydon

Pre-requisites for the chapter: the reader should have an understanding of:

- The physiological changes occurring during pregnancy in all major bodily systems.
- The definition and classification of obesity.
- Risk factors associated with obesity in the general population.
- Interprofessional team learning and working.
- The midwife's role and statutory responsibilities in the identification and management of childbearing women and their babies considered to be at risk.
- Local NHS Trust Clinical Governance and Risk Management procedures relating to the reporting of critical incidents and Clinical Negligence Scheme for Trusts (CNST) requirements.

Pre-reading self-assessment

1 How is Body Mass Index (BMI) calculated?
2 What are the causes of obesity in the general population?
3 What are the long-term health consequences of being obese?
4 Outline the risk management policy currently used in your local maternity unit for the safe management of mothers and babies.

Recommended prior reading

Centre for Maternal and Child Enquiries (CMACE) (2010) *Maternal Obesity in the UK: Findings from a National Project*. London: CMACE.

Centre for Maternal and Child Enquiries (CMACE) and the Royal College of Obstetricians and Gynaecologists (2010) *Management of Women with Obesity in Pregnancy: Joint Guideline*. London: CMACE/RCOG.

National Health Service Litigation Authority (NHSLA) (2011) *Clinical Negligence Scheme for Trusts: Maternity Clinical Risk Management Standards, Version 1, 2011/12*. London: NHSLA.

BACKGROUND

It is acknowledged that the modern world has become increasingly risk averse. Individuals believe they can prevent, manage and control risk and risky situations; if they fail, they seek legal redress (Bryers and van Teijlingen 2010). Developments throughout the twentieth century, e.g. medical, economic and socio-political reforms, coupled with the introduction of Clinical Negligence Scheme for Trusts (CNST), mean the concept of risk and risk management has become a central principle of care. In addition, there appears to be a public expectation that every pregnancy will result in a normal healthy baby, and when the outcome is not as expected, this can result in disappointment, complaint and sometimes litigation (Wilson and Symon 2002). Consequently, midwifery and obstetric practice in the NHS have become driven by clinical governance through risk assessment systems. It is essential therefore that student midwives have a good understanding of the concept of risk and engage in risk management processes wherever it is appropriate.

Although childbirth is a physiological process in the majority of cases, there are factors that arise in pregnancy and childbirth that can affect the health and well-being of the woman and her baby. Identifying such factors with timely referral to medical colleagues/other appropriate health professionals is fundamental to the statutory role of the midwife (NMC 2004). Symon (2006), however, affirms that in the context of maternity care, risk is a contentious issue, often being used as a label that denotes suitability for a particular model of care. It is important that the concept of risk and risk management is put into perspective in respect of the challenges that today's student midwives face when attempting to empower women into making choices. This is necessary when promoting normality and midwife-led care: the focus of current maternity service policy in the UK (Department of Health 2010).

Following an examination of the concept of risk and risk management theory, this case study will explore the potential risks obesity poses to the childbearing woman and her unborn baby in order to assist the reader in applying the theoretical principles to midwifery practice.

THE CONCEPT OF RISK

Every individual takes risks each day in their daily lives. Some risks carry a high penalty and others less so, thus accepting the level of risk despite the potential consequences could at worst result in death, or even serious injury. However, if sufficient care is taken, the chance of something adverse happening is very low. When a risk is evaluated, two factors are taken into account:

- the *probability* of something adverse happening; and
- the *consequences* if it does.

Moreover, identifying, evaluating and understanding risks are very important aspects of organizational management, especially within health care as most people generally associate the word *risk* with health risks, injury and death.

It is useful to think of risks to an individual or to the environment as falling into two categories:

1 risk of *harm*;
2 risk of *detriment* to the individual.

In the context of maternity care, the risk of *harm* would include injury to a woman and/or her baby during childbirth or to a health professional engaged in providing maternity care. On the other hand, the risk of *detriment* means some form of economic/social loss, which might indeed include a valuation of harm to living things but which also includes damage of a much wider kind, such as bad publicity for the local maternity services. Health service managers are expected to be conversant in risk management theory, and be able to identify and manage risks so that the probability of harm or detriment occurring is lessened and the consequences of risk are reduced. It is therefore expected that such organizations will adhere to the legislation pertaining to health and safety in the workplace and other legal principles such as *the duty of care* to both the public and employees as part of the risk management strategy. RCOG (2009a) summarizes basic questions that can be addressed by risk management, as shown in Table 2.1.

RISK MANAGEMENT THEORY AND LITIGATION

Risk management is the systematic identification, analysis and control of any potential and actual risk and of any circumstances that put individuals at risk of harm. The concept of risk management was first introduced in the NHS in the mid-1990s with the prime aim of reducing litigation risks. The Department of Health (DH) attributed the majority of mistakes in the NHS as being caused by a systems failure rather than any one individual, e.g. communication, supervision, checking equipment and staffing levels (DH 2000a). In addition, the Department of Health entrusted the CEO in each Trust with the overall legal accountability for ensuring that there were sufficient risk management systems in place to deliver all services in compliance with relevant statutory requirements, NHSLA standards and the Care Quality Commission's essential standards of quality and safety: the essence of clinical governance (DH 2000b). Risk management should therefore be used positively to deliver quality health care rather than focusing on countering the threat of litigation.

The NHS in 2010/2011 paid out over £900 million in litigation costs, of which some 50 per cent arose from midwifery/obstetric claims (NHSLA 2011a). Working in an area of health care with the highest litigation risk, however, does not mean that there are any more

Table 2.1 Basic questions addressed by risk management

Question	Risk management
What could go wrong?	Risk identification
What are the chances of it going wrong and what would be the impact?	Risk analysis and evaluation
What can we do to minimize the chance of this happening or to mitigate damage when it has gone wrong?	Risk treatment: the cost of prevention compared with the costs of getting it wrong
What can we learn from things that have gone wrong?	Risk control: sharing and learning

Source: RCOG 2009a.

claims in maternity than in other health services. Nonetheless, as the compensation payable often involves 24-hour care for the claimant for the rest of their life, the cost implications are vast.

Clinical Negligence Scheme for Trusts (CNST)

Clinical Negligence Scheme for Trusts (CNST) is a voluntary risk-pooling scheme for clinical negligence claims arising out of incidents occurring after 1 April 1995 and is administered by the NHSLA. All NHS Trusts, Foundation Trusts and Primary Care Trusts in England subscribe to CNST and pay an insurance premium based on their individual compliance to certain general standards. Risk management is therefore an essential activity with significant funding implications for all NHS Trusts striving for excellence.

There is a special standard for maternity services that Trusts have to achieve, relating to the following five standards (NHSLA 2011b):

1 organization
2 clinical care
3 high risk conditions
4 communication
5 postnatal and neonatal care.

CNST have issued a set of additional criteria and minimum requirements for specific maternity situations that are being piloted during 2011/2012 (NHSLA 2011b). Table 2.2 highlights the criterion and the minimum requirement specifically for *obesity*.

Table 2.2 CNST Maternity Clinical Risk Management: *Pilot Criterion* 2011/2012

Criterion	Minimum requirement	
3.10: Obesity	c.	Calculation of BMI and recording of it in the electronic patient information system.
	g.	An obstetric anaesthetic management plan for labour and birth should be discussed with the woman and documented in the health record.
	h.	All women with a BMI $\geq$ 30 kg/m^2 should have an antenatal consultation with an obstetric consultant to discuss possible intrapartum complications: the discussion must be documented in the health record.
	j.	Women with a booking BMI of $\geq$ 40kg/m^2 to have an individual documented assessment in the third trimester of pregnancy by an appropriately qualified professional to determine manual handling requirements for childbirth and consider tissue viability issues.

Source: NHSLA 2011b.

Risk is best managed within a framework that integrates all aspects of clinical governance, including clinical audit, education and training, complaints and claims handling, health and safety, research and service development, rather than in isolation. RCOG (2009a) refers to the **RADICAL** framework for management of risk in health care to fulfil this purpose:

- **R**aise Awareness.
- **D**esign for safety.
- **I**nvolve users.
- **C**ollect and **A**nalyse safety data.
- **L**earn from patient safety incidents.

RCOG (2009a) affirms that the organization should nurture a safety culture where there is strong leadership, teamwork, communication, user involvement and training. These themes are further addressed by the Royal Colleges (2007) in their joint publication, *Safer Childbirth*.

By using a simple risk management model, as shown in Figure 2.1, midwives and other health professionals can be effective in minimizing risk and optimizing outcome in the provision of maternity care. This generic model encourages a proactive approach to risk management: identifying and managing risks *before* they occur, so as to avoid harm. In the model there are two feedback loops, of which the first requires the midwife to determine whether the response to the original risk has created any additional risk. The second feedback loop provides an opportunity for all involved in the risk management process to learn and evaluate performance to further improve the standard of maternity care for future childbearing women and their families.

RISK ASSESSMENT, CLINICAL GUIDELINES AND PATHWAYS OF CARE

Risk assessment specifically refers to the process of determining the level of risk that a hazard poses in combination with the likelihood of its occurrence. Clinical guidelines can be

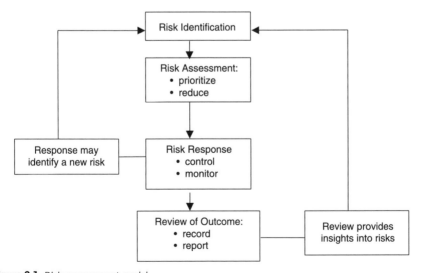

Figure 2.1 Risk management model

used to support health professionals, especially midwives, whose role is crucial in making an initial assessment of each childbearing woman. It is vital to establish any potential risk factors and promptly refer to appropriate members of the multidisciplinary team. As part of the CNST standards, it is mandatory that maternity units have up-to-date evidence-based multidisciplinary guidelines/pathways of care (NHSLA 2011b) for most critical or common conditions to promote an efficient and effective maternity service. CMACE/RCOG (2010) classify obesity as one of the high risk conditions requiring the use of a local multidisciplinary guideline in all maternity units. The specific content of the guideline is detailed in Table 2.3.

RECOMMENDATIONS FROM CMACE, DH AND NICE

The risk of dying during childbirth in the UK is low, with the latest maternal mortality figures being 11.39 per 100,000 maternities (CMACE 2011). The number of direct deaths has fallen from 6.24 per 100,000 maternities in the triennium 2003–2005, to 4.67 per 100,000 in the latest report from 2006–2008 (CMACE 2011). This decline has been attributed to the reduction in venous thromboembolism (VTE) and to haemorrhage, both being co-morbidities of pregnant women who are obese.

Since the Seventh Confidential Enquiry into Maternal Deaths in the UK (Lewis 2007) reported a number of deaths where early warning signs of impending maternal collapse went unrecognized, there has been a significant increase in the use of EWS systems within obstetric-led maternity units. Lewis (2007), CMACE (2011), DH (2009a) and NICE (2007a) endorse the use of the Modified Early Obstetric Warning Score (MEOWS) in improving the recognition of early warning signs of those women identified at risk of developing serious complications and life-threatening conditions to prompt earlier initiation of high level care and more senior involvement in care planning and management.

THE USE OF MODIFIED EARLY OBSTETRIC WARNING SCORE AND SITUATION, BACKGROUND, ASSESSMENT AND RECOMMENDATION (SBAR) TOOLS

EWS

Although most women cope well with pregnancy and labour, there is a significant minority who do not: of these, a small proportion will develop critical illness severe enough to require admission to ICU (see Case 1). Assessing the well-being of the childbearing woman and her fetus, and identifying any risk factors and subsequent deviations from the physiological

Table 2.3 Contents of multidisciplinary guidelines for pregnant women with a booking BMI of $\geq$ 30 kg/m^2

Referral criteria	Care in pregnancy
Facilities and equipment	Place of birth and care in labour
Provision of anaesthetic services	Postnatal advice
Management of obstetric emergencies	

Source: CMACE/RCOG 2010.

changes that should be occurring at each stage of the childbirth process, is a vital role of every midwife. Part of this role involves accurate and appropriately timed recording of clinical observations which is crucial for the prevention of maternal morbidity and mortality.

The first EWS system was developed by Morgan et al. (1997) and was based on a system of weighted physiological variables. It was then modified by Stenhouse et al. (1999) with the inclusion of urine output and deviations from the individual's normal blood pressure, resulting in the Modified Early Warning Score (MEWS). The MEOWS is a further modification that includes physiological factors specific to pregnancy, such as liquor and lochia (see Figure 2.2 for an example). EWS relies on observations of the physiological status of the individual, reflecting a clinical evaluation of oxygen delivery and organ perfusion. Of all the parameters, respiratory rate is probably the most sensitive indicator of an individual's physiological well-being as this reflects both respiratory and cardiac function (see Case 1).

Studies have shown that physiological deterioration usually precedes critical illness and that the EWS is a useful tool as it draws attention to vital signs of deterioration before it manifests (Baines and Kanagasundaram 2008). Cullinane et al. (2005) and Burch et al. (2008) have found that abnormalities of basic physiological observations are present in patients before they are admitted to the ICU. In Figure 2.2, either when one observation falls into the darker shaded section or two observations fall into the lighter shaded section, immediate actions are triggered, including referral to experienced senior clinicians. The early detection of severe illness in childbearing women, however, remains a challenge to all involved in their care as serious complications are relatively rare, and this, combined with the normal physiological changes associated with pregnancy and childbirth, can compound the problem (NCEPOD 2005).

Check point

The reasons for using MEOWS are:

- to improve the quality of physiological observation and monitoring;
- to provide a good indication of physiological trends;
- to provide a sensitive indicator of abnormal physiology;
- to improve the communication within the multidisciplinary team;
- to support good clinical judgement;
- to promote clear referral pathways and treatment/care plans;
- to allow for timely admission to intensive care.

Think

MEOWS is NOT:

- a predictor of outcome;
- a comprehensive clinical assessment tool;
- a replacement for clinical judgement.

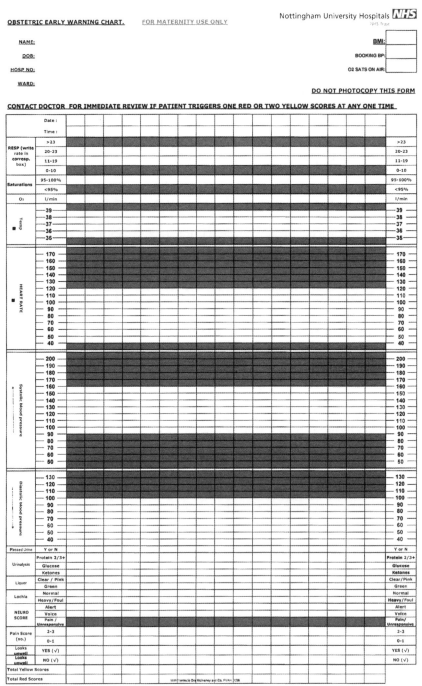

Figure 2.2 NUH Modified Early Obstetric Warning Score chart

SBAR

The NHS is often criticized for poor communication but there are few tools that actively focus on how to improve communication, in particular, verbal communication. The SBAR tool (NHS Institute for Innovation and Improvement 2008), however, is an easy-to-remember mechanism that can be used to frame clinical conversations, especially critical ones, requiring immediate attention and action. It enables the clarification of which information should be communicated between members of the team, and helps to develop teamwork and foster a culture of safety (RCOG 2009a). The SBAR tool can be used in all clinical conversations, such as face-to-face or telephone conversations between individual team members (see Case 3) or through collaboration at multidisciplinary team meetings.

The tool consists of standardized prompt questions in four steps (see Table 2.4) to ensure that health professionals are assertively and effectively sharing concise and focused information,

Table 2.4 Steps in the SBAR process

Step	Action
1 Situation	Identify yourself and the area/ward you are calling from. Identify the woman by name and the reason for your report/referral. Describe your concerns and provide details of their vital signs.
2 Background	State the reason for the woman's admission. Explain the significant medical history. Provide the woman's background: <ul><li>admitting diagnosis</li><li>date of admission</li><li>prior procedures</li><li>current medications</li><li>allergies</li><li>pertinent laboratory results</li><li>other relevant diagnostic results collected from observation charts and records.</li></ul>
3 Assessment	State your assessment of the situation by critically considering the underlying cause for the woman's condition having reviewed your findings and consolidating them with other objective indicators, e.g. laboratory results: e.g. *'I think she may have had a pulmonary embolus'* or if you do not have an assessment, *'I am not sure what the problem is, but I am very concerned.'*
4 Recommendation	Explain what you need/recommend, being specific about your request and the time-frame. Make suggestions about the course of action and subsequent care. Repeat your request/recommendation to ensure clarity and accuracy (especially if calling a sleeping senior colleague about care and management as it may take some time for them to absorb the facts and respond).

Source: NHS Institute for Innovation and Improvement 2008.

reducing the need for repetition. Incorporating SBAR may seem simple, but it may take consider-able effort for it to be effective as it can be very difficult to change the way people communicate, particularly with senior colleagues. Less experienced clinicians may find making recommenda-tions a challenge which is an important stage of the SBAR process, as it clearly describes the action the messenger needs. The NHS Institute for Innovation and Improvement (2008) suggests that where individuals are anxious about giving recommendations, trying out the tool with supportive colleagues is a useful strategy to adopt in order to improve their confidence.

INTERPROFESSIONAL COLLABORATION

It is imperative that there is always effective team working and good communication between the midwife and the multidisciplinary team in the management of risk in order to minimize adverse outcomes (Lewis and Drife 2004; Lewis 2007; NICE 2007a; NPSA 2007; RCOG 2009a; CMACE 2011). Clear, concise record keeping is essential in detailing the specific management decisions that are made with the interests of the woman and her baby being at the forefront to ensure the optimal outcome (NMC 2004, 2010).

Supervisors of midwives can support midwives in identifying childbearing women and/or their babies presenting with potential risk and any education and training needs required in relation to risk management strategies. Furthermore, as part of CNST standards, all health professionals working in maternity care should have training in risk management strategies including incident reporting and complaints/claims management (NPSA 2004, 2005; NHSLA 2011b) which can be facilitated through interprofessional working and learning (DH 2001). Table 2.5 highlights CNST Standard 1, Criterion 8 (NHSLA 2011b) that sets out the requirements of the reporting system for maternity care. In addition, student midwives

Table 2.5 Standard 1 – Criterion 8: Incidents, Complaints and Claims

The maternity service has an approved system for ensuring local and organizational learning occurs following all grades and types of incidents, complaints and claims that is implemented and monitored.

Approved documentation as a minimum must include a description of the following:

- Maternity-specific data set for incident reporting.
- Maternity service's process for learning from experience, including case reviews.
- Arrangements for the regular review and discussion of all incidents, complaints and claims by the relevant local committee/group.
- Arrangements for ensuring that all serious untoward incidents (SUIs) undergo a root cause analysis, involving as appropriate unbiased external input.
- Arrangements for ensuring that lessons learnt from all incidents, complaints and claims are actively disseminated to all staff.
- Process for providing board assurance that lessons learnt from SUIs are implemented and monitored.
- Process for monitoring compliance with all of the above requirements, review of results and subsequent monitoring of action plans.

Source: NHSLA 2011b.

should also be familiar with local Trust strategy pertaining to women's safety and incident reporting through engaging with their mentors and members of the multidisciplinary team in the care of high risk pregnancies.

CASE STUDY

Kelly is 24 years of age and is in a stable relationship with her partner David. At 8 weeks she discovers that she is pregnant: the couple are delighted with the news. They begin looking forward to the birth of their first baby in the local free-standing midwife-led unit where most of Kelly's family has given birth. Kelly and David attend the midwife's booking clinic two weeks later. At this first meeting, the midwife takes details of Kelly's medical, family and social history and ascertains there is nothing of any significance to note. Kelly is generally fit and well and has never been admitted to hospital for any reason.

The midwife examines Kelly and finds her blood pressure and urinalysis assessments are within the normal range. Venepuncture is performed for Hb estimation. The midwife notes that Kelly is overweight for her height, having calculated that her BMI is 36.2 kg/m^2, which, according to CMACE (2010), means that Kelly is obese.

1 **What is the purpose of the booking visit?**

A The prevalence of obesity (BMI $\geq$ 30 kg/m^2) in the general population in England has markedly increased since the early 1990s and currently affects an estimated 25 per cent of adults and 18.5 per cent of women of childbearing age (CMACE 2010). As a consequence, midwives are increasingly coming into contact with pregnant women such as Kelly, who are obese. The booking visit provides an ideal opportunity for the midwife to undertake an overall clinical assessment of Kelly in order to plan the optimal care for her during pregnancy. This first encounter is vitally important to the establishment of a good relationship between the midwife and Kelly so that she feels respected and not stigmatized due to her weight. Lewis (2007) reports two morbidly obese women who died in the first trimester, one of whom actively avoided attending antenatal appointments. This highlights that such women may find it difficult to talk to clinicians for fear of stigmatization.

2 **What advice should the midwife give Kelly regarding weight assessment and management?**

A It is recommended by CMACE (2010) that the midwife should ask Kelly to be weighed and measured in order to calculate her BMI, rather than base BMI calculations on self-reported weights and heights. Nawaz et al. (2001) and Gorber et al. (2007) have provided evidence that women are likely to over-estimate their height and under-estimate their weight with the degree of under-reporting weight being more frequent with increasing BMI. As the booking visit takes place in the midwife's clinic, it would be expected that there would be access to reliable equipment with appropriate working loads to make such an assessment, compared to the visit taking place at Kelly's home.

The midwife has a duty of care to inform Kelly of the potential health risks of having a raised BMI of 36.2 kg/m^2 when pregnant, although a raised BMI in itself is not a direct cause of maternal death, as there are usually other causative factors such as specific health problems and social deprivation. At this first meeting, the midwife should advise Kelly of possible planned management strategies to minimize risk throughout pregnancy, labour and the puerperium based on the Care Pathway for Women with Obesity in Pregnancy produced by CMACE/RCOG (2010) (see Figure 2.3). All weight measurements and details of the discussions should be clearly documented in Kelly's hand-held maternity records and the electronic patient information system (NMC 2004, 2010). Furber and McGowan (2011) state that health professionals should be more aware of the psychological effects of being obese and recommend that communication strategies about a pregnant woman's care should be clear, honest and conveyed in a sensitive manner. All written comments related to Kelly's size that are included in her hand-held records should be explained by the midwife and all other health professionals at the time of writing.

All pregnant women should receive nutritional advice *prior* to conception from appropriately trained health professionals which could be from a dietician, a nutritionist or the midwife if she has undergone further training in this area (CMACE 2010). It is important that the midwife establishes whether Kelly has been taking folic acid supplementation to minimize the risk of congenital abnormalities, particularly neural tube defects. With a BMI of $\geq$ 30 kg/m^2, the recommended daily dose would be 5 mg daily a month before conception and during the first trimester (see Figure 2.3). CMACE/RCOG (2010) also recommend that Kelly should take 10 mcg vitamin D supplementation daily during pregnancy and while breastfeeding as she and her baby have an increased risk of vitamin D deficiency compared to a pregnant woman with a healthy weight (BMI < 25 kg/m^2).

The advice given to Kelly regarding weight management and physical activity during and after pregnancy should be based on the recommendations within the NICE (2010) framework. This framework is also supportive of *The Pregnancy Book* (DH 2009b) and the Eat Well website (www.eatwell.gov.uk) as additional sources of advice to avoid excessive weight gain during pregnancy.

3   **What are the potential risks to Kelly and her pregnancy of being obese?**

A   Having a raised BMI at booking puts Kelly at risk of pregnancy complications such as an increased likelihood of miscarriage, pre-eclampsia, gestational diabetes/type 2 diabetes, cardiac problems, VTE, induced labour, caesarean section anaesthetic complications, wound infections and postpartum haemorrhage (PPH) (CMACE 2010). Amir and Donath (2007) have found that women with obesity are also less likely to initiate or maintain breastfeeding. It is recognized that as the BMI increases, the risks of fetal demise or neonatal death also increase; however, the biomechanisms for fetal/neonatal death in association with maternal obesity are poorly understood. According to Callaway et al. (2006) and Leddy et al. (2008), high maternal weight is associated with fetal macrosomia, shoulder dystocia, preterm birth, admission to NICU and jaundice.

During the booking visit, the midwife should inform Kelly of additional care that will be offered due to the risks associated with a raised BMI. This should include increased surveillance for pre-eclampsia and oral glucose tolerance testing at 24–28 weeks (PRECOG Development Group 2004; NICE 2008a; CMACE/RCOG 2010).

Check point

- An appropriate size of arm cuff should be used for blood pressure measurements taken at booking and subsequent antenatal consultations.
- The cuff size should be documented in the woman's records.

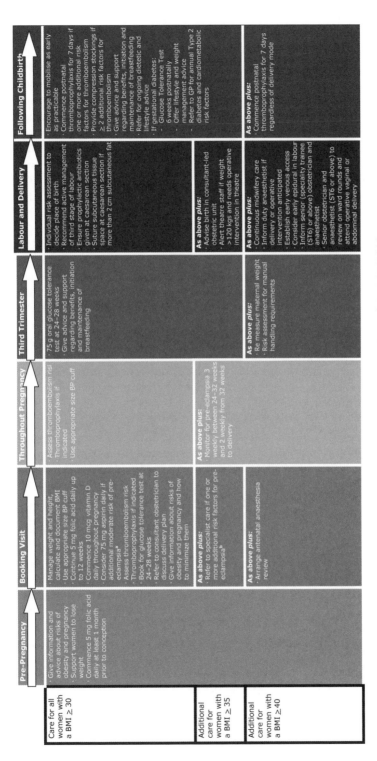

Figure 2.3 Pre-pregnancy, antenatal, labour and postnatal care pathway for women with obesity © CMACE/RCOG. 2010.

a first pregnancy, previous pre-eclampsia, ≥ 10 years since last baby, family history of pre-eclampsia, booking diastolic ≥ 80 mmHg, booking proteinuria ≥ 1+ on more than one occasion or ≥ 0.3 g/24 hours, multiple pregnancy, and certain underlying medical conditions such as antiphospholipid antibodies or pre-existing hypertension, renal disease or diabetes.

b first pregnancy, maternal age > 40 years, family history of pre-eclampsia, multiple pregnancy

In respect of assessing Kelly's risk of VTE, the midwife should be conversant with the RCOG (2009b) Green Top Guideline No. 37a (see Case 4). Drife (2011) draws attention to the fact that obesity remains the most important risk factor for VTE, with 14 women of the 18 maternal deaths in the latest triennial report being classed as over weight (BMI $\geq$ 25 kg/m^2), 11 of whom had a BMI of $\geq$ 30 kg/m^2 and three with a BMI of $\geq$ 40 kg/m^2. RCOG (2009b) recommend that if women present with three risk factors, they should be prescribed prophylactic low molecular weight heparin (LMWH) throughout pregnancy, i.e. enoxaparin, dalteparin and tinzaparin. However, at this stage, Kelly is only presenting with one risk factor and would not warrant this intervention. The midwife, nevertheless, should be alert to Kelly developing complications throughout pregnancy, in particular, thrombophlebitis/deep vein thrombosis (DVT) or any chest symptoms and act promptly, referring to specialist services for a thromboprophylaxis review.

4   **At what stage in the pregnancy would a consultant review be appropriate?**

A   The BMI should be considered in the context of Kelly's full psychosocial, medical and obstetric history rather than in isolation. However, as this is Kelly's first pregnancy and she has a BMI $\geq$ 30 kg/m^2, in accordance with NICE (2008b) and CMACE/RCOG (2010) guidance, the midwife should use her professional judgement and refer her to consultant obstetrician care due to presenting at booking with one or more additional risk factors for pre-eclampsia (NMC 2004).

Drife (2011) recommends that as all women are at risk of VTE from the very beginning of pregnancy to the end of the puerperium, risk assessment in early pregnancy is a key factor in reducing mortality and referral to a consultant obstetrician is advocated for women with a BMI of $\geq$ 35 kg/m^2. This, however, does not mean that the care cannot still be shared with the community midwife as long as Kelly remains well during pregnancy.

Prior to the onset of labour, Kelly should be referred to the consultant obstetrician to discuss how potential intrapartum risks may be minimized. The decision for mode of birth should only be taken after careful consideration of Kelly's individual circumstances and in conjunction with the full multidisciplinary team and Kelly and David (CMACE/RCOG 2010).

5   **Which other health professionals should be involved in Kelly's care?**

A   Oates et al. (2011) reinforce the fact that in order to complete the most comprehensive history of a pregnant woman, there should be good communication between midwife and GP with local auditable robust systems in place to enable two-way flow of information throughout pregnancy and the puerperium. This is particularly important should midwifery services be offered in a range of locations, e.g. Children's Centres. It is recommended that not only should the midwife notify the GP that Kelly is pregnant and seek additional information if risk factors are identified, but the GP should also inform the midwife if Kelly has any medical or mental health problems.

During pregnancy, continuing risk assessment of women who are obese is vital. Should Kelly develop complications associated with her obesity (CMACE/RCOG 2010), referral may be made to a range of specialists such as the haematologist, cardiologist, diabetic consultant and neonatologist. Consequently details of any referrals and the subsequent management strategies, including an appropriate intrapartum care plan, should be clearly identified in Kelly's records to ensure all members of the multidisciplinary team involved in her care are well informed of the plan (CMACE 2011).

Women with obesity often present anaesthetic difficulty and have a much higher rate of intervention such as caesarean section requiring anaesthesia (CMACE 2010). It would be appropriate for Kelly to see a consultant anaesthetist during the third trimester of pregnancy to identify any anaesthetic challenges in advance that are likely to impact on her care plan. In the CMACE (2010) national report, it was found that while such anaesthetic review was available to pregnant women who had a high BMI, this was taken up in < 50 per cent of the cases. However, although this may reflect selection of those at highest risk, the importance of anaesthetic review should still be highlighted for service provision.

Rasmussen and Yaktine (2009) recommend that women who are obese with a BMI of ≥ 30 kg/m^2, should gain only between 5–9 kg in total during pregnancy in order to improve maternal and fetal outcomes, compared to a woman of normal weight gaining between 11.4–18.2 kg. Studies by Keil et al. (2007) and Cedergren (2006) have reported that a low pregnancy weight gain of < 8 kg was associated with significantly lower risk of pre-eclampsia, caesarean section and pre-term birth in women with a BMI of ≥ 25 kg/m^2. Olson et al. (2009) found that excess weight gain in pregnancy is also associated with the child being overweight at 3 years, with the impact being greater in mothers with increased BMI. If general healthy eating advice is not sufficient in preventing Kelly from gaining unnecessary weight, referral to a dietician or nutritionist for more detailed advice about portion size and exercise would be appropriate.

As Kelly's pregnancy continues, she may experience increasing breathlessness due to reduced lung capacity with movement and mobility becoming more difficult. NICE (2010) recognize the importance of all women maintaining a simple exercise regime during pregnancy and in Kelly's case this would help in reducing her risk of VTE and need for thromboprophylaxis. Referral to a physiotherapist or health and fitness adviser in the local community could also be considered to advise Kelly on techniques to improve her fitness and lung capacity that can also be beneficial to her in labour.

6 **What options are available to Kelly regarding choice of place of birth?**

A The midwife will be aware of Kelly's intent to give birth in the local free-standing midwife-led unit, but should also be aware of the possible intrapartum complications and adverse pregnancy-related outcomes associated with increasing BMI. It is therefore recommended by CMACE (2010), CMACE/RCOG (2010) and NICE (2007b) that women with a BMI ≥ 35 kg/m^2, such as Kelly, should give birth in a consultant-led obstetric unit with appropriate neonatal services, so that immediate intervention is available in the event of intrapartum and postpartum complications and emergencies. Providing Kelly and David with an opportunity to articulate their rationale for birthing in the free-standing midwife-led unit would help the midwife to explore alternative intrapartum support strategies that the couple may find acceptable.

In this situation, the midwife could offer to attend Kelly in labour and provide the intrapartum care and one-to-one support within the consultant-led obstetric unit. The birth outcome and the health of Kelly and her baby will determine at what point they can transfer back home to the care of the community team. The supervisor of midwives should be aware of Kelly's case so she can support the midwife in the plan of action for midwifery care that is ultimately determined. Details of these discussions should all be documented in Kelly's records (NMC 2004, 2010).

7 **What are the possible risks that Kelly may face during labour and birth?**

A The midwife and members of the multidisciplinary team should consider the potential risks that Kelly may experience during labour and birth to then prepare an appropriate care plan for optimal maternal and fetal outcome. Table 2.6 lists these risks with the associated pathophysiology and consequences.

Table 2.6 Intrapartum and birthing risks associated with women who have a BMI of ≥ 35 kg/m²

Risk	Associated pathophysiology and consequences
Respiratory problems	Decrease in total lung capacity, vital capacity, inspiratory capacity and expiratory reserve leading to maternal hypoxaemia that can compromise fetal oxygenation.
Cardiovascular problems	Cardiac output is considerably increased to help maintain adequate oxygenation, leading to an increase in coronary artery disease. Increase in stomach volume and increased acidity of gastric contents can lead to heartburn in pregnancy and intrapartum aspiration of gastric contents.
Fetal size: Macrosomia	Large babies associated with women with diabetes mellitus and gestational diabetes; can lead to induction of labour, prolonged labour, shoulder dystocia, birth injuries and caesarean section.
IUGR	Associated with woman who have hypertension/pre-eclampsia.
Fetal compromise/ perinatal mortality	Associated link to fetal compromise, meconium aspiration, stillbirth and neonatal death due to maternal co-morbidities.
	External fetal monitoring in labour can be difficult due to maternal size and can increase intervention rate, e.g. ARM and FSE.
Induction of labour	Obesity is not an indication for induction of labour (IOL) alone, but does increase intervention rate such as epidural and operative birth.
Anaesthesia	Epidural analgesia may prove technically difficult to administer and general anaesthesia carries a higher risk to the woman of airway complications, cardiopulmonary dysfunction and perioperative morbidity/mortality.
Postpartum haemorrhage	Achieving haemostasis and minimizing thrombosis risk is critical. Balancing the risk of bleeding due to lax abdominal muscles and excess adipose tissue with thrombosis is a challenge.
Wound healing/ pressure ulcers	Wound dehiscence and infection are increased due to excess adipose tissue, poor mobility, ischaemia to the wound and co-morbidities delaying wound healing, e.g. gestational diabetes.
Thromboembolism	Immobility, haemodynamic instability, compromised respiratory and cardiac function increase the risk of VTE.

8 **What are the actions that can be taken to ensure the optimal outcome for Kelly and her baby?**

A CMACE (2010) found in their study that < 50 per cent of women with a BMI ≥ 40 kg/m^2 had a written obstetric management plan for labour and birth, and < 30 per cent had documented evidence of information given antenatally about potential intrapartum complications related to obesity. Similarly, when admitted for labour and birth, it was noted that improvements could also be made in alerting an obstetrician of appropriate seniority as well as theatre and anaesthetic staff. Such a strategy is reinforced by CMACE/RCOG (2010) and should be identified in local guidance pertaining to the intrapartum care of the pregnant woman who is obese, to minimize the risks.

It is vital that Kelly has continuous one-to-one midwifery care during her labour and that MEOWS and SBAR are used by the midwife and the multidisciplinary team to ensure that her well-being and vital signs are closely monitored. Any early signs of deterioration should be promptly identified and acted upon as Lewis (2007) affirms that obesity can mask the clinical symptoms of critical illness.

With regard to equipment, it is important that Kelly is assessed regarding manual handling so that the unit where she is to labour and birth her baby, has appropriate equipment such as extra-wide chairs, beds and theatre tables with appropriate working loads should they be required. The lack of such an assessment and availability of equipment would pose a risk to Kelly and her carers and it is critical that this equipment is readily available for emergency situations with health professionals being trained and competent in its use (CMACE 2010). In addition, CMACE/RCOG (2010) endorse that all maternity units should have documented environmental risk assessment regarding the availability of facilities for pregnant women with a booking BMI of ≥ 30 kg/m^2.

Check point

The environmental risk assessment should address:

- circulation space
- accessibility: doorway width and thresholds
- appropriate size theatre gowns
- equipment storage
- transportation
- staffing levels
- availability of and procurement process for specific equipment:
  - large BP cuffs
  - sit-on weighing scales
  - large chairs without arms
  - large wheelchairs
  - ultrasound scan couches
  - ward and birthing beds
  - theatre trolleys and operating theatre beds
  - moving and handling aids including lateral transfer equipment.

Part of the midwife's role is to prepare Kelly for labour and birth through the facilitation of antenatal classes within the local community (NMC 2004). This will also provide Kelly with an opportunity to undertake gentle exercise, develop breathing techniques and increase her awareness of the labour process, analgesia and positions for labour and birth.

Although Arrowsmith et al. (2011) found in their study that induction of labour (IOL) for prolonged labour in women who are obese was a reasonable and safe management option, spontaneous labour would be the preferred option in Kelly's case to minimize intervention and facilitate a physiological birth. As immobility and obesity are independently associated with VTE, in combination, they can pose a much greater risk to Kelly during labour and following the birth of her baby. Kelly should therefore be encouraged to be mobile as much as possible during labour, i.e. using a birthing ball, adopting upright or all-fours positions, and as early as is practicable following her baby's birth (depending on the mode of birth), to reduce the risk of VTE (see Case 4). In addition, being upright and mobile would also help improve Kelly's lung capacity and oxygen perfusion, minimize fetal compromise, encourage the descent of the presenting part and reduce any pressure ulcers developing.

During pregnancy it is recommended that women with a high BMI have regular ultrasound scan (USS) in order to assess fetal growth (Rajasingam and Swamy 2010). However, this evidence is unreliable as USSs are less efficacious in assessing fetal anomaly and growth in the presence of obesity. Nevertheless as an adjunct to care, it should help in estimating fetal weight and confirming fetal lie and presentation as determining these by abdominal palpation can sometimes be a challenge for midwives and obstetricians. The most appropriate means of assessing fetal well-being in labour will be determined by a number of factors, but due to the potential risks associated with maternal obesity, electronic fetal monitoring (EFM) via a fetal scalp electrode (FSE) may be necessary. If there is any risk of shoulder dystocia, the midwife should be familiar with the local procedure to deal with this emergency should it arise and seek support from experienced colleagues, including a paediatrician, in order to minimize trauma to Kelly and her baby (see Case 14). Kelly would be advised to have an active management of the third stage of labour in order to minimize the risk of postpartum haemorrhage (PPH) (see Case 8) (CMACE/RCOG 2010).

If Kelly requires an instrumental vaginal or caesarean section birth, as these births could prove technically difficult due to her obesity, appropriately experienced clinicians should be present to perform or supervise such procedures, including an anaesthetist and neonatologist. Prophylactic antibiotics would be administered at the time of surgery to minimize the risk of wound infection and thromboembolic deterrent (TED) stockings applied to reduce the risk of VTE. In addition, if there is > 2 cm subcutaneous fat, the subcutaneous space should also be sutured in order to reduce the risk of wound infection and dehiscence (NICE 2004).

CASE REVIEW

Kelly went into spontaneous labour at 38 weeks and, as recommended, gave birth in the consultant-led obstetric unit to a baby girl, Chloe, who weighed 4.10 kgs with David and her community midwife in attendance. According to CMACE/RCOG (2010) guidance, Kelly was encouraged to mobilize as soon as possible after the birth and to prevent dehydration in order to reduce the risk of VTE and the need for thromboprophylaxis. She was transferred home to the care of the midwife and G P after three days and referred for ongoing dietetic and lifestyle advice to reduce her weight and B M I prior to contemplating another pregnancy.

Summary of key points

- Obesity impacts adversely on a woman's health throughout her life and can lead to the development of type 2 diabetes and coronary heart disease.
- Outcomes for pregnant women who are obese and their babies can be significantly improved with early and appropriate care interventions.
- The problem of obesity can be best addressed *before* pregnancy as some of the risks such as miscarriage and fetal abnormalities occur during the first trimester.
- Risk assessment is vital at all stages of the childbirth continuum with timely referral to determine appropriate care pathways and management.
- The responsibility to improve the pregnancy outcome lies with all services who encounter women with obesity, such as primary care, family planning and diabetic services.
- Appropriate standards of care/care pathways for the management of women with obesity in pregnancy should be based on best practice and national guidance.
- Local guidelines and risk management systems are essential in supporting the multidisciplinary team to promptly recognize signs of critical illness and act effectively to minimize further risks and morbidity in the pregnant woman who is obese.

REFERENCES

Amir, L.H. and Donath, S. (2007) A systematic review of maternal obesity and breastfeeding intention, initiation and duration, *BMC Pregnancy and Childbirth*, 7(9).

Arrowsmith, S., Wray, S. and Quenby, S. (2011) Maternal complications following induction of labour in prolonged labour, *BJOG: An International Journal of Obstetrics and Gynaecology*, 118(5): 578–88.

Baines, E. and Kanagasundaram, N.S. (2008) Early warning scores, *Student BMJ*, 16: 294–336.

Bryers, H.M. and van Teijlingen, E. (2010) Risk, theory, social and medical models: a critical analysis of the concept of risk in maternity care, *Midwifery*, 5(26): 488–96.

Burch, V.C., Tarr, G. and Morroni, C. (2008) Modified early warning score predicts the need for hospital admission and in-hospital mortality, *Emergency Medical Journal*, 25: 674–8. DOI:10.1136/emj.2007.057661.

Callaway, L.K., Prins, J.B., Chang, A.M. and McIntyre, H.D. (2006) The prevalence and impact of overweight and obesity in an Australian obstetric population, *Medical Journal of Australia*, 184(2): 56–9.

Cedergren, M. (2006) Effects of gestational weight gain and body mass index on obstetric outcome in Sweden, *International Journal of Gynecology and Obstetrics*, 93(3): 269–74.

Centre for Maternal and Child Enquiries (CMACE) (2010) *Maternal Obesity in the UK: Findings from a National Project*. London: CMACE.

Centre for Maternal and Child Enquiries (CMACE) (2011) *Saving Mothers' Lives: Reviewing Maternal Deaths to Make Motherhood Safer: 2006–2008. The Eighth Report of the Confidential Enquiries into Maternal Deaths in the United Kingdom*. Ed. G. Lewis. *BJOG*, 118 (Suppl. 1): 1–203.

Centre for Maternal and Child Enquiries (CMACE) and the Royal College of Obstetricians and Gynaecologists (2010) *Management of Women with Obesity in Pregnancy: Joint Guideline*. London: CMACE/RCOG.

Cullinane, M., Findlay, G., Hargraves, C. and Lucas, S. (2005) *An Acute Problem*. London: National Confidential Enquiry into Patient Outcome and Death.

Department of Health (2000a) *An Organization with a Memory: Report of an Expert Group on Learning from Adverse Events in the NHS*. London: HMSO. Available at: http://www.dh.gov.uk

Department of Health (2000b) *The NHS Plan: A Plan for Investment, a Plan for Reform*. London: HMSO.

Department of Health (2001) *Working Together, Learning Together: A Framework for Lifelong Learning in the NHS*. London: HMSO.

Department of Health (2009a) *Competencies for Recognising and Responding to Acutely Ill Patients in Hospital*. Available at: http://www.dh.gov.uk/en/Publicationsandstatistics/Publications/Publications PolicyAndGuidance/DH_096989 (accessed 1 August 2011).

Department of Health (2009b) *The Pregnancy Book*. London: Department of Health.

Department of Health (2010) *Maternity and Early Years: Making a Good Start to Family Life*. London: Department of Health. Available at: http://www.dh.gov.uk/en/Publicationsandstatistics/Publications/ PublicationsPolicyAndGuidance/DH_114023 (accessed 1 August 2011).

Drife, J. (2011) Thrombosis and thromboembolism, in Centre for Maternal and Child Enquiries, *Saving Mothers' Lives: Reviewing Maternal Deaths to Make Motherhood Safer: 2006–2008. The Eighth Report on Confidential Enquiries into Maternal Deaths in the United Kingdom*. Ed. G. Lewis. *BJOG:* 118 (Suppl. 1): 57–65.

Furber, C.M. and McGowan, L. (2011) A qualitative study of the experiences of women who are obese and pregnant in the UK, *Midwifery*, 27(4): 437–44.

Gorber, S.C., Tremblay, M., Moher, D. and Gorber, B. (2007) A comparison of direct vs. self-report measures for assessing height, weight and body mass index: a systematic review, *Obesity Reviews*, 8(4): 307–26.

Keil, D.W., Dodson, E.A., Artal, R., Boehmer, T.K. and Leet, T.L. (2007) Gestational weight gain and pregnancy outcomes in obese women: how much is enough? *Obstetric Gynecology*, 110(4): 752–8.

Leddy, M.A., Power, M.L. and Schulkin, J. (2008) The impact of maternal obesity on maternal and fetal health, *Reviews in Obstetrics and Gynaecology*, 1(4): 170–8.

Lewis, G. (ed.) (2007) *The Confidential Enquiry into Maternal and Child Health (CEMACH). Saving Mothers' Lives: Reviewing Maternal Deaths to Make Motherhood Safer, 2003–2005. The Seventh Report on Confidential Enquiries into Maternal Deaths in the United Kingdom*. London: CEMACH.

Lewis, G. and Drife, J. (eds) (2004) *Why Mothers Die, 2000–2002. The Sixth Report of the Confidential Enquiries into Maternal Deaths in the United Kingdom*. London: RCOG.

Morgan, R.J.M., Williams, F. and Wright, M.M. (1997) An early warning scoring system for detecting developing critical illness, *Clinical Intensive Care*, 8(2): 100.

National Confidential Enquiry into Patient Outcome and Death (2005) *An Acute Problem*. London: NCEPOD. Available at http://www.ncepod.org.uk/2005aap.htm

National Health Service Litigation Authority (2011a) *Risk Management*. Available at: http://www.nhsla.com/riskmanagement (accessed 1 August 2011).

National Health Service Litigation Authority (2011b) *Clinical Negligence Scheme for Trusts Maternity Clinical Risk Management Standards Version 1 2011/12*. London: NHSLA. Available at: http://www.nhsla.com

National Health Service Institute for Innovation and Improvement (2008) *SBAR: Situation, Background, Assessment and Recommendation Tool*. Available at http://www.institute.nhs.uk (accessed 12 January 2011)

National Institute for Health and Clinical Excellence (2004) *Caesarean Section*. London: RCOG Press. Available at: http://www.nice.org.uk/Guidance/CG13

National Institute for Health and Clinical Excellence (2007a) *Acutely Ill Patients in Hospital: Recognition of and Response to Acute Illness in Adults in Hospital*. London: NICE.

National Institute for Health and Clinical Excellence (2007b) *Intrapartum Care: Care of Healthy Women and Their Babies during Childbirth*, London: NICE. Available at: http://www.nice.org.uk/Guidance/CG55

National Institute for Health and Clinical Excellence (NICE) (2008a) *Diabetes in Pregnancy: Management of Diabetes and Its Complications from Pre-Conception to the Postnatal Period*. London: NICE. Available at: http://www.nice.org.uk/Guidance/CG63

National Institute for Health and Clinical Excellence (NICE) (2008b) *Antenatal Care: Routine Care for the Healthy Pregnant Woman*. London: NICE. Available at: http://www.nice.org.uk/guidance/CG62

National Institute for Health and Clinical Excellence (NICE) (2010) *Dietary Interventions and Physical Activity Interventions for Weight Management Before, During and After Pregnancy*. London: NICE. Available at: http://www.nice.org.uk/guidance/PH27

National Patient Safety Agency (2004) *Seven Steps to Patient Safety*. London: NPSA. Available at: http://www.npsa.nhs.uk

National Patient Safety Agency (2005) *Building a Memory: Preventing Harm, Reducing Risks and Improving Patient Safety. The First Report of the National Reporting Learning System and the Patient Safety Observatory*. London: NPSA. Available at: http://www.npsa.nhs.uk

National Patient Safety Agency (2007) *Safer Care for the Acutely Ill Patient: Learning from Serious Incidents*. London: NPSA. Available at: http://www.npsa.nhs.uk/nrls/alerts-and-directives/directives-guidance/acutely-ill-patient/

Nawaz, H., Chan, W., Abdulrahman, M., Larson, D. and Katz, D.L. (2001) Self-reported weight and height for obesity research, *American Journal of Preventative Medicine*, 20(4): 294–8.

Nursing and Midwifery Council (2004) *Midwives Rules and Standards*. London: NMC.

Nursing and Midwifery Council (2010) *Record Keeping: Guidance for Nurses and Midwives*. London: NMC.

Oates, M., Harper, A., Shakespeare, J. and Nelson-Percy, C. (2011) Back to basics, in Centre for Maternal and Child Enquiries, *Saving Mothers' Lives: Reviewing Maternal Deaths to Make Motherhood Safer: 2006–2008. The Eighth Report on Confidential Enquiries into Maternal Deaths in the United Kingdom*. Ed. G. Lewis. *BJOG:* 118 (Suppl. 1): 16–21.

Olson, C.M., Strawderman, M.S. and Dennison, B.A. (2009) Maternal weight gain during pregnancy and child weight at age 3 years, *Maternal and Child Health Journal*, 13(6): 839–46.

PRECOG Development Group (2004) *Pre-eclampsia Community Guideline (PRECOG)*. Leicester: Action on Pre-eclampsia (APEC). Available at: http://www.apec.org.uk

Rajasingam, D. and Swamy, S. (2010) Intrapartum care of obese women, in Y. Richens and T. Lavender (eds) *Care for Pregnant Women Who Are Obese*. Huntingdon: Quay Books, pp. 117–31.

Rasmussen, K.M. and Yaktine, A.L. (eds) (2009) *Weight Gain During Pregnancy: Re-examining the Guidelines*. Washington, DC: Institute of Medicine and National Research Council of the National Academies, The National Academies Press.

Royal College of Obstetricians and Gynaecologists (2009a) *Improving Patient Safety: Risk Management for Maternity and Gynaecology: Clinical Governance Advice 2*. London: RCOG Press.

Royal College of Obstetricians and Gynaecologists (2009b) *Thrombosis and Embolism during Pregnancy and the Puerperium: Reducing the Risk:* Green Top Guideline 37a. London: RCOG Press.

Royal College of Obstetricians and Gynaecologists, Royal College of Midwives, Royal College of Anaesthetists, Royal College of Paediatrics and Child Health (2007) *Safer Childbirth: Minimum Standards for the Organisation and Delivery of Care in Labour*. London: RCOG Press.

Stenhouse, C., Coates, S., Tivey, M., Allsop, P. and Parker, T. (1999) Prospective evaluation of a Modified Early Warning Score to aid earlier detection of patients developing critical illness on a general surgical ward, *British Journal of Anaesthesia*, 84: 663.

Symon, A. (2006) The risk-choice paradox, in A. Symon, *Risk and Choice in Maternity Care: An International Perspective*. Edinburgh: Churchill Livingstone, Elsevier, pp. 1–11.

Wilson, J.H. and Symon, A. (2002) *Clinical Risk Management in Midwifery: The Right to a Perfect Baby*. Oxford: Books for Midwives.

ANNOTATED FURTHER READING

Centre for Maternal and Child Enquiries (CMACE) (2011) *Saving Mothers' Lives: Reviewing Maternal Deaths to Make Motherhood Safer: 2006–2008. The Eighth Report on Confidential Enquiries into Maternal Deaths in the United Kingdom*. Ed. G. Lewis. *BJOG:* 118 (Suppl. 1): 1–203.

Provides an insight into the extent that obesity contributed to the 261 maternal deaths during 2006–2008 with recommendations for best practice for the multidisciplinary team to take heed of.

Richens, Y. and Lavender, T. (eds) (2010) *Care for Pregnant Women Who Are Obese*. Huntingdon: Quay Books.

The first book to focus on the growing epidemic of obesity and its effect on the care of pregnant women, the health of their babies and the maternity services.

USEFUL WEBSITES

www.cmace.org.uk	Centre for Maternal and Child Enquiries
www.cqc.org.uk	Care Quality Commission
www.dh.gov.uk	Department of Health
www.eatwell.gov.uk	Eat Well
www.ihi.org	Institute for Healthcare Improvements
www.institute.nhs.uk	NHS Institute for Innovation and Improvement
www.ncepod.org.uk	National Confidential Enquiry into Patient Outcome and Death
www.nhsla.com	National Health Service Litigation Authority
www.nice.org.uk	National Institute for Health and Clinical Excellence
www.npsa.nhs.uk	National Patient Safety Agency
www.nrls.npsa.mhs.uk	National Reporting and Learning Service
www.rcog.org.uk	Royal College of Obstetricians and Gynaecologists

Pre-eclampsia, eclampsia and HELLP syndrome

Jayne E. Marshall and Margaret M. Ramsay

Pre-requisites for the chapter: the reader should have an understanding of:

- The physiological changes occurring in the cardiovascular, haematological (including the coagulation pathway or clotting cascade) and renal systems during pregnancy.
- Risk factors associated with hypertensive disease.
- Skills of adult and neonatal basic and advanced life support.
- Fetal monitoring and cardiotocography interpretation skills.
- Normal values for umbilical cord blood acid base analysis.
- The Modified Early Obstetric Warning Scoring System (MEOWS).
- Interprofessional team learning and working.
- The midwife's role and statutory responsibilities in the management of maternity complications/emergencies.
- Local National Health Service (NHS) Trust medicine code and clinical governance/risk management procedures.

Pre-reading self-assessment

1 What is blood pressure?
2 What are plasma proteins?
3 What is the function of anti-diuretic hormone (ADH)?
4 What are osmo-receptors?
5 How is volume homeostasis maintained?
6 What is the significance of the renin-angiotensin-aldosterone system in electrolyte balance?
7 What is haemolysis?
8 What are the functions of platelets?
9 Which of the substances produced in the liver are involved in the clotting of blood?
10 What are the functions of the liver and the liver enzymes?
11 What are bilirubin and biliverdin?

(Continued overleaf)

Recommended prior reading

National Institute for Health and Clinical Excellence (2010) *Hypertension in Pregnancy: The Management Of Hypertensive Disorders During Pregnancy*. Clinical Guideline No. 107. London: NICE. Available at: http://www.nice.org.uk

NHS Institute for Innovation and Improvement (2008) *SBAR: Situation, Background, Assessment, Recommendation*. Available at: http://www.institute.nhs.uk. (accessed 12 January 2011)

CASE STUDY: PART 1

Elizabeth, a 44-year-old woman, and her husband John were delighted to find a positive pregnancy test after the third cycle of IVF. Donor eggs had been used and the scan performed at the local IVF clinic showed a singleton pregnancy. When she was 9 weeks pregnant, Elizabeth visited the local health centre for her first appointment with the midwife to discuss the plan of care for her first pregnancy in respect of antenatal visits and place of birth. Her BP on this occasion was 125/75 mmHg and the urine sample was clear of any abnormalities.

At 12 weeks, Elizabeth attended the consultant clinic at the local hospital. A nuchal translucency scan was undertaken which gave a low risk for trisomy 21, much to Elizabeth's relief. A detailed scan of fetal anatomy was undertaken at 20 weeks: her BP was 120/62 mmHg and urine showed no abnormalities. An appointment was made to see the consultant at 28 weeks to review fetal growth.

Elizabeth remained well and the fetus active. At 24 weeks, she visited the community midwife where her BP was 130/80 mmHg and her urine was clear of any abnormalities. Elizabeth said she was looking forward to going on holiday to Italy with John for a couple of weeks as she was beginning to feel exhausted by work in the office. On the last day of her holiday, Elizabeth mentioned to John that she was still feeling tired and had been struggling to get rid of a migrainous headache. She went to bed early, but did not feel much better when she awoke the next day. During the flight home, Elizabeth complained of nausea and upper abdominal pain and upon arrival at the airport terminal, rushed to the restroom and started to vomit. John rang the local maternity unit and arranged to take Elizabeth there, rather than going home.

On admission to the triage unit of the maternity unit, Elizabeth's BP was found to be 180/115 mmHg and her urine sample contained 4+ protein. From the certain dates of embryo transfer, Elizabeth was 27 weeks pregnant. The midwife referred Elizabeth to the obstetrician on call for his opinion. At this point Elizabeth's BP had increased to 230/120 mmHg with moderate epigastric tenderness on palpation of the abdomen. The symphysis pubis fundal height (SPFH) measured 23 cm and the tendon reflexes were brisk with 5 beats of clonus.

About an hour later Elizabeth's blood results were found to be as shown in Results Chart 3.1. Other renal and liver function tests and the clotting screen were within the normal range for pregnancy.

1 **Identify the risk factors that Elizabeth may have and outline the plan of care for subsequent antenatal visits.**

A As Elizabeth and John have undergone infertility treatment to achieve a successful pregnancy, it is expected that they are well aware of how fertility and pregnancy outcomes change with

Results Chart 3.1

Blood test	Result	Normal range
Haemoglobin	16.3 g/dL	10.5–13.5 g/dL
Platelets	165 × 10⁹/L	150–400 × 10⁹/L
White cell count	14.8 × 10⁹/L	6–16 × 10⁹/L
Creatinine	80 micromol/L	40–70 micromol/L
Urea	4.5 mmol/L	2.5–4.5 mmol/L
Uric acid	283 micromol/L	150–300 micromol/L
Alanine transferase	678 U/L	< 40 U/L
Bilirubin	15 micromol/L	< 15 micromol/L
Albumin	28 g/L	25–35 g/L

age. Biologically, the optimum period for childbearing is between 20–35 years of age when most women will get pregnant. Leridon (2004) states that during this age period, 75 per cent of women aged 30 and 66 per cent of women aged 35 will conceive naturally within a year and have a baby. After this age it is increasingly difficult to become pregnant, with a higher chance of miscarriage occurring. As with Elizabeth and John, at this stage, fertility treatment may be considered, sometimes with multiple embryo implantations or donor eggs from younger women to improve the pregnancy success rate. According to the HFEA (2010), figures show that the live birth rate for women aged less than 35 undergoing IVF is 33.1 per cent with the rate falling to 2.5 per cent for women over the age of 44 years.

Reviewing Elizabeth's history at this first antenatal visit, the midwife would be fully aware that for Elizabeth and John this first pregnancy would be full of a range of emotions. They would be delighted that after years of infertility treatment they had finally succeeded in achieving a pregnancy, but may be anxious that due to Elizabeth's advanced age, she would remain well and have a healthy baby at term. It is well documented that adverse pregnancy outcomes also rise with age, and women over 40 years are considered to be at a higher risk of pregnancy complications, including fetal chromosomal abnormalities (Hoffman et al. 2007; Luke and Brown 2007; Delpisheh et al. 2008; Khoshnood et al. 2008). However, in Elizabeth and John's case, the pregnancy had been achieved with younger donor eggs so the aging effects associated with chromosomal defects would be reduced.

In view of Elizabeth's infertility treatment, advanced age and potential risk of developing complications of pregnancy such as pre-eclampsia and diabetes, the midwife should inform Elizabeth that her care will be planned in collaboration with the consultant obstetrician at the local hospital. While surveillance of blood pressure and urinalysis could remain in the community setting, additional antenatal surveillance of maternal and fetal well-being would be undertaken by the hospital obstetric team. The place of birth would be determined by the health and well-being of both Elizabeth and her unborn baby, but at this early stage of pregnancy, all available options should be considered: home, birth centre and hospital (DH 2007). The details of these discussions relating to the care plan should be clearly documented by the midwife in Elizabeth's maternity records according to the NMC (2004, 2010) *Midwives Rules and Standards* and guidance on record keeping.

2 **Why is the precise determination of diastolic pressure critically important in pregnancy?**

A In early pregnancy, there is a marked decrease in diastolic BP but little change in systolic pressure. As a result of reduced peripheral vascular resistance, the systolic BP falls an average of 5–10 mmHg below baseline levels with the diastolic BP decreasing 10–15 mmHg by 24 weeks gestation. From this time, the BP gradually rises, returning to pre-pregnancy levels at term. It is therefore important that BP is assessed as early as possible in pregnancy in order to establish a baseline that is as near to a pre-pregnancy level as is possible to make clear comparisons throughout pregnancy. This will then serve in the prompt identification of any hypertensive disease of pregnancy which is the second major cause of maternal death in the UK, according to the latest triennial report (Lewis 2011).

Compression of the inferior vena cava and lower aorta by the enlarging uterus from the late second trimester results in reduced venous return which in turn decreases stroke volume and cardiac output. In addition, posture can have a major effect on the BP with the supine position decreasing cardiac output by as much as 25 per cent. Elizabeth may suffer from supine hypotensive syndrome which consists of hypotension, bradycardia, dizziness, light-headedness and even syncope, should she remain in the supine position too long. Encouraging her to move onto her left side will enable the cardiac output to be instantly restored.

3 **Which Korotkoff sound is used as standard practice to measure the diastolic pressure more accurately in pregnancy?**

A As hypertensive disease remains a major contributor to maternal and perinatal morbidity and death, the accurate measurement of maternal BP is vitally important. Blood pressure should not be assessed after a woman has undertaken any exercise, experienced anxiety or pain or has smoked. In such circumstances, it is recommended that a 10-minute rest period is observed before measuring the BP. NICE (2010a, 2010b), PRECOG Development Group (2004) and Williams et al. (2004) have summarized the guidance regarding the standard for BP assessment in pregnancy which is identified in Box 3.1.

Box 3.1 Blood pressure measurement by standard mercury sphygmomanometer or semi-automated device

The woman should be seated or lying in the left lateral position at an angle of 45°.
Remove tight clothing, ensure arm is relaxed and supported at heart level.
Use a properly maintained, calibrated, and validated device.
Avoid talking during procedure.
Use cuff of appropriate size: length of bladder should be at least 80 per cent of arm circumference (35 cm = standard size, 41 cm = large size, > 42 cm = thigh size).
Inflate cuff to 20–30 mmHg above palpated systolic BP.
Lower column slowly, by 2 mmHg per second or per beat.
Read blood pressure to nearest 2 mmHg (do NOT round up).

Measure diastolic blood pressure as disappearance of sounds (Korotkoff Phase V).
Take the mean of at least two readings if marked differences between initial measure-
ments are found.
Do not treat on the basis of an isolated reading.

(Williams et al. 2004; NICE 2010a, 2010b;
PRECOG Development Group 2004).

Think

- Some automated blood pressure monitoring systems *underestimate* the systolic
  blood pressure in pre-eclampsia.

The use of Korotkoff Phase V where the audibility of the heart sounds disappears as a measure
of the diastolic BP has been found to be easier to obtain, more reproducible and closer to the
intra-arterial pressure in pregnancy. This reading should always be used unless the sound is
near to zero, in which case the muffling sound of Korotkoff Phase IV should also be observed
(PRECOG Development Group 2004) and then recorded (NMC 2010).

4 **What could be the possible causes of Elizabeth's symptoms at 27 weeks of
pregnancy?**

A The cause of any deterioration in maternal health should be thoroughly investigated as there
may be underlying disorders or pathology such as diabetes or cardiomyopathy which may
affect normal organ function. The differential diagnoses that should be considered by the
midwife are listed in Table 3.1.

In the latest triennial report of the Confidential Enquiries into Maternal Deaths, 2006–
2008, Neilson (2011) states that there has been no reduction in the number of mortalities
relating to pre-eclampsia and eclampsia (Lewis 2011) in that there were a total of 19 deaths,
8 of which had also developed HELLP syndrome (see Table 3.2). It is therefore important for
midwives at the front-line of maternity care to be fully aware of symptoms women may
present with that could be signs of developing pre-eclampsia to ensure that appropriate and
prompt referral is made to the obstetric team (NMC 2004).

5 **What should be the triage midwife's actions on discovering such observations in
respect of determining Elizabeth's subsequent management and care?**

A Having undertaken an antenatal examination followed by auscultation of the fetal heart
(FH) to assess fetal well-being along with the BP and urinalysis results, the midwife
should recognize her professional responsibility and the need to alert the obstetric team of
Elizabeth's admission realizing that the severity of her condition could be significant of

Table 3.1   Differential diagnoses to explain Elizabeth's symptoms within the context of the given scenario

Symptom	Differential diagnosis	
Tiredness/exhaustion	Anaemia	
	Cardiac disease	
	Hypothyroidism	
Migraine/persistent headache	Anaemia	
	Heat stroke	
	Pre-eclampsia	
Nausea/vomiting	Urinary tract infection, pyelonephritis	
	Thyroid disorders	
	Gastroenteritis	
	Heat stroke	
	Pre-eclampsia	
Upper abdominal pain	*Pregnancy specific*	
	Physiological	*Pathological*
	Heartburn	Spontaneous miscarriage
	Vomiting	Pre-term labour
	Constipation	Placental abruption
	Braxton Hicks contractions	Uterine fibroids
	Round ligament pain	Severe pre-eclampsia
		H E L L P syndrome
		Uterine rupture
	Incidental causes	
	Common pathology	*Rare pathology*
	Appendicitis	Rectus haematoma
	Urinary tract infection, pyelonephritis	Porphyria
		Arteriovenous haemorrhage
	Acute cholecystitis	Malignant disease
	Ovarian pathology, e.g. torsion	
	Gastro-oesophageal reflux/ peptic ulcer disease	
	Acute pancreatitis	
	Inflammatory bowel disease	
	Intestinal obstruction	
	Malaria	
	Tuberculosis (also associated with HIV)	

pre-eclampsia. Table 3.2 reflects the classification of hypertensive disease as identified by NICE (2010a).

In addition, the Guideline Development Group (GDG) has defined mild, moderate and severe hypertension to help with the implementation of NICE (2010a) guidance which is highlighted as follows in Box 3.2.

Table 3.2 Definitions of hypertensive disease related to pregnancy

Chronic hypertension is hypertension that is present at the first antenatal visit or before 20 weeks if the woman is already taking antihypertensive medication when referred to the maternity services. It can be primary or secondary in aetiology.

Gestational hypertension is new hypertension in pregnancy presenting after 20 weeks without significant proteinuria.

Significant proteinuria is if the protein: creatinine ratio is > 30 mg/mmol or a validated 24 hour urine collection result shows > 300 mg protein.

Pre-eclampsia is new hypertension presenting after 20 weeks with significant proteinuria.

Severe pre-eclampsia is pre-eclampsia with severe hypertension and/or biochemical and/or haematological impairment.

HELLP syndrome is haemolysis, elevated liver enzymes and low platelet count.

Eclampsia is a convulsive condition associated with pre-eclampsia.

Source: NICE 2010a.

Box 3.2 Degrees of hypertension (NICE 2010a)

Mild hypertension: diastolic blood pressure 90–99 mmHg and systolic blood pressure 140–149 mmHg.
Moderate hypertension: diastolic blood pressure 100–109 mmHg and systolic blood pressure 150–159 mmHg.
Severe hypertension: diastolic blood pressure 110 mmHg or greater and systolic blood pressure 160 mmHg or greater.

The midwife would be wise to consider the SBAR (Situation, Background, Assessment, Recommendation) tool (NHS Institute for Innovation and Improvement 2008) as discussed in Case 2 to guarantee that her communication with other members of the multiprofessional team is effective in ensuring Elizabeth's management and subsequent care are both appropriate and prompt. The following example provides a typical script to the obstetrician that the midwife might employ using the SBAR tool:

- *Situation*: This is Helen, midwife in triage. I have Elizabeth Brown, a 44-year-old primigravida who is booked for midwife-led care and has been experiencing frontal headaches, upper abdominal pain and nausea and vomiting. On admission, her BP was 180/115 mmHg and her urine sample contained 4+ protein.
- *Background*: Elizabeth is 27 weeks pregnant with an IVF pregnancy by donor eggs. She came directly from the airport following a holiday in Italy, having felt generally unwell and tired for the past few weeks. Prior to this point, she had been well with no significant medical history and fetal growth was within the normal range for gestational age. There is no vaginal bleeding evident or any signs of labour. She is not taking any medication and has no known allergies.

- *Assessment*: I have undertaken an antenatal examination and find the pregnancy to be smaller than the gestational age (about 24 weeks), and have commenced a CTG which so far is reactive with good baseline variability. I have already started a fluid balance chart to monitor renal function. Based on her history, presentation and the fact she is experiencing epigastric pain, I feel she is showing signs of pre-eclampsia.
- *Recommendation*: Would you like me to organize transfer to the obstetric critical care unit or do you want to review Elizabeth here on triage? In the meantime do you want me to insert an indwelling urinary catheter and get IV access? I have got all the blood profile forms ready for you. When are you likely to get here to see Elizabeth?

In addition to the midwife's findings from assessing Elizabeth's condition, it is important that she also clearly documents her dialogue and discussions with the obstetrician as well as Elizabeth and John, within Elizabeth's maternity records (NMC 2010).

6   **What is the significance of tendon reflexes in the assessment of Elizabeth's condition?**

A   Prolonged clonus (4 or more beats) is an indication of cerebral irritability and indicates that seizures may soon occur.

7   **Identify the probable diagnosis and subsequent actions/investigations that should be undertaken at this point.**

A   In the context of hypertension with proteinuria occurring during pregnancy, prolonged clonus is a strong pointer to the diagnosis of severe pre-eclampsia, with eclamptic seizures imminent. It is crucial that IV access is established promptly and blood tests taken from Elizabeth for full blood count, renal function, liver function, clotting and to group and save blood. It is important to gain control of the very high BP, using agents such as IV hydralazine given in small doses (2.5–5 mg) and repeated every 20 minutes, aiming to suppress the BP to ≤ 160/105 mmHg. Alternatively, IV labetalol could be used, given as slow injections of 20 mg, repeated every 10 minutes. To protect Elizabeth from experiencing eclamptic seizures, magnesium sulphate should be given by an IV loading dose of 4 g over 20 minutes, followed by a constant infusion of 1 g/hr (Magpie Trial Collaborative Group 2002). A urinary catheter should be inserted into Elizabeth's bladder and hourly urine measurements monitored and recorded on a fluid balance chart. A cardiotocograph (CTG) should also be commenced to assess the well-being of Elizabeth's baby as at 27 weeks the pregnancy is over the legal viability age.

8   **What are the potential risks involved to the well-being of Elizabeth and the fetus?**

A   Pre-eclampsia has the potential of causing serious maternal complications, including cerebral haemorrhage, seizures, coagulopathy, renal or hepatic derangement (Haddad et al. 2000; Vigil-De 2001; Deruelle et al. 2006). The blood tests sent must be studied for abnormalities at first presentation and then repeated at intervals where there are marked features of systemic illness. Early birth of Elizabeth's baby is likely so it would be wise to administer corticosteroids such as 12 mg betamethasone or dexamethasone IM to assist fetal lung maturity and reduce respiratory distress syndrome in the pre-term infant (Roberts and Dalziel 2006). It is thought that the maximum effect from steroids on promoting fetal lung maturity takes 48 hours, but on balance they should be given, even if it seems unlikely that the birth of Elizabeth's baby could be withheld for that time. There would also seem to be chronic placental insufficiency with pre-eclampsia, causing IUGR as the fundal height measured only 23 cm at 27 weeks (comparable with the size of a 24-week pregnancy). Fetal compromise (hypoxaemia) may be precipitated by decreasing maternal BP as antihypertensives are given, altering uterine blood flow. A further risk to Elizabeth and her fetus is that of acute compromise due to placental abruption.

9 **What is the significance of Elizabeth's latest blood results when compared with the normal pregnancy range?**

A Overall, the blood results point to multiple organ dysfunction, which, in addition to the documented hypertension and proteinuria, show that Elizabeth has severe pre-eclampsia. The significance of the results is shown in Table 3.3.

Table 3.3 Significance of elevated results

Result	Significance
Elevated haemoglobin/haemoconcentration	Plasma volume loss into peripheral tissues leading to oedema
Elevated creatinine	Impaired renal clearance function
Elevated alanine transferase	Liver cell damage

CASE STUDY: PART 2

At this point the CTG had a baseline fetal heart rate (FHR) of 145–155 beats/min. with a variability of 5–10 beats/min. Although some accelerations were evident, there were also frequent variable decelerations, without any evidence of uterine activity. Repeated doses of hydralazine (totalling 20 mg) were required as Elizabeth's BP remained very high and labile. In the first 6 hours following admission, her urine output was only 140 mL. During this time she had drunk 1500 mL of clear fluids and had been receiving 50 mL/hr of intravenous fluid with the magnesium sulphate infusion.

Blood tests were repeated 6 hours after admission and the following results were obtained (Results Chart 3.2). Other renal and liver function tests and the clotting screen were within the normal range for pregnancy.

Results Chart 3.2

Blood test	Results (on admission)	Results (6 hours later)
Haemoglobin	16.3 g/dL	15.8 g/dL
Platelets	165 × 10⁹/L	70 × 10⁹/L
White cell count	14.8 × 10⁹/L	16.5 × 10⁹/L
Creatinine	80 micromol/L	83 micromol/L
Urea	4.5 mmol/L	4.9 mmol/L
Uric acid	283 micromol/L	325 micromol/L
Alanine transferase	678 U/L	787 U/L
Bilirubin	15 micromol/L	38 micromol/L
Albumin	28 g/L	27 g/L

It was evident by this time that the situation was deteriorating as Elizabeth's BP remained dangerously high and difficult to control, there was oliguria and increasing concerns about fetal well-being. The consultant obstetrician, who had been informed at various stages during the night of developments by midwifery and obstetric staff, came into the hospital to see Elizabeth and review her condition. Birth by caesarean section was promptly advised. Prior to transferring Elizabeth to the operating theatre a portable ultrasound scan showed an extended breech presentation with a fundal placenta.

A general anaesthetic was given to Elizabeth following the administration of additional doses of IV labetalol and hydralazine to reduce the BP to 109/96 mmHg. The tissues of the abdominal wall were found to be oedematous and there was free peritoneal fluid. The lower uterine segment at 27 weeks was adequate for a transverse incision. The baby was born in the amniotic sac, but the membranes burst as the buttocks were born. The baby boy, Henry, was handed to attending neonatologists; he weighed 0.89 kg and was taken to the NICU. His umbilical venous pH was 7.20 and base deficit 4.7. Once the placenta and membranes were expelled, the wound and abdominal layers were closed, ensuring that haemostasis had occurred.

Elizabeth returned to the obstetric critical care unit from theatre. IV fluids were restricted to 80 mL/hr, with oral fluids being offered as and when Elizabeth could tolerate them. The midwife made hourly observations of P, BP, RR and urine output. Elizabeth was given 50 mg of oral atenolol and IV bolus doses of labetalol when her BP exceeded 170/100 mmHg. The IV infusion of magnesium sulphate continued. Initially on return from theatre, her urine output was 30–35 mL/hr, but after 6 hours the volumes were increasing to 80 mL/hr; according to Miller et al. (2009) the normal urine output should be a minimum of 0.5 mL/kg/hr.

10   **Comparing the two sets of blood results, on admission and then 6 hours later, what trends are developing?**

A   The most important changes are decreasing platelet count, increasing alanine transferase and elevated bilirubin. The decreasing Hb may be within laboratory measuring error, but in the context of elevated bilirubin could indicate red cell destruction, i.e. haemolysis. The trends point to severe pre-eclampsia of the HELLP syndrome variety (Haemolysis, Elevated Liver enzymes, Low Platelets).

11   **What do you consider to be the potential risks/dangers to Elizabeth and the fetus?**

A   The potential risks to Elizabeth are that she may develop a significant coagulopathy due to rapidly deteriorating liver function and consumption of platelets; this could even result in her having spontaneous bleeding or bruising. Since her BP is extremely high, she is at significant risk of intracerebral haemorrhage. She may become rapidly anaemic due to red cell haemolysis. There is also risk of deteriorating renal function and, given the rapidly changing picture indicating a very severe form of pre-eclampsia, she is at risk of progressing to eclamptic seizures.

The potential risks to the fetus are those of acute-on-chronic hypoxaemia: the growth-restricted fetus is likely to already have a poorly functioning placenta and any change in placental perfusion, such as may occur with maternal BP changes, could critically compromise placental gas exchange (Rath et al. 2000). There are also risks of placental abruption with such high maternal BP which could suddenly cause catastrophic fetal compromise. Fetal death *in utero* is a possibility under these circumstances.

12   **What are the factors that would determine the timing and mode of birth?**

A   The only 'cure' for pre-eclampsia is expediting the birth of the fetus and placenta. In severe cases, birth is indicated for maternal health reasons: inability to gain control of hypertension, rapidly deteriorating liver function, rapidly developing coagulopathy, rapidly deteriorating renal function (especially if there is oliguria with < 30 mL/hr urine output). Although there are significant risks for the fetus of being born very prematurely, it may be in its best interests, should there be features to suggest hypoxaemia *in utero*.

There needs to be clear decision making at very premature gestations as to whether or not the fetus has a chance of survival should the birth be expedited. This is judged by gestational age and predicted body weight. If there is no realistic chance of survival, then it is better not to undertake electronic fetal monitoring. If the fetus is judged to be potentially viable, then CTG features such as recurrent decelerations, poor heart rate variability and baseline tachycardia, can all point to hypoxaemia and acidaemia and should be used as triggers to provoke birth in the interest of the fetus. Ideally, as stated previously, at premature gestations, time should be allowed for maternally-administered steroids to promote fetal lung maturity (i.e. 48 hours from the first dose) but when there is rapid deterioration in maternal or fetal health, then the birth of the baby must be considered sooner than this.

The mode of birth at very premature gestations with an extremely sick woman and/or fetus is of necessity by caesarean section. In Elizabeth's case, it would be extremely difficult to induce labour at 27 weeks as the process would take too long, maternal health would deteriorate and it is unlikely that the fetus would survive the additional stresses of labour. It is also likely that the caesarean would require a vertical or 'classical' uterine incision, as the lower uterine segment may be poorly formed in the early third trimester.

13   **What are the particular risks of anaesthesia and major surgery in Elizabeth's case?**

A   Regional anaesthetic techniques, such as spinal or epidural anaesthesia are associated with risks for haematoma formation around the needle entry site in women with significant coagulopathy (such as is indicated by a platelet count of 70×10^9/L). A haematoma close to the spinal cord could cause nerve root or cord compression. A general anaesthetic requires orotracheal intubation, which always provokes a pressor response, i.e. a surge in BP. This is potentially dangerous when maternal BP is already high and might provoke an intracerebral haemorrhage. It is important to give additional antihypertensive drugs prior to induction of anaesthesia, to minimize this pressor response.

Surgery in women with coagulopathy due to low platelet counts brings increased risks for bleeding within the operative field. Such bleeding may be controlled with surgical haemostatic techniques (occlusive sutures, cauterization) but may require the infusion of additional clotting factors (fresh frozen plasma, cryoprecipitate, platelets). In the case of the birth of Elizabeth's very small pre-term baby, an experienced obstetrician would be required to manage potential intra-operative difficulties such as determining the most appropriate uterine incision, achieving haemostasis and to be familiar with the gentle handling of pre-term babies.

14   **Where should Elizabeth's care and management take place following the birth of baby Henry?**

A   Elizabeth would be transferred back to the obstetric critical care unit (NICE 2010a) where she should receive one-to-one specialist care by experienced midwives trained in critical care/high dependency skills to closely monitor her condition and recovery from the surgery and general anaesthesia.

15   **What observations would you undertake to minimize further risk to Elizabeth's health and well-being?**

A   Using the Modified Early Obstetric Warning Scoring system (MEOWS) (see Case 2) to record all observations undertaken on Elizabeth in the immediate postoperative/postnatal period will enable the midwife to promptly report any deviation from normality. Such a document provides effective communication within the multiprofessional team to ensure that clear referral pathways and treatment/care plans are mobilized when necessary. Elizabeth's condition should be closely monitored for at least the first 24–72 hours as there is still a risk of her developing eclampsia. The midwife should therefore be alert to the following signs developing, shown in Table 3.4.

The AVPU Scale (Greater Manchester Critical Care Skills Institute 2002) can be used to assess Elizabeth's conscious level in terms of her being **A**lert and conscious, responsive to **V**oice and **P**ain or whether she is **U**nresponsive, noting that **P** and **U** scores should be promptly reported to the anaesthetic and obstetric team (see Case 1).

Table 3.4 Signs and symptoms of impending eclampsia and associated pathophysiology

Sign and symptom	Pathophysiology
Sharp rise in blood pressure.	Dilatation of the spiral arterioles in the placental bed by the stripping away of their muscle coating around the second trimester leading to the physiological fall in blood pressure, fails to occur. The blood pressure is raised as it is forced through constricted arterioles.
Headache: usually severe, persistent and frontal in location (cerebral vasospasm).	There is generalized endothelial dysfunction leading to increased vascular tone, vasospasm and disturbances of maternal microcirculation. Consequently, there is hypoperfusion and vasoconstriction in the maternal brain, kidneys and liver and in the placenta (Walker 2000).
Visual disturbances: blurring of vision or flashing lights (cerebral vasospasm) Drowsiness or confusion (cerebral vasospasm).	
Diminished urine output ± increase in proteinuria (renal failure).	
Epigastric pain (liver oedema) ± nausea and vomiting.	
Intrauterine growth restriction.	

Source: NICE 2010a, 2010b.

When assessing Elizabeth's pain, the midwife should also be alert to this extending from the abdomen to the neck and shoulder as being a serious complication of HELLP syndrome, indicating subcapsular haematoma of the liver that has the potential to rupture. Furthermore, as this condition can also include clotting abnormalities such as DIC (see also Case 5), observation of the lochia and caesarean section wound to ensure haemostasis is vital.

It is also important for the midwife to be alert to Elizabeth's psychological state following the birth and provide care that is sensitive and empathetic to her needs and that of her husband John. Couples who have experienced infertility can also encounter difficulties adjusting to parenthood especially when their baby is being cared for by competent health professionals within the NICU. Elizabeth and John may value an opportunity to talk with the midwife about their feelings of events surrounding the pre-term birth and their anxieties about Henry and their ability to care for him. NICE (2007) recommend that midwives and health care professionals should draw on the support of family and friends rather than offering single session formal debriefing sessions to talk over birth events as there is no reliable data to support the latter format in reducing postnatal emotional distress. Once Elizabeth's condition improves, the midwife should negotiate with the staff on the NICU a suitable time for her to visit Henry.

16 **What are the benefits and risks of magnesium sulphate in cases such as Elizabeth's?**

A Magnesium sulphate has been shown in a large randomized controlled trial to be the best agent for preventing eclamptic seizures (Magpie Trial Collaborative Group 2002), without serious harmful effects to childbearing women or babies. It also probably reduces the risk for maternal death in women with severe pre-eclampsia. In women who have already experienced an eclamptic seizure, magnesium sulphate is the best agent for preventing further seizures and controlling an acute seizure (the Eclampsia Trial Collaborative Group 1995).

CASE STUDY: PART 3

The following day, Elizabeth's condition had greatly improved and her BP was in the range of 150–179 mmHg systolic and 89–100 mmHg diastolic. Her urine output varied between 40–500 mL/hr. In the whole 24-hour period, her total fluid input was 3250 mL and output 5130 mL. There was still 4+ proteinuria, but this had diminished to 2+ proteinuria by the evening. Her abdomen was soft and the wound only minimally bruised when the pressure dressing was removed.

Elizabeth's blood results 24 hours following the birth can be seen in Results Chart 3.3. Other liver function tests were normal.

Henry did very well, but spent several weeks in the NICU until ready for discharge home to Elizabeth and John. Elizabeth's BP remained well controlled on a combination of one daily dose of 50 mg atenolol and twice daily doses of 30 mg nifedipine. She was transferred home on this medication and her GP reduced it slowly over the following 6 weeks. At the time of her hospital postnatal examination at 7 weeks post-birth, Elizabeth had discontinued all antihypertensive therapy and her BP was 117/56 mmHg. The urine tested negative for protein. Her Hb level was 13 g/dL and platelet count 298 × 10⁹/L. Considering the severity of pre-eclampsia and HELLP syndrome, the obstetrician discussed the management of future pregnancies with Elizabeth and John.

Results Chart 3.3

Blood test	Result (on admission)	Result (6 hours later)	Result (24 hours following birth)
Haemoglobin	16.3 g/dL	15.8 g/dL	13.0 g/dL
Platelets	165×10^9/L	70×10^9/L	43×10^9/L
White cell count	14.8×10^9/L	16.5×10^9/L	14.6×10^9/L
Creatinine	80 micromol/L	83 micromol/L	78 micromol/L
Urea	4.5 mmol/L	4.9 mmol/L	6.9 mmol/L
Uric acid	283 micromol/L	325 micromol/L	292 micromol/L
Alanine transferase	678 U/L	787 U/L	341 U/L
Bilirubin	15 micromol/L	38 micromol/L	14 micromol/L
Albumin	28 g/L	27 g/L	21 g/L
Sodium	133 mmol/L	129 mmol/L	127 mmol/L
Potassium	4.4 mmol/L	4.9 mmol/L	4.8 mmol/L

17   **How would you interpret these latest results when comparing them with Elizabeth's previous results and the normal pregnancy range?**

A   The most striking feature of these results is the low platelet count, which is very much to be expected in a woman with HELLP syndrome. Typically, platelet counts reach their nadir 48 hours post-birth. There are signs of improving liver function (alanine transferase decreasing and bilirubin now back to normal range) and stable renal function. The decrease in Hb is consistent with recent surgery. There is no ongoing evidence of haemolysis, since bilirubin levels are normal. The sodium level is low, indicating some derangement of renal tubular function. Albumin levels are lower than previously, indicating that there has been more protein loss (in the urine) than production (in the liver).

18   **How could the low sodium, albumin and platelet levels be improved?**

A   The low sodium, albumin and platelet levels just need time to correct themselves; no specific actions are required. If there was ongoing bleeding (e.g. from the surgical incision site) or spontaneous bruising, it would be necessary to administer a platelet transfusion. The sodium level is not dangerously low, so will correct itself as renal function normalizes given adequate dietary salt intake. The albumin levels will improve as urinary proteinuria diminishes and liver function normalizes.

19   **Considering the risk factors apparent in Elizabeth's case post-birth, when would you consider she could be safely transferred to the postnatal ward?**

A   Elizabeth should not be transferred to the postnatal ward until she is showing signs of sustained improvement from pre-eclampsia. This will be evidenced by her BP decreasing (including a lessening of her need for antihypertensive drug treatment), her urine output improving and the proteinuria diminishing. Typically, the post-birth diuresis is exaggerated in women with pre-eclampsia, as they have a lot of tissue oedema which is mobilized back into the plasma and then eliminated via the kidneys. One of the pathophysiological processes in pre-eclampsia is that endothelial cells (which line all blood vessels, including the glomeruli of the kidneys) are malfunctioning. This leads to a failure of regulation of local vascular tone and increased capillary permeability. As endothelial cell function normalizes after the baby is born, the tendency to vascular spasm and hypertension recovers and fluid is correctly partitioned between intravascular and extravascular compartments. The risk for eclamptic seizures remains while Elizabeth still has symptoms of headaches, epigastric pain or visual disturbances, and also while she shows signs of hyper-reflexia or sustained clonus. While Elizabeth is showing any of these signs or symptoms, she will require a transfusion of magnesium sulphate for at least 24 hours after birth. As NICE (2010a) advocate, BP should be monitored at least 4 times a day while Elizabeth is hospitalized and then every 1–2 days for up to 2 weeks when transferred home to community midwifery/GP care until medication is withdrawn and there is no evidence of any hypertension.

Think

- Elizabeth should not be transferred to the postnatal ward while receiving magnesium sulphate.

---

20 **What are Elizabeth's risks of developing pre-eclampsia in a subsequent pregnancy?**

A According to NICE (2010a), women such as Elizabeth who have a history of severe pre-eclampsia and HELLP syndrome leading to birth before 28 weeks have a 1 in 2 risk (55 per cent) of developing severe pre-eclampsia, HELLP syndrome or eclampsia in a future pregnancy. This risk, however, is lessened to 1 in 4 pregnancies (25 per cent) should the birth have occurred before 34 weeks. While it is acknowledged that in cases of pre-eclampsia *without* HELLP syndrome or eclampsia, the risk of pre-eclampsia recurring in a future pregnancy is about 1 in 6 (16 per cent) pregnancies with no additional risk, should the interval before the next pregnancy be less than 10 years (NICE 2010a). As there is no consensus of opinion as to the optimal interval between pregnancies following caesarean section, the obstetrician should provide Elizabeth and John with advice that is relevant to their individual situation so they are enabled to make an informed decision about when to contemplate another pregnancy.

Studies by Manten et al. (2007) and Wilson et al. (2003) have identified that women such as Elizabeth have an increased risk of developing hypertension and cardiovascular disease in later life. However, as Elizabeth had no proteinuria and no hypertension at the postnatal review, the obstetrician should therefore inform her that although the relative risk of end-stage renal disease is increased, the absolute risk is low and no further follow-up would be indicated.

NICE (2010a, 2010b) and Milne et al. (2005) provide a list of factors that the obstetrician and midwife should consider in assessing Elizabeth's risk of the development of pre-eclampsia in a subsequent pregnancy, as shown in Table 3.5.

21 **What could be done to reduce such risks?**

A In the UK, it is recognized by the NMC (2004) that part of the midwife's role is to offer sound family planning and pre-conception advice to couples regarding subsequent pregnancies based on their individual health risks and personal circumstances. Although it is appreciated that

Table 3.5 Factors associated with the risk of pre-eclampsia

Moderate risk	*High risk*
First pregnancy	Hypertensive disease during previous pregnancy
Age ≥ 40 years	Chronic hypertension
Pregnancy interval > 10 years	Chronic renal disease
BMI ≥ 35 kg/m² at first visit	Autoimmune disease such as systemic lupus
Family history of pre-eclampsia	erythematosus or antiphospholipid syndrome
Multiple pregnancy	Type 1 or type 2 diabetes

Source: Milne et al. 2005; NICE 2010a, 2010b.

Elizabeth and John have experienced fertility problems in the past, there is always a chance of a subsequent natural conception while ovulation is still occurring, albeit may be infrequently. Elizabeth and John will probably be fully aware of assessing the time of optimal fertility (Frank-Herrmann et al. 2007) and should be advised to continue using this method but combine it with a barrier method such as a condom when most fertile for the first few months until ready to attempt another pregnancy. This would enable Elizabeth to further improve her health status before becoming pregnant for a second time.

Following a caesarean section, it is recommended that Elizabeth should be advised to maintain her BMI within the healthy range before becoming pregnant again (18.5–24.9 kg/m²) as stated by NICE (2006, 2010c) in order to minimize subsequent health risks. This may involve a critical review of Elizabeth's diet and physical exercise regime with appropriate health advisors as well as the midwife. It is common practice to inform all prospective parents that daily folic acid supplementation of 400 micrograms should be taken prior to conception and then for up to 12 weeks of pregnancy to reduce the risk of neural tube defects, such as anencephaly and spina bifida, occurring (DH 2000).

It is also recommended that women who have a moderate to high risk of developing pre-eclampsia should take 75 mg of aspirin each day from 12 weeks of pregnancy until the baby is born to minimize the risk of any potential complications (NICE 2010a). A recent systematic review by Palacios and Pena Rosas (2010) that considered 12 randomized controlled trials of 15,528 women, found that calcium supplementation reduces the risk of hypertension and pre-eclampsia during pregnancy. However, as most of these studies assessed only nulliparous or primiparous women and women at low risk of hypertension, NICE (2010a) advise caution to the widespread use of calcium supplementation in pregnancy until further studies have been conducted to examine risk reduction in women at moderate and high risk of pre-eclampsia. Until this time, NICE is reluctant to recommend national guidance on the use of calcium supplementation. Furthermore, as calcium inhibits the absorption of iron, the timing of the supplementation should be separated during the day from the recommended daily iron and folic acid supplementation.

22   **Should Elizabeth and John achieve another pregnancy, what advice would you give them as a midwife about antenatal surveillance?**

A   The midwife should advise Elizabeth and John that in a subsequent pregnancy, the antenatal care package would be integrated between the community midwifery team and the specialist antenatal surveillance services within the local hospital. Such a care plan should be clearly documented in Elizabeth's records (NMC 2010) taking into account her individual emotional, cultural, health and midwifery needs that embraces continuity of care. As in Elizabeth's first pregnancy, a combined test (nuchal translucency, beta-human chorionic gonadotropin and pregnancy-associated plasma protein A) would be recommended between 11 weeks and 13 weeks and 6 days of pregnancy to assess chromosomal abnormality risk in view of Elizabeth's age. Milne et al. (2005) suggest that an early referral, before 20 weeks of pregnancy, to specialist services that include biochemical, haematological and clinical assessment is also important to determine risk.

From Elizabeth's past history, there is evidence that pre-eclampsia developed around 25 weeks of pregnancy; it would therefore be advisable that Elizabeth should attend the hospital at least two weeks before the previous gestational onset (i.e. at 22–23 weeks) for a further review with the consultant and/or physician to determine that her health and that of the fetus remains optimal. NICE (2010a) recommend that ultrasound fetal growth and amniotic fluid volume assessment and umbilical artery Doppler velocimetry should be undertaken at this point and repeated 4 weeks later in cases where there has been previous severe pre-eclampsia requiring birth before 34 weeks with the baby weighing less than the 10th centile for gestational age. Depending on the results, this will determine the pattern of subsequent antenatal visits. In the meantime, the midwife should inform Elizabeth of the need to seek immediate advice from a health care professional if she experiences any of the symptoms associated with pre-eclampsia as detailed in Table 3.4.

Due to Elizabeth's ill health around the time of Henry's birth and the fact that he spent several weeks in the NICU, she had experienced very little involvement in his initial care and may be anxious about what would be expected of her in a subsequent pregnancy. It is vital that the midwife acknowledges this anxiety and clearly documents this in her records to reassure Elizabeth and John that every effort would be made by health care professionals to support them with the care and feeding of any subsequent baby (NMC 2010).

Summary of key points

- Pre-eclampsia may occur at very early gestation with sudden and rapidly deteriorating features and remains a challenge to health care professionals working in maternity services (Lewis 2011).
- Accurate assessment and documentation of maternal blood pressure and urinary protein are vital in recognizing women at risk of developing pre-eclampsia.
- Midwives should be conversant with the clinical features and first-line management of impending pre-eclampsia to effect prompt referral to the multi-professional team.
- Adequate control of maternal blood pressure is vital to avoid cerebral haemorrhage.
- Magnesium sulphate protects from eclamptic seizures and improves maternal and fetal outcomes.
- The only 'cure' for pre-eclampsia/HELLP syndrome/eclampsia is the birth of the fetus and placenta.

REFERENCES

Delpisheh, A., Brabin, L., Attia, E. and Brabin, B.J. (2008) Pregnancy late in life: a hospital-based study of birth outcomes, *Journal of Women's Health*, 17(6): 965–70.

Department of Health (DH) (2000) *Folic Acid and the Prevention of Disease: Report of the Committee on Medical Aspects of Food and Nutrition Policy*. London: HMSO.

Department of Health (DH) (2007) *Maternity Matters: Choice, Access and Continuity of Care in a Safe Service*. London: HMSO.

Deruelle, P., Coudoux, E., Ego, A., Houfflin-Debarge, V., Codacioni, X. and Subtil, D. (2006) Risk factors for post-partum complications occurring after pre-eclampsia and HELLP syndrome: a study of 453 consecutive pregnancies, *European Journal of Obstetrics and Gynaecology and Reproductive Biology*, 125(1): 59–65.

Eclampsia Trial Collaborative Group (1995) Which anticonvulsant for women with eclampsia? Evidence from the Collaborative Eclampsia Group, *The Lancet*, 345(8963): 1455–63.

Frank-Herrmann, P., Heil, J., Gnoth, C., Toledo, E., Baur, S., Pyper, C., Jenetzky, E., Strowitzki, T. and Freundl, G. (2007) The effectiveness of a fertility awareness based method to avoid pregnancy in relation to a couple's sexual behaviour during the fertile time: a prospective longitudinal study, *Human Reproduction*, 22(5): 1310–19.

Greater Manchester Critical Care Skills Institute (2002) *Acute Illness Management. AIM Course Manual*, 3rd edn. Manchester: Greater Manchester Critical Care Skills Institute.

Haddad, B., Barton, J.R., Livingston, J.C., Chahine, R. and Sibai, B.M. (2000) Risk factors for adverse maternal outcomes among women with HELLP (haemolysis, elevated liver enzymes and low platelet count) syndrome, *American Journal of Obstetrics and Gynecology*, 183(2): 444–8.

Hoffman, M.C., Jeffers, S., Carter, J., Duthely, L., Cotter, A. and Gonzalez-Quintero, V.H. (2007) Pregnancy at or beyond age 40 years is associated with an increased risk of foetal death and other adverse outcomes, *American Journal of Obstetrics and Gynecology*, 196(5): 11–13.

Human Fertilisation and Embryology Authority (2010) *Fertility Facts and Figures 2008*. London: HFEA.

Khoshnood, B., Bouvier-Colle, M.H., Leridon, H. and Blondel, B. (2008) Impact of advanced maternal age on fecundity and women's and children's health, *Journal de Gynécologie, Obstétrique et Biologie de la Reproduction*, 37(8): 733–47.

Leridon, H. (2004) Can assisted reproductive technology compensate for the natural decline in fertility with age? A model assessment, *Human Reproduction*, 19(7): 1549–54.

Lewis, G. (2011) The women who died, in Centre for Maternal and Child Enquiries (CMACE) *Saving Mothers' Lives: Reviewing Maternal Deaths to Make Motherhood Safer: 2006–2008. The Eighth Report on Confidential Enquiries into Maternal Deaths in the United Kingdom*. Ed. G. Lewis. BJOG: 118 (Suppl. 1): 30–56.

Luke, B. and Brown, M.B. (2007) Elevated risks of pregnancy complications and adverse outcomes with increasing maternal age, *Human Reproduction*, 22(5): 1264–72.

Magpie Trial Collaborative Group (2002) Do women with pre-eclampsia, and their babies, benefit from magnesium sulphate? The Magpie Trial: a randomised placebo-controlled trial, *The Lancet*, 359(9321): 1877–90.

Manten, G.T., Sikkema, M.J., Voorbij, H.A., Visser, G.H., Bruinse, H.W. and Franx, A.I. (2007) Risk factors for cardiovascular disease in women with a history of pregnancy complicated by pre-eclampsia or intra-uterine growth restriction, *Hypertension in Pregnancy*, 26(1): 39–50.

Miller, R.D., Eriksson, L.I., Fleisher, L.A., Wiener-Kronish, J.P. and Young, W.L. (2009) *Miller's Anesthesia*, 7th edn. Philadelphia, PA: Churchill Livingstone, Elsevier.

Milne, F., Redman, C., Walker, J., Baker, P., Bradley, J., Cooper, C., de Swiet, M., Fletcher, G., Jokinen, M., Murphy, D., Nelson-Piercy, C., Osgood, V., Robson, S., Shennan, A., Tufnel, L.A., Twaddle, S. and

Waugh, W. (2005) The pre-eclampsia community guideline (PRECOG): how to screen for and detect onset of pre-eclampsia in the community, *British Medical Journal*, 330(7491): 576–80.

National Health Service Institute for Innovation and Improvement (2008) *SBAR: Situation, Background, Assessment and Recommendation Tool*. Available at: http://www.institute.nhs.uk (accessed January 2011).

National Institute for Health and Clinical Excellence (2006) *Obesity*. Clinical Guideline No. 43. London: NICE.

National Institute for Health and Clinical Excellence (2007) *Antenatal and Postnatal Mental Health: Clinical Management Service Guideline*. Clinical Guideline No. 45. London: NICE.

National Institute for Health and Clinical Excellence (2010a) *Hypertension in Pregnancy: The Management of Hypertensive Disorders During Pregnancy*. Clinical Guideline No. 107. London: NICE.

National Institute for Health and Clinical Excellence (2010b) *Antenatal Care: Routine Care for the Healthy Pregnant Woman*. Clinical Guideline No. 62. London: NICE.

National Institute for Health and Clinical Excellence (2010c) *Dietary Interventions and Physical Activity Interventions for Weight Management Before, During and After Pregnancy: Public Health Guideline 27*. London: NICE.

Neilson, J. (2011) Pre-eclampsia and eclampsia, in Centre for Maternal and Child Enquiries (CMACE) *Saving Mothers' Lives: Reviewing Maternal Deaths to Make Motherhood Safer: 2006–2008. The Eighth Report on Confidential Enquiries into Maternal Deaths in the United Kingdom*. Ed. G. Lewis. *BJOG:* 118 (Suppl. 1): 66–70.

Nursing and Midwifery Council (2004) *Midwives Rules and Standards*. London: NMC.

Nursing and Midwifery Council (2010) *Record Keeping: Guidance for Nurses and Midwives*. London: NMC.

Palacios, C. and Pena-Rosas, J.P. (2010) Calcium supplementation during pregnancy for preventing hypertensive disorders and related problems: RHL commentary, *The WHO Reproductive Health Library*. Geneva: World Health Organization.

PRECOG Development Group (2004) *Pre-eclampsia Community Guideline (PRECOG)*. Leicester: Action on Pre-eclampsia (APEC). Available at: http://www.apec.org.uk

Rath, W., Faridi, A. and Dudenhausen, J.W. (2000) HELLP syndrome, *Journal of Perinatal Medicine*, 28(4): 249–60.

Roberts, D. and Dalziel, S.R. (2006) Antenatal corticosteroids for accelerating fetal lung maturation for women at risk of pre-term birth, *Cochrane Database of Systematic Reviews*, Issue 3, Art. No.: CD004454. DOI: 10.1002/14651858.CD004454.pub2.

Vigil-De, G.P. (2001) Pregnancy complicated by pre-eclampsia: eclampsia with HELLP syndrome, *International Journal of Obstetrics and Gynaecology*, 72(1): 17–23.

Walker, J. (2000) Severe eclampsia and eclampsia, *Ballière's Best Practice: Clinical Obstetrics and Gynaecology*, 14(1): 57–71.

Williams, B., Poulter, N.R., Brown, M.J., Davis, M., McInnes, G.T., Potter, J.P., Sever, P.S. and Thom, S. McG (2004) The BHS Guidelines Working Party Guidelines for Management of Hypertension: Report of the Fourth Working Party of the British Hypertension Society: BHS IV, *Journal of Human Hypertension*, 18: 139–85.

Wilson, B.J., Watson, M.S., Prescott, G.L., Sunderland, S., Campbell, D.M., Hannaford, P., Cairns, W. and Smith, S. (2003) Hypertensive disease of pregnancy and risk of hypertension and stroke in later life: results from a cohort study, *British Medical Journal*, 326(7394): 845–85.

ANNOTATED FURTHER READING

Linheimer, M., Roberts, J. and Cunningham, F. (2009) *Chesley's Hypertensive Disorders in Pregnancy*, 3rd edn. Waltham, MA: Academic Press, Elsevier.

This text differs from other texts devoted to pre-eclampsia, as it covers the whole range of disorders associated with high blood pressure, specifically focusing on prediction, prevention, and best evidence management for clinicians.

Neilson, J. (2011) Pre-eclampsia and eclampsia, in Centre for Maternal and Child Enquiries (CMACE) *Saving Mothers' Lives: Reviewing Maternal Deaths To Make Motherhood Safer: 2006–2008. The Eighth Report on Confidential Enquiries into Maternal Deaths in the United Kingdom*. Ed. G. Lewis. *BJOG:* 118 (Suppl. 1): 66–70.

Provides scrutiny of the 19 maternal deaths that occurred directly as a result of pre-eclampsia and eclampsia in the triennium, 2006–2008, offering good practice recommendations to further reduce morbidity and mortality in this area.

USEFUL WEBSITES

www.apec.org.uk	Action on Pre-eclampsia
www.bhsoc.org	British Hypertension Society
www.cmace.org.uk	Centre for Maternal and Child Enquiries
www.hfea.gov.uk	Human Fertilisation and Embryology Association
www.institute.nhs.uk	National Health Service Institute for Innovation and Improvement
www.nice.org.uk	National Institute for Health and Clinical Excellence
www.npeu.ox.ac.uk	National Perinatal Epidemiology Unit
www.npsa.nhs.uk	National Patient Safety Agency
www.rcog.org.uk	Royal College of Obstetricians and Gynaecologists

Thromboembolism

Jayne E. Marshall and Margaret M. Ramsay

Pre-requisites for the chapter: the reader should have an understanding of:

- The haematological changes that occur during pregnancy.
- Risk factors associated with thromboembolic disease.
- Skills of adult and neonatal basic and advanced life support.
- The safe administration of medicines in line with statutory and local Trust code, policies and guidelines.
- The Modified Early Obstetric Warning Scoring (MEOWS) system and SBAR tool.
- Effective interprofessional team learning and working.
- The midwife's role and statutory responsibilities in the management of maternity complications/emergencies.
- Clinical governance and risk management procedures.

Pre-reading self-assessment

1 Which four substances must be present for blood to clot?
2 What are the three main stages of blood clotting?
3 What effect does vitamin K have on blood clotting?
4 What is fibrinolysis and how does this occur?
5 What is the significance of varicosities?
6 What is thrombophlebitis?
7 What is a positive Homan's sign?
8 What are the differences between heparin and warfarin?

Recommended prior reading

Drife, J. (2011) Thrombosis and Thromboembolism, in Centre for Maternal and Child Enquiries (CMACE) *Saving Mothers' Lives: Reviewing Maternal Deaths To Make Motherhood Safer: 2006–2008. The Eighth Report on Confidential Enquiries into Maternal Deaths in the United Kingdom*. Ed. G. Lewis. *BJOG:* 118 (Suppl. 1): 57–65.

National Institute for Health and Clinical Excellence (2010) *Venous Thromboembolism: Reducing the Risk of Venous Thromboembolism (Deep Vein Thrombosis and Pulmonary Embolism) in Patients Admitted to Hospital.* Clinical Guideline No. 92. London: NICE.

CASE STUDY

Alison, a 20-year-old multigravida, was admitted to the maternity ward at 10 weeks gestation with a 3-day history of vomiting, and had been unable to tolerate food and fluids. There had been no diarrhoea. Her previous two pregnancies had also been complicated by vomiting. On admission, Alison complained of constant left iliac fossa pain that worsened on climbing stairs. An ultrasound scan was performed and it confirmed a viable singleton intrauterine pregnancy, with normal maternal ovaries. Alison was prescribed IV fluids and anti-emetics.

Two days later, the vomiting had settled down and Alison was beginning to eat and drink a little. However, she was awakened in the night with left leg pain, mainly in the buttock and posterior thigh. The midwife noted that Alison's leg was diffusely swollen from the feet up to the groin. The leg felt warm to touch and was extremely tender over the calf and shin. There were no varicosities and no evidence of cellulitis. Deep vein thrombosis (DVT) was suspected and upon referral to the obstetrician Alison was commenced on full dose low molecular weight heparin (LMWH): enoxaparin 1 mg/kg 12-hourly. Given her booking weight of 45 kg, doses of 40 mg twice a day were administered.

Leg Doppler studies found occlusive thrombus in the left superficial femoral veins, extending to the left common iliac vein. The inferior vena cava was free of thrombus. The veins of the right leg outlined normally. Alison found her leg very painful and she had difficulty in mobilizing. After 3 days of full anticoagulation, her symptoms improved and she was discharged home. She continued to self-administer BD injections of enoxaparin.

The following week, Alison was reviewed in the combined obstetric haematology clinic. She reported that her leg was much more comfortable. A blood test was taken to measure the anti-Xa activity, 3 hours after her dose of enoxaparin. This gave a result of 0.37 iu/mL, which was less than the desired therapeutic range of 0.5–1.0 iu/mL. Alison was therefore asked to increase her dose of enoxaparin to 60 mg BD and advised to wear full-length grade 2 graduated compression stockings, to make her left leg more comfortable, and reduce the residual swelling in it. At 24 weeks gestation, when Alison had received 3 months of full anticoagulation, the haematologist advised her to reduce the dose to a daily prophylactic dose of 60 mg enoxaparin. This dose was prescribed for the remainder of the pregnancy.

At 38 weeks Alison was seen in the antenatal clinic where a vaginal examination (VE) and membrane sweep was undertaken by the obstetrician. At this stage, the cervix was 1 cm long and 2 cm dilated. Alison was keen on a vaginal birth, having had two previous babies without any difficulty. However, an induction of labour (IOL) was planned for the following week should labour have not commenced spontaneously.

The following week, Alison was induced by amniotomy followed by an intravenous infusion (IVI) of Syntocinon after 2 hours. Throughout labour, Alison wore thromboembolic deterrent (TED) stockings and anticoagulant therapy was withdrawn as Alison requested an epidural for analgesia. After 3 hours and a short second stage of labour, Alison gave birth to a healthy baby girl, Abigail, weighing 3.1 kgs. Anticoagulant therapy was recommended 12 hours following the birth and Alison was transferred home with Abigail to community midwifery care after 48 hours.

1   **What risk factors does Alison have for deep vein thrombosis?**

A   The risk of thrombosis is present in all pregnant women from the first trimester until at least 6 weeks postpartum. The factors that promote venous thromboembolism (VTE) are stasis of blood flow, alteration of the constituents of the blood (hypercoagulability) and abnormalities/

damage to the vessel wall, all of which are affected by pregnancy. Pressure of the gravid uterus on the inferior vena cava and pelvic veins, an increase in coagulation factors with decrease in natural inhibitors to anticoagulation and reduced venous tone all predispose to VTE (Elliott and Pavord 2008). Furthermore, if left untreated, 25 per cent of DVT will be complicated by pulmonary embolism (PE) where a fragment of thrombus breaks away and travels through the right side of the heart to lodge in the pulmonary circulation. Elliott and Pavord (2008) confirm that the risk of PE is higher with femoral or ileofemoral thrombus than for distal DVT.

In the latest triennial report in the UK from 2006–2008, Drife (2011) reports on 18 maternal deaths from thrombosis and/or VTE of which three women had excessive vomiting and two died after prolonged immobility. This is a marked decline, however, from the 41 deaths reported in the previous triennium, 2003–2005 (Lewis 2007). The risk factors for VTE are highlighted in Table 4.1, which in Alison's case are hyperemesis gravidarum and dehydration, with accompanying immobility due to hospitalization, suggesting that she is at risk of developing VTE in her pregnancy.

Table 4.1 Risk factors for VTE in pregnancy

Low risk ≥ 3 factors/2 if admitted	Intermediate risk	High risk
Age > 35 years	Single previous VTE with no family history or thrombophilia	Single previous VTE + – thrombophilia or family history – unprovoked/oestrogen-related
Obesity (BMI > 30 kg/m²)	Thrombophilia + no VTE	Previous recurrent VTE (> 1)
Parity ≥ 3		
Smoker	Medical co-morbidities heart or lung disease – SLE	
Gross varicose veins	– cancer – inflammatory conditions	
Current systemic infection	– nephrotic syndrome – sickle cell disease	
Immobility – paraplegia – SPD	Intravenous drug user	
	Surgical procedure – appendicectomy	
Long-distance travel		
Pre-eclampsia		
Dehydration/hyperemesis gravidarum/OHSS		
Multiple pregnancy or ART		

ART – assisted reproductive therapy; OHSS – ovarian hyperstimulation syndrome; SLE–systemic lupus erythematosus; SPD – symphysis pubis dysfunction.
Source: RCOG 2009.

RCOG (2009), NICE (2010) and SIGN (2010) recommend that all pregnant women have a thrombotic risk assessment at the first antenatal visit, taking into account their personal and family history, the presence of any risk factors and any known thrombophilia balancing with the risk of bleeding (see Tables 4.2 and 4.3). This assessment should be repeated throughout pregnancy if circumstances change, such as excessive weight gain, immobility or vomiting with dehydration. Further to the RCOG (2009) guidance on thrombo-

Table 4.2 Risk assessment for venous thromboembolism

Pre-existing risk factors	Tick	Score
Previous recurrent VTE		3
Previous VTE – unprovoked or oestrogen-related		3
Previous VTE – provoked		2
Family history of VTE		1
Known thrombophilia		2
Medical comorbidities		2
Age (> 35 years)		1
Obesity		1/2[a]
Parity ≤ 3		1
Smoker		1
Gross varicose veins		1

Obstetric risk factors	Tick	Score
Pre-eclampsia		1
Dehydration/hyperemesis/OHSS		1
Multiple pregnancy or ART		1
Caesarean section in labour		2
Elective caesarean section		1
Mid-cavity or rotational forceps		1
Prolonged labour (> 24 hours)		1
PPH (> 1 litre or transfusion)		1

Transient risk factors	Tick	Score
Current systemic infection		1
Immobility		1
Surgical procedure in pregnancy or ≤ 6 weeks postpartum		2
TOTAL SCORE		

Thromboprophylaxis with LMWH should be considered if:

≥ *three* risk factors antenatally and managed as an outpatient

≥ *two** risk factors antenatally and managed as an inpatient or any postnatal woman who is within 6 weeks of delivery

For women with an identified bleeding risk, the balance of risks of bleeding and clotting should be discussed in consultation with a haematologist with experience of thrombosis and bleeding in pregnancy

*NICE (2010) recommend ≥ *one* risk factor(s)

Note: [a] Score 1 for BMI > 30 kg/m^2; 2 for BMI > 40 kg/m^2 (BMI based on booking weight).

Source: RCOG 2009; NICE 2010; SIGN 2010.

Table 4.3 Bleeding risk

Haemophilia or other known bleeding disorder (e.g. von Willebrand's disease or acquired coagulopathy).

Active antenatal or postpartum bleeding.

Women considered at increased risk of major haemorrhage (e.g. placenta praevia).

Thrombocytopenia (platelet count <75 x 10^9/L).

Acute stroke in previous 4 weeks (haemorrhagic or ischaemic).

Severe renal disease (glomerular filtration rate < 30 mL/minute/1.73m^2).

Severe liver disease (prothrombin time above normal range or known varices).

Uncontrolled hypertension (blood pressure > 200 mmHg systolic or > 120 mmHg diastolic).

prophylaxis (identified in Table 4.2), NICE (2010) have revised the recommendations. All women who are pregnant or have given birth within the previous 6 weeks and are admitted to hospital but are not undergoing surgery, should be considered for pharmacological VTE prophylaxis with low molecular weight heparin (LMWH) (or unfractionated heparin (UFH) for those with renal failure) if they have *one* or more risk factors.

2 **What preventative measures could have been taken?**

A On admission with severe hyperemesis gravidarum and dehydration, Alison also complained of constant left iliac fossa pain that worsened on climbing stairs. A full risk assessment for VTE would have indicated the possibility of a DVT further exacerbated by reduced mobility associated with IV therapy and accompanying bed rest. This therefore places Alison at an *intermediate risk* where thromboprophylaxis with LMWH should be considered upon collaboration with the Trust specialists in thrombosis in pregnancy including consultant obstetrician and haematologist (RCOG 2009; NICE 2010; SIGN 2010; Drife 2011). In addition, it would have been prudent at this point for leg Doppler studies to have been undertaken, especially as DVTs commonly occur in the leg veins. Chan et al. (2010) conducted a systematic review and found of the 124 DVTs occurring in childbirth, 88 per cent presented in the left leg and that proximal DVT restricted to the femoral or iliac veins is also more common in > 60 per cent of cases.

There is much debate about the use of graduated compression stockings in the management of VTE, their function being to increase the mean blood flow velocity in the leg veins and reduce venous stasis (SIGN 2010). Compression hosiery may be considered to assist in reducing Alison's risk of developing post-thrombotic syndrome following DVT, the risk of which can be as high as 50 per cent (Gorman et al. 2000). In the American College of Chest Physicians (ACCP) guideline, Bates et al. (2008) recommend compression hosiery during pregnancy and in the puerperium for all women with a previous DVT and for women considered to be at high risk of VTE after caesarean section until mobility improves. However, hydrostatic pressures on standing appear to overcome venous compression from TEDS (Lord and Hamilton 2004; Partsch and Partsch 2005) and thus stockings may be of less benefit once Alison becomes more ambulant. Furthermore, studies comparing thigh-length and knee-length stockings have been too few to determine whether or not they are equally effective,

Table 4.4 Contraindications for and application of TEDS

Contraindications	Application
Massive leg oedema	Select correct size
Severe peripheral neuropathy	Do not fold down
Pulmonary oedema (e.g. heart failure)	Apply carefully, aligning toe hole under toe
Major leg deformity	Remove daily for no more than 30 minutes
Severe peripheral arterial disease	Check fitting daily for change in leg
Dermatitis	circumference
	Grade 2 graduated compression stockings should be worn during the day with an ankle pressure gradient of 30–40 mmHg for two years to prevent post-thrombotic syndrome (*if symptomatic*)

although a meta-analysis suggested no major difference in efficacy in surgical patients (Sajid et al. 2006). However, it should be taken into consideration that in pregnant women most DVTs are ileofemoral and as a consequence, thigh-length thromboembolic deterrent stockings (TEDS) should be worn as a preventative measure. Table 4.4 highlights the contraindications and application of TEDS.

3   **What treatment should be given?**

A   The treatment for acute thromboembolism in pregnancy is heparin, as it does not cross the placenta. LMWHs are used most widely as they are easier to use and associated with lower haemorrhagic risk than UFHs as well as being efficacious (Greer and Nelson-Piercy 2005; RCOG 2010). Warfarin is not used for the reasons stated below (*see answer to Question 7*). In pregnancy, there is the most experience with enoxaparin, dalteparin and tinzaparin. According to RCOG (2010), suitable dose schedules are:

>   enoxaparin: 1 mg/kg twice daily,

>   dalteparin: 100 units/kg twice daily and

>   tinzaparin: 175 units/kg once daily (RCOG, 2010).

These dose schedules are different to those used for non-pregnant adults, as they should be sufficient to allow for the increased renal clearance of LMWH during pregnancy. There is no need for routine monitoring of anti-Xa levels in women taking LMWH, but these are useful in the extremes of body weight (< 50 kg or > 90 kg) or in women with poor renal function. If levels are assessed, then the peak anti-Xa, 3 hours post-injection should be in the range 0.5–1.2 u/mL for greatest efficacy (RCOG 2010).

4   **What is the purpose of such treatment?**

A   Anticoagulants are given to prevent formation of further blood clots in other locations, to allow the existing clots to stabilize and to prevent fragmentation and embolization of clots.

Pulmonary embolism from DVT remains the leading direct cause of maternal death (Drife 2011). Vessels partly occluded by blood clots become re-canalized, with the clot being incorporated into the vessel wall. As this process happens, the localized pain and swelling associated with thombosis should diminish.

5 **What advice should you give to Alison regarding the effects and safety to her and her baby of administering LMWH?**

A Alison needs to be taught how to administer the LWMH injections into her subcutaneous fat. She should be advised to rotate the injection sites, with those most convenient being in her lower lateral abdomen and thighs. She should anticipate a stinging sensation upon injecting and that there might be a slight bruise at the injection site. Occasionally, Alison may find a larger bruise occurring and should report persisting redness or itching at injection sites to the midwife. Moreover, the midwife should reassure Alison that LMWH does not cross the placenta and thus will not have any adverse effect on her baby (RCOG 2009, 2010).

6 **How long should treatment continue?**

A Anticoagulation treatment should be given for the duration of the pregnancy and for at least 6 weeks into the puerperium. In pregnancy, many coagulation factors are increased and remain so for several weeks following the birth of the baby. Global assessment of coagulation with thromboelastography also demonstrates hypercoagulability persisting for at least 4 weeks postpartum (Ramsay 2010). Thus there remains an ongoing risk for further thromboembolism during this time.

7 **Are there any oral anticoagulants that can be used safely in pregnancy?**

A Warfarin and other vitamin K antagonists (VKA) freely cross the placenta (RCOG 2009). Their use in pregnancy is associated with increased risk of miscarriage, teratogenic effects in the first trimester and haemorrhagic complications in the fetus at any stage of pregnancy. Thus none of the VKAs can be considered safe to use in pregnancy, although warfarin is safe to use while breast-feeding (RCOG 2009).

8 **What advice would you give to Alison regarding labour and birth?**

A RCOG (2009) consider that it is desirable to continue LMWH during the intrapartum period in women such as Alison, who are receiving antenatal therapeutic thromboprophylaxis with LMWH due to the increase in risk for thrombosis unless regional analgesia is requested. However, there are also associated risks of bleeding and, as a consequence, careful assessment of Alison's individual risks should be considered when discussing her plan for labour and birth. This plan of management and care should involve the consultant obstetrician, consultant haematologist and consultant anaesthetist and be carefully documented in Alison's maternity records (NMC 2004, 2010). The midwife should advise Alison that, depending on her haematological status, it would be anticipated that she commences labour spontaneously so as to minimize obstetric intervention.

It is important that Alison remains hydrated during labour and that the length of her labour is not prolonged so as not to further increase thrombotic risk. As Alison had developed her DVT early in pregnancy, she had been given many weeks of full therapeutic doses of LMWH which after three months, had been converted to a lower dose of LMWH.

In someone whose DVT had occurred later in pregnancy, or who was known to have a particularly high risk of recurrent VTE, it may be prudent for the LMWH to be converted to IV UFH to allow more flexibility in controlling anticoagulation and minimize the time with trough levels.

For the second and third stages of labour, the administration of heparin would need to be temporarily interrupted to reduce bleeding, with active management of the third stage of labour being undertaken to reduce the risk of postpartum haemorrhage (PPH) (see Case 8). The midwife should be aware that oxytocic drugs should only be administered by IV to Alison to avoid haematomas associated with intramuscular (IM) routes. If it is considered unsuitable to temporarily interrupt the use of heparin during labour, and if Alison requires a caesarean section, she should be informed that general anaesthesia may be necessary despite it being associated with a higher thrombosis risk due to immobility. A summary of the midwifery management and care that should be considered in Alison's case is shown in Box 4.1.

Box 4.1 Intrapartum midwifery management and care of women with VTE risks

- Recommend use of TEDS while hospitalized.
- Encourage mobility/frequent change of position.
- Keep hydrated/IV fluids if necessary.
- Encourage leg exercises if woman has epidural.
- Avoid prolonged use of lithotomy position if instrumental birth/perineal suturing required.
- Active management of third stage of labour with IV oxytocin.
- Prompt suturing of perineal tears/episiotomy.
- Accurate assessment and concise documentation of maternal and fetal well-being using MEOWS system if high risk.

---

9   **What are Alison's options for pain relief during labour while anticoagulated?**

A   Discussion about pain relief in labour should be undertaken by the midwife in advance of labour commencing in order to ascertain Alison's wishes alongside the options available such as gas and air, pethidine and epidural. According to local obstetric anaesthetic protocols (RCOG 2010), there should be collaboration with an experienced obstetrician, haematologist and anaesthetist if regional analgesia or anaesthesia is to be sited to minimize or prevent the risk of significant spinal bleeding and epidural haematoma. This collaboration should be undertaken at the antenatal anaesthetic clinic where available.

> **Check points**
>
> - Regional analgesia/anaesthesia techniques should not be used until at least 12 hours following the previous *prophylactic* dose of LMWH.
> - Regional analgesia/anaesthesia techniques should not be used for at least 24 hours after the last *therapeutic* dose of LMWH.
> - LMWH should not be given for 4 hours after use of spinal anaesthesia or after the epidural catheter has been removed: the epidural catheter should not be removed within 10–12 hours of the most recent injection.
>
> (Horlocker et al. 2003)

If Alison should present in spontaneous labour having self-administered LMWH within the last 12 hours, it would be inappropriate for an epidural catheter to be sited and so she should be offered alternatives such as gas and air or an opiate-based analgesia such as pethidine. On the other hand, a decision was made to induce Alison's labour, which assisted in planning thromboprophylaxis around the induction process (RCOG 2009) and her request for epidural analgesia. This would mean Alison taking the last dose of enoxaparin on the morning prior to induction of labour and an early elective epidural being sited the next day when it would be 24 hours since her last dose of LMWH.

10 **What advice should be given to Alison following the birth of Abigail regarding postnatal care and subsequent risk of VTE?**

A The pregnancy-associated prothrombotic changes in the coagulation system are maximal immediately following birth and do not revert completely back to normal until several weeks after birth (Ramsay 2010). Indeed, the time of greatest risk for VTE associated with pregnancy is the early puerperium and, although most VTE occurs antenatally, the risk is greatest in the weeks immediately after birth with a 25-fold increase in risk of thrombosis (Pabinger et al. 2005; De Stefano et al. 2006). It is therefore important that there is a clearly defined plan of postnatal care for Alison documented with frequent risk assessment and observations of her well-being using the MEOWS system. Particular vigilance should be given to leg care, hydration, mobility, use of TEDS, and consideration of the most suitable form and length of postpartum anticoagulant therapy.

RCOG (2009) recommend that the first dose of LMWH be given as soon as possible after the baby's birth, provided that there is no PPH. However, as Alison had epidural analgesia during labour, the midwife should advise her that LMWH will recommence after the epidural catheter has been removed which is usually 10–12 hours after the most recent injection (Horlocker et al. 2003).

All women with a previous history of confirmed VTE should be offered thromboprophylaxis with LMWH for at least 6 weeks postpartum, regardless of the mode of birth; this is particularly important for women, such as Alison, who have had thrombosis during pregnancy. Women can be given the choice following the birth of remaining on LMWH during the puerperium or changing to oral warfarin. If the latter option is chosen, then they will be required to have regular blood tests. If Alison chose to change to warfarin, she would require information about the safety of warfarin due to its interaction with certain drugs such as antibiotics and foods rich in vitamin K, namely, green leafy vegetables (e.g. broccoli, cauliflower, cabbage, brussels sprouts, kale, spinach, etc.), green tea, cranberry products, caffeine beverages and certain vitamin supplements.

Think

Alison should be advised that breastfeeding Abigail is *not* contraindicated with either heparin or vitamin K antagonist therapy (RCOG 2009).

Contraceptive options should be discussed with Alison prior to transferring home with Abigail (NICE 2006). The combined oral contraceptive pill should be avoided where there is a history of VTE as oestrogen increases blood clotting; however, Depo-Provera, the progesterone-only pill and barrier methods (diaphragms and/or condoms) with the addition of spermicides may be considered (Elliott and Pavord 2008). Intra-uterine contraceptive devices (IUCDs) including intra-uterine progesterone-only devices are also suitable, albeit should not be inserted in the immediate postnatal period. However, in cases where warfarin is being administered, oral contraception should be avoided as oestrogen and progesterone antagonize the anticoagulant effect.

Follow-up appointments should be arranged with the consultant obstetrician and haematologist, including testing for thrombophilia to determine Alison's long-term management and well-being. If Alison is on warfarin therapy and decides to become pregnant again, the teratogenic effects of this anticoagulant should be conveyed to her. RCOG (2009) note that warfarin is known to cross the placenta, causing limb and facial structural abnormalities in about 5 per cent of fetuses exposed between 6–12 weeks gestation with increased risk of spontaneous miscarriage, stillbirth and fetal and maternal haemorrhage during pregnancy. It is therefore advisable that Alison seeks medical advice pre-conceptually, or as soon as possible and within two weeks following a first missed menstrual period if she suspects that she may be pregnant.

Summary of key points

- Risk assessment and early recognition of VTE are vital throughout pregnancy and the puerperium.
- Outcomes for childbearing women with VTE can be significantly improved with early and appropriate care interventions.
- Comprehensive management and care plans should be clearly documented in the woman's maternity records following discussion with all members of the multidisciplinary team.
- Full dose LMWH is safe and effective treatment for acute VTE in pregnancy. Smaller doses of LMWH can also be used for thromboprophylaxis in women with a prior history or increased risk of developing VTE.
- The combined oral contraceptive pill should be avoided in women with a history of VTE.
- Women should be counselled about the risks of long-term warfarin therapy in terms of drug and food interactions and teratogenicity if taken early in a subsequent pregnancy.

REFERENCES

Bates, S.M., Greer, I.A., Pabinger, I., Sofaer, S. and Hirsh, J. (2008) Venous thromboembolism, thrombophilia, antithrombotic therapy, and pregnancy: American College of Chest Physicians Evidence-Based Clinical Practice Guidelines, 8th edn, *Chest*, 6 (Suppl.): 844S–6S.

Chan, W.S., Spencer, F.A. and Ginsberg, J.S. (2010) Anatomic distribution of deep vein thrombosis in pregnancy, *Canadian Medical Association Journal*, 182(7): 657–60.

De Stefano, V., Martinelli, I., Rossi, E., Battaglioli, T., Za, T., Mannuccio Mannucci, P. and Leone, G. (2006) The risk of recurrent venous thromboembolism in pregnancy and puerperium without antithrombotic prophylaxis, *British Journal of Haematology*, 135(3): 386–91.

Drife, J. (2011) Thrombosis and Thromboembolism, in Centre for Maternal and Child Enquiries (CMACE) *Saving Mothers' Lives: Reviewing Maternal Deaths To Make Motherhood Safer: 2006–2008: The Eighth Report on Confidential Enquiries into Maternal Deaths in the United Kingdom*. Ed. G. Lewis. *BJOG:* 118 (Suppl. 1): 57–65.

Elliott, D. and Pavord, S. (2008) Thrombo-embolic disorders, in S.E. Robson and J. Waugh (eds) *Medical Disorders in Pregnancy: A Manual for Midwives*. Oxford: Blackwell Publishing, pp. 185–94.

Gorman, W.P., Davis, K.R. and Donnelly, R. (2000) ABC of arterial and venous disease: swollen lower limb – 1: general assessment and deep vein thrombosis, *British Medical Journal*, 320(7247): 1453–6.

Greer, I.A. and Nelson-Piercy, C. (2005) Low molecular weight heparins for thromboprophylaxis and treatment of venous thromboembolism in pregnancy; a systematic review of safety and efficacy, *Blood*, 106(2): 401–7.

Horlocker, T.T., Wedel, D.J., Benzon, H., Brown, D.L., Enneking, F.K., Heit, J.A., Mulroy, M.F., Rosenquist, J., Rowlingson, J., Tryba, M. and Yuan, C.S. (2003) Regional anesthesia in the anticoagulated patient: defining the risks (the second ASRA Consensus Conference on Neuraxial Anesthesia and Anticoagulation), *Regional Anaesthesia Pain Medicine*, 28(3): 172–97.

Lewis, G. (ed.) (2007) *The Confidential Enquiry into Maternal and Child Health (CEMACH). Saving Mothers' Lives: Reviewing Maternal Deaths to Make Motherhood Safer, 2003–2005. The Seventh Report on Confidential Enquiries into Maternal Deaths in the United Kingdom*. London: CEMACH.

Lord, R.A. and Hamilton, D. (2004) Graduated compression stockings (20–30 mmHg) do not compress leg veins in the standing position, *Australian and New Zealand Journal of Surgery*, 74(7): 581–5.

National Institute for Health and Clinical Excellence (2006) *Postnatal Care: Routine Postnatal Care of Women and Their Babies*. Clinical Guideline No. 37. London: NICE.

National Institute for Health and Clinical Excellence (2010) *Venous Thromboembolism: Reducing the Risk of Venous Thromboembolism (Deep Vein Thrombosis and Pulmonary Embolism) in Patients Admitted to Hospital*. Clinical Guideline No. 92. London: NICE.

Nursing and Midwifery Council (2004) *Midwives Rules and Standards*. London: NMC.

Nursing and Midwifery Council (2010) *Record Keeping: Guidance for Nurses and Midwives*. London: NMC.

Pabinger, I., Grafenhofer, H., Kaider, A., Kyrle, P.A., Quehenberger, P., Mannhalter, C. and Lechner, K. (2005). Risk of pregnancy-associated recurrent venous thromboembolism in women with a history of venous thrombosis, *Journal of Thrombosis and Haemostasis*, 3(5): 949–54.

Partsch, B. and Partsch, H. (2005) Calf compression pressure required to achieve venous closure from supine to standing positions, *Journal of Vascular Surgery*, 42(4): 734–8.

Ramsay, M.M. (2010) Normal haematological changes during pregnancy and the puerperium, in Pavord, S. and Hunt, B. (eds) *The Obstetric Haematology Manual*. Cambridge: Cambridge University Press, pp. 3–12.

Royal College of Obstetricians and Gynaecologists (2009) *Thrombosis and Embolism during Pregnancy and the Puerperium: Reducing the Risk*. Green Top Guideline No. 37a. London: RCOG Press.

Royal College of Obstetricians and Gynaecologists (2010) *The Acute Management of Thrombosis and Embolism during Pregnancy and the Puerperium: Acute Management.* Green Top Guideline No. 37b. London: RCOG Press.

Sajid, M.S., Tai, N.R.M., Goli, G., Morris, R.W., Baker, D.M. and Hamilton, G. (2006) Knee versus thigh length graduated compression stockings for prevention of deep venous thrombosis: a systematic review, *European Journal of Vascular and Endovascular Surgery*, 32(6): 730–6.

Scottish Intercollegiate Guidelines Network (2010) *Prevention and Management of Venous Thromboembolism: A National Clinical Guideline No. 122.* Edinburgh: SIGN.

ANNOTATED FURTHER READING

Bombeli, T. and Spahn, D.R. (2004) Updates in perioperative coagulation: physiology and management of thromboembolism and haemorrhage, *British Journal of Anaesthesia*, 93(2): 275–87.

Provides an overview of various diagnostic coagulation tests and antithrombotic and haemostatic drugs available for the treatment/prophylaxis of thromboembolic disease and the treatment of bleeding.

Royal College of Obstetricians and Gynaecologists (2009) *Thrombosis and Embolism during Pregnancy and the Puerperium: Reducing the Risk.* Green Top Guideline No. 37a. London: RCOG Press.

A comprehensive guide for all health professionals involved in the prevention and management of women at risk of VTE in pregnancy and the puerperium. Clinical algorithms are particularly useful in the initial and continued risk assessment of childbearing women.

USEFUL WEBSITES

www.bcshguidelines.com	British Committee for Standards in Haematology
www.b-s-h.org.uk	British Society for Haematology
www.cmace.org.uk	Centre for Maternal and Child Enquiries
www.dh.gov.uk	Department of Health
www.nice.org.uk	National Institute for Health and Clinical Excellence
www.rcog.org.uk	Royal College of Obstetricians and Gynaecologists
www.sign.ac.uk	Scottish Intercollegiate Guidelines Network

CASE STUDY 5
Disseminated intravascular coagulation (DIC)
Jayne E. Marshall and
Margaret M. Ramsay

Pre-requisites for the chapter: the reader should have an understanding of:

- The haematological changes that occur during pregnancy.
- Risk factors associated with coagulation disorders.
- Content pertaining to Case 3: Pre-eclampsia, eclampsia and H E L L P syndrome and Case 4: Thromboembolism.
- Skills of adult and neonatal basic and advanced life support.
- The safe administration of medicines in line with statutory and local Trust Code, policies and guidelines.
- Serious Hazards of Transfusion (www.shotuk.org).
- The Modified Early Obstetric Warning Score system (M E O W S).
- Effective interprofessional team learning and working.
- The midwife's role and statutory responsibilities in the management of maternity emergencies.
- Clinical governance and risk management procedures.

Pre-reading self-assessment

1 What is ischaemia?
2 What are fibrin degradation products?
3 What is antithrombin?
4 What is the significance of Protein C and Protein S?
5 What is central venous pressure?
6 What are the types of blood products currently available for transfusion?

Recommended prior reading

Dawson, A. (2011) Amniotic fluid embolism, in Centre for Maternal and Child Enquiries *Saving Mothers' Lives: Reviewing Maternal Deaths to Make Motherhood Safer: 2006–2008. The Eighth Report on Confidential Enquiries into Maternal Deaths in the United Kingdom.* Ed. Lewis. G. *BJOG:* 118 (Suppl. 1): 77–84.

(Continued overleaf)

Norman, J. (2011) Haemorrhage, in Centre for Maternal and Child Enquiries *Saving Mothers' Lives: Reviewing Maternal Deaths to Make Motherhood Safer: 2006–2008. The Eighth Report on Confidential Enquiries into Maternal Deaths in the United Kingdom.* Ed. G. Lewis. *BJOG:* 118 (Suppl. 1): 71–6.

CASE STUDY

Deborah, a 30-year-old woman in her seventh pregnancy, had experienced five miscarriages; four in the first trimester and one at 18 weeks. Her only successful pregnancy had been induced at 36 weeks due to pre-eclampsia and intra-uterine growth restriction (IUGR), resulting in the birth of her daughter Amy, who weighed 1.72 kg. Deborah presented initially at the midwives' clinic when she was approximately 8 weeks pregnant.

Deborah had already undergone investigations to establish a cause for the recurrent miscarriages, including thrombophilia screening; the outcome of which was positive for the lupus anticoagulant (LA) and anticardiolipin antibodies (aCL). These tests had been repeated at the beginning of her current pregnancy and Deborah had been advised that she had antiphospholipid syndrome (APS).

At the 12-week hospital antenatal appointment, Deborah was prescribed a daily dose of 75 mg aspirin by the doctor. She attended for follow-up appointments at 20 and 28 weeks and was informed that the baby was growing well and that her BP and urine tests were normal. However, at 32 weeks of pregnancy, Deborah suddenly experienced heavy vaginal bleeding with blood clots. She became pale, but remained alert and complained of severe pain. Her husband, Robert, called for the emergency ambulance.

The paramedic attending Deborah sited a large-bore IV cannula and undertook venepuncture prior to transferring Deborah from her remote farmhouse to the labour ward of the local maternity unit, leaving Robert behind until Deborah's mother arrived to look after Amy. On admission to the labour ward, the midwife assessed Deborah and found her BP to be 84/48 mmHg with a pulse of 112 bpm. Fresh vaginal bleeding with blood clots was persisting and the uterus was tense and tender, SPFH measured 36 cm. The fetal heart could not be located with a Pinard stethoscope or a fetal ultrasonic monitor, so the midwife referred Deborah to the obstetrician on duty, who organized a portable ultrasound scan (USS). Sadly, this confirmed an intra-uterine fetal death (IUFD).

Another large-bore IV cannula was sited and further venepuncture undertaken, with samples being sent urgently to the laboratory along with those taken by the paramedic crew about an hour and a half earlier. The blood transfusion laboratory was asked to cross-match six units of blood and instructed to send two units of O–negative blood to labour ward urgently for Deborah to be transfused. The results of the blood tests, comparing the earlier samples taken by the paramedics with those by the obstetrician on labour ward, were as follows (see Results Chart 5.1).

With Deborah's consent, the obstetrician undertook a vaginal examination (VE) and performed an amniotomy having found a 1 cm dilated, partially effaced cervix. An intravenous infusion (IVI) of Syntocinon was commenced. Deborah was given a patient-controlled analgesia (PCA) of diamorphine to help ease the pain along with Entonox. Intramuscular injections of opioids were avoided, due to the coagulopathy and potential

Results Chart 5.1

Blood test	At home (paramedic)	On admission to labour ward
Haemoglobin	10.5 g/dL	8.5 g/dL
Platelets	169 × 10⁹/L	137 × 10⁹/L
White cell count	16.7 × 10⁹/L	16.5 × 10⁹/L
APTT	26 sec. (control 31)	33 sec. (control 31)
Thrombin time	11 sec. (control 10)	11 sec. (control 10)
INR	0.98	1.11
Fibrinogen	3.35 g/L	1.61 g/L
Creatinine	44 micromol/L	49 micromol/L
Urea	3.0 mmol/L	3.2 mmol/L
Sodium	137 mmol/L	136 mmol/L
Potassium	4.8 micromol/L	4.8 micromol/L

for severe bruising at injection sites. As the pain eased, Deborah's BP and pulse stabilized. She had received three units of blood IV but had only passed 150 mL urine since admission at this point. The obstetrician discussed Deborah's blood results with a consultant haematologist who advised administering 10 units of cryoprecipitate and 15 units of platelets.

Blood tests were repeated two hours after Deborah was admitted to the labour ward and the results were as follows (as shown in Results Chart 5.2).

Results Chart 5.2

Blood test	On admission to labour ward	Two hours later
Haemoglobin	8.5 g/dL	11.2 g/dL
Platelets	137 × 10⁹/L	98 × 10⁹/L
White cell count	16.5 × 10⁹/L	13.4 × 10⁹/L
APTT	33 sec. (control 31)	34 sec. (control 31)
Thrombin time	11 sec. (control 10)	12 sec. (control 10)
INR	1.11	1.14
Fibrinogen	1.61 g/L	1.27 g/L

Once Deborah's mother had arrived at their home to care for Amy, Robert drove to the labour ward to be with Deborah. A further VE was undertaken by the obstetrician and the cervix was found to be 2–3 cm dilated but still only partially effaced. Slight but persistent fresh vaginal bleeding was evident. Discussion between the obstetric, haematological and anaesthetic consultants took place regarding the management of Deborah's coagulopathy, sharing their concerns with Deborah, Robert and the attending midwives. The blood tests indicated disseminated intravascular coagulation (DIC), and as it appeared that it might be some time before Deborah would give birth vaginally, by which time her coagulation status would have further deteriorated, the decision was made to perform a caesarean section. The haematologist advised that an IVI of cryoprecipitate should be administered with a view to keeping the measured fibrinogen above 1 g/L and that 15 units of platelets should be transfused just prior to surgery.

At surgery, a couvelaire uterus was identified, which bled profusely as the lower segment was incised. There were no difficulties delivering the baby boy, who weighed 1.67 kg, showing no signs of life. The remaining liquor in the amniotic sac was clear, but there were old retroplacental clots totalling 300 mL. The placenta was small and had pale areas underneath the adherent blood clots. The uterine cavity was confirmed to be empty and the uterus was sutured closed. The anaesthetist gave 1 mL Syntometrine prior to the placenta being removed, followed by an IVI of Syntocinon at 10 units/hr. In total, approximately 1500 mL of blood were lost during surgery. Intraoperatively, 3 more units of blood were transfused, totalling 6 units since admission.

Deborah was transferred from the operating theatre to the obstetric critical care area. Her initial observations were: BP 120/60 mmHg, CVP +7 cm H_2O and pulse 95 beats/min. Her urine output had only been 720 mL since admission, with 120 mL in the last hour. Deborah's condition was continuously assessed each hour by the attending midwife to ensure there was no further deterioration. Blood tests were repeated 4 hours post-operatively and the results were as follows (see Results Chart 5.3).

Results Chart 5.3

Blood test	On admission to labour ward	Two hours later	Four hours post-operatively
Haemoglobin	8.5 g/dL	11.2 g/dL	9.8 g/dL
Platelets	137 × 10⁹/L	98 × 10⁹/L	82 × 10⁹/L
White cell count	16.5 × 10⁹/L	13.4 × 10⁹/L	12.9 × 10⁹/L
APTT	33 sec. (control 31)	34 sec. (control 31)	31 sec. (control 31)
Thrombin time	11 sec. (control 10)	12 sec. (control 10)	12 sec. (control 10)
INR	1.11	1.14	0.92
Fibrinogen	1.61 g/L	1.27 g/L	2.08 g/L
Creatinine		49 micromol/L	42 micromol/L
Urea		3.2 mmol/L	2.9 mmol/L
Sodium		136 mmol/L	135 mmol/L
Potassium		4.8 micromol/L	4.0 micromol/L

In the first 12 hours post-operatively, Deborah's BP was low but stable averaging 90/50 mmHg with a pulse of 60–75 beats/min, CVP +7 cmH$_2$0 and transcutaneous oxygen saturation in the range of 95–98 per cent. Her urine output was 65–200 mL/hr which improved as she began to drink oral fluids. She had been given approximately 100 mL/hr of IV crystalloid fluid since admission. Blood tests were repeated 12 hours post-operatively and the results can be seen in Results Chart 5.4.

By the following day, Deborah was feeling much better, although emotionally still very traumatized. Her platelet count was 109 × 10⁹/L and haemoglobin 11.0 g/dL. She was transferred home after four days with plans for further review with the obstetrician and haematologist. By this stage, her platelet count was 180 × 10⁹/L and haemoglobin 11.6 g/dL. Discussion took place with Deborah about future pregnancies in view of her obstetric history and having APS.

Results Chart 5.4

Blood test	On admission to labour ward	Two hours later	Four hours post-operatively	Twelve hours post-operatively
Haemoglobin	8.5 g/dL	11.2 g/dL	9.8 g/dL	10.6 g/dL
Platelets	137 × 10⁹/L	98 × 10⁹/L	82 × 10⁹/L	73 × 10⁹/L
White cell count	16.5 × 10⁹/L	13.4 × 10⁹/L	12.9 × 10⁹/L	13.4 × 10⁹/L
APTT	33 sec.	34 sec.	31 sec.	30 sec.
	(control 31)	(control 31)	(control 31)	(control 31)
Thrombin time	11 sec.	12 sec.	12 sec.	11 sec.
	(control 10)	(control 10)	(control 10)	(control 10)
INR	1.11	1.14	0.92	0.85
Fibrinogen	1.61 g/L	1.27 g/L	2.08 g/L	2.74 g/L
Creatinine		49 micromol/L	42 micromol/L	49 micromol/L
Urea		3.2 mmol/L	2.9 mmol/L	2.2 mmol/L
Sodium		136 mmol/L	135 mmol/L	135 mmol/L
Potassium		4.8 micromol/L	4.0 micromol/L	3.7 micromol/L

1 **Identify the risk factors that Deborah initially presents with at the midwives' clinic and the plan of care for subsequent antenatal care.**

A The first visit at the midwives' clinic provides an ideal opportunity for the midwife to take a thorough obstetric and medical history from Deborah in addition to undertaking an overall clinical assessment in order to plan the most appropriate care for her throughout pregnancy. In addition, this first encounter is vitally important to the establishment of a good relationship between the midwife and Deborah, although she may already know the midwife/local midwifery team from her last pregnancy.

Based on her history, the risk factors that Deborah presents with at this first visit to the midwives' clinic are as follows:

- Recurrent pregnancy loss at < 10 weeks of pregnancy.
- Death of an apparently normal fetus at > 10 weeks of pregnancy.
- Previous pre-eclampsia.
- Previous pre-term birth.
- Baby with IUGR.
- Diagnosis of APS.

Bearing in mind all these risk factors associated with poor pregnancy outcome, the midwife should promptly refer Deborah for consultant-led care within a unit where there is a specialist maternal medicine clinic (NMC 2004).

> **Think**
>
> In this high risk clinical situation Deborah should still have midwifery contact to ensure her psycho-social and emotional needs are being met.

It is essential that there should be collaboration with haematologists and immunologists in conjunction with the community midwife and GP to ensure the optimum care and treatment plan is determined for Deborah. This would involve an early dating ultrasound scan (USS) to check the viability of the pregnancy followed by regular/serial scans to detect signs of intra-uterine growth restriction (IUGR). Throughout pregnancy there should be continuous risk assessment (see Case 2), including monitoring antiphospholipid antibody titres to determine the course of treatment. Khare and Nelson-Piercy (2003) state that fetal loss is directly related to the antibody titre, in that where women with APS are treated with antithrombotics in pregnancy, the chance of a live birth increases to 70 per cent compared to untreated cases where a live birth is around 20 per cent. In addition, regular assessment of BP is essential to monitor the development of pre-eclampsia especially around the mid-trimester as even with treatment for APS, Deborah is still susceptible to pre-eclampsia and IUGR (see Case 3). The midwife should also advise Deborah to be alert for any signs of infection as this could trigger secondary antiphospholipid syndrome (SAPS) if left untreated (NMC 2004). Prompt identification and early treatment are therefore essential.

As pregnancy progresses, Deborah and Robert should be involved in discussions with the multidisciplinary team to plan the intrapartum care and management required that is based on the best possible evidence and clearly documented in Deborah's maternity records (NMC 2010). In addition, it may be considered appropriate for Deborah and Robert to have further counselling about the risks that APS could pose on her health and that of her unborn baby in terms of the prognosis of the pregnancy, the possibility of pre-term birth and potential for further medical complications.

2   What is antiphospholipid syndrome (APS)?

A   APS is an autoimmune disorder that was originally observed in individuals with systemic lupus erythematosus (SLE) and first described by Graham Hughes (1984); consequently it is also known as Hughes Syndrome. It is associated with thromboembolic disorders, recurrent miscarriages (as in Deborah's case) and neurological disorders, such as cerebral vascular accident (CVA), and mainly presents in young and middle-aged adults with a prevalence of 2–4 per cent. However, in 30 per cent of cases, APS is found in conjunction with SLE.

Phospholipid is a component of cell membranes and, in APS, antiphospholipid antibodies (APA) are produced. APA constitutes either the presence of one or both of two autoantibodies: lupus anticoagulant (LA) and anticardiolipin antibodies (aCL). It is known that aCL occur five times more often than LA in individuals with APS. Robson and Hodgett (2008) warn that as cardiolipin is a component of the Wesserman reaction which tests for syphilis, individuals with APS may also get a false positive in areas where this test is still used. The autoantibodies LA and/or aCL bind to phospholipid-binding proteins and the organ or vessel in the body can be affected and predisposes an individual to thrombotic disorders. If blood platelets are involved, a state of hypercoagulability results and the individual is known colloquially to have *sticky blood*. There are three forms of APS (Table 5.1) which can manifest in one of three ways.

In individuals with an initial presentation of primary APS, around 10 per cent will eventually be diagnosed with an autoimmune disorder such as SLE or a mixed connective tissue disorder.

3   What are the pregnancy risks associated with APS?

A   According to Khare and Nelson-Piercy (2003), the risks of APS (Table 5.2) to a pregnant woman are vast in terms of fetal and maternal morbidity, especially if not treated.

Table 5.1 Manifestation of thrombotic disease in antiphospholipid syndrome

Primary APS (PAPS)	Secondary APS (SAPS)	Catastrophic APS (CAPS)
Occurs in isolation and manifests as one of: – arterial/venous thrombo-embolic disease, – endocarditis, – recurrent pregnancy failure associated with thrombocyto-penia in 20–40% of cases	Associated with infection or autoimmune disease, e.g. SLE and thrombocytopenia and manifests as PAPS	This is rare, but develops rapidly with small vessel thrombosis causing multi-organ failure, VTE, PE and CVA resulting in a high mortality rate

Table 5.2 Risks associated with APS

Maternal risks associated with APS	Fetal risks associated with APS
VTE/thrombosis in any organ/tissue Pre-eclampsia/HELLP syndrome Placental insufficiency Placental abruption Treatment side effects, e.g. osteoporosis risk with LMWH	Miscarriage Pre-term infant IUGR IUFD/NND

4 **What treatment strategies can be used for APS in pregnancy?**

A The therapeutic use of antithrombotics such as aspirin and LMWH in recurrent pregnancy loss is controversial and there has been little research to substantiate the benefit of one treatment over another until recently (RCOG 2011a). A Cochrane Review of anticoagulants for non-APS recurrent pregnancy loss by Kaandorp et al. (2009) identified only two studies of 189 women. Neither study showed a benefit of one treatment over another, concluding that there was no evidence for this practice and identifying the urgent need for further trials in this area. Although in the case of APS and recurrent pregnancy loss, Empson et al. (2005) had found no benefit in an analysis of three trials of aspirin compared with placebo, RCOG (2011a) still recommend the use of aspirin and heparin to reduce platelet clot formation in cases such as Deborah's. Should LMWH be prescribed for Deborah, anti-factor Xa activity may need to be monitored to adjust the dose accordingly.

Where there is a history of thrombotic complications, it is usual for LMWH or second/third trimester warfarin to be administered in order to prevent VTE (see Case 4). In some specialist centres, Khare and Nelson-Piercy (2003) suggest that immunoglobulin as IVIG might be given to women with previously poor obstetric outcomes on aspirin and LMWH to improve the autoimmune effects of pregnancy.

5 **What could be the possible cause of Deborah's symptoms at 32 weeks of pregnancy?**

A At 32 weeks of pregnancy, the sudden onset of heavy vaginal bleeding with evidence of clots accompanied by severe abdominal pain would be indicative of Deborah experiencing a placental abruption. Although the cause of placental separation cannot always be satisfactorily explained, there appears to be an association with defective trophoblast invasion, similar to that found in pre-eclampsia. Furthermore, Ananth et al. (2007) state that women who have experienced pre-eclampsia, placental abruption, or IUGR have an increased risk of developing any of these complications in a subsequent pregnancy. All three conditions have been found by Brenner (2004) to be associated with thrombophilias such as APS that have an increased propensity for abnormal coagulation within the placenta. Consequently it is believed that a significant proportion of these three conditions belong to a spectrum of ischaemic placental disease and share a common aetiology, particularly when seen in pre-term gestations (Brenner 2004; Ananth et al. 2007). However, ACOG (2010) has released a guideline recommending that thrombophilias are no longer tested for after placental abruption, as they do not appear to increase the risk of abruption.

6 **What would be the immediate management of these symptoms?**

A As Deborah is experiencing severe pain with the heavy vaginal bleeding, her skin will probably appear pale and moist, significant of shock and it is vital she is transferred to hospital as an emergency. Deborah's temperature, pulse, respirations (TPR) and BP should be assessed and recorded using MEOWS, noting any hypotension, tachycardia and tachypnoea which would be associated with signs of underlying critical illness and hypovolaemic shock (Mitchell 2010; NMC 2010). Hypovolaemia can lead to impaired perfusion of vital organs and tissue hypoxaemia with severe consequences (Carrington and Down 2009) (see Cases 1 and 12). Adopting a left-lateral position or lying with a pillow or towel wedged under the right hip to achieve a slight pelvic tilt will prevent Deborah from supine hypotensive syndrome (Crafter 2009).

When bleeding is also concealed behind the placenta and within the uterine wall, as in Deborah's case, the uterus appears large for dates and is firm and tender upon touch. Although abdominal palpation should be kept to a minimum in order to avoid further pain and damage, it may in fact be difficult to palpate fetal parts or hear the FH with a Pinard stethoscope and a hand-held Doppler should be used (if available). As pain exacerbates shock, then Deborah may be given an analgesic, such as an opiate before her arrival at the hospital. This should be clearly documented to alert those attending her of its administration (Crafter 2009). A VE should *NOT* be undertaken, until the placental location is confirmed by USS in case it is lying in the lower segment.

All soiled sanitary pads and clothing should be saved to allow accurate measurement of blood loss and its colour noted: fresh blood loss is bright red whereas blood that has been retained in utero for any length in time is a darker brown colour. It should be borne in mind that as the true blood loss may be far greater than that observed visually, it may be necessary to implement the local NHS Trust guidelines for major obstetric haemorrhage (Addo et al. 2008; RCOG 2011b) (see Case 8).

7 **What blood tests should be taken in Deborah's case? State the rationale for them being undertaken.**

A The following blood tests would need to be taken to assess Deborah's health and well-being and plan subsequent management (Ramsay 2010) (see Table 5.3).

8 **What may have contributed to the vaginal bleeding?**

A The fact that Deborah had been taking low-dose aspirin (75 mg daily) may possibly have contributed to her vaginal bleeding, although will not have caused it. At these low doses, aspirin affects platelet function by inhibiting the production of the platelet-aggregating agent thromboxane A_2

Table 5.3 Blood tests and their rationale

Blood test	Rationale for test
FBC	Hb and platelet level to assess severity of haemorrhage (which may or may not be revealed)
Coagulation screen and fibrinogen level	Level of clotting factors to assess the risk of bleeding tendency
U & Es and creatinine levels	To assess renal function in hypotensive state
Blood group and antibody studies	Cross-match blood for transfusion

that causes platelet adhesion and clumping, the consequential effect being the platelet contribution to a fibrin mesh–platelet clot is reduced. Rutherford (2009) asserts that aspirin exerts its anti-platelet effect for around 10 days after administration and may prolong the bleeding time, hence Deborah should be advised to discontinue taking any further aspirin.

9 **What is the significance to Deborah's health and well-being of the blood test results taken by the paramedic and those taken on admission to the labour ward? (Results Chart 5.1)**

A The blood results indicate a significant fall in haemoglobin levels over the short time period between the two tests (approx. 90 minutes). In addition, the platelet count has decreased. The earlier blood clotting studies are normal for pregnancy, but the second set show low fibrinogen levels and prolongation of activated partial thromboplastin time (APTT) and International Normalized Ratio (INR) (expressing the prothrombin time versus control serum). These tests reflect the length of time taken for intrinsic and extrinsic coagulation pathways to form a fibrin clot and show that, at the time of the second blood tests, Deborah's blood clotting is deranged (Lefkou and Hunt 2010; Ramsay 2010). The fall in fibrinogen and the low platelet count indicate that the cause is likely to be consumption of clotting factors in that there is a large blood clot somewhere that has used up a significant quantity of Deborah's blood clotting factors. The inference is that Deborah has a considerable amount of concealed uterine haemorrhage in addition to the blood loss that has been seen. Her renal function tests, however, are normal at both these time points, indicating that the kidneys are being appropriately perfused and functioning well.

The picture of low fibrinogen, low platelets and prolongation of coagulation tests is known as *consumptive coagulopathy* or DIC. At this point, the coagulation screen results are only slightly prolonged, but if the processes continue, then it would be expected that the fibrinogen and platelet counts would fall further and the APTT and INR would be further prolonged. A further confirmatory test of DIC is to look for fibrin degradation products (FDP), which are the result of clot destruction (Lefkou and Hunt 2010). Essentially, DIC is the process of inappropriate clot formation and destruction within the circulation, which eventually exhausts the raw materials of clots, i.e. fibrin and platelets, and can have major consequences on Deborah's well-being if left untreated.

10 **What would be the subsequent management of Deborah once diagnosed with DIC?**

A The management of DIC is to treat the underlying cause or trigger and also to replace the deficient haemostatic components to support clotting pathways. All the obstetric causes of

DIC (pre-eclampsia, placental abruption, amniotic fluid embolism, IUFD, sepsis and septic abortion) require urgent birth of the fetus and placenta as their definitive management (Lefkou and Hunt 2010). Replacement of haemostatic factors involves the use of various blood products: platelets, fresh frozen plasma (rich in all the clotting factors), cryoprecipitate (rich in fibrinogen) and red cells. These will be issued by the blood transfusion service, in response to discussion between the consultant obstetrician and consultant haematologist about Deborah's circumstances and results of the coagulation tests. Repeat coagulation tests and fibrinogen levels can also be used to monitor success of the replacement therapy and guide further administration of blood products.

11   **Comparing the blood tests taken 2 hours later with those on admission to labour word, what conclusions can you draw about Deborah's coagulation status and subsequent management? (Results Chart 5.2)**

A   The repeat coagulation tests show further deterioration in Deborah's blood coagulation status, with lower platelet count and more prolonged APTT, INR and thrombin times. The fibrinogen level remains low, despite the recent administration of IV cryoprecipitate. Deborah's management and care need to be escalated as her measured blood coagulation parameters indicate the situation is worsening (Lefkou and Hunt 2010; Ramsay 2010). The definitive cure in Deborah's case would be to expedite the birth of the fetus and placenta and to implement the Trust's major obstetric haemorrhage protocol (Addo et al. 2008; RCOG 2011b) (see Case 8).

12   **What are the particular risks of anaesthesia and major surgery in Deborah's case?**

A   There should be collaboration with an experienced obstetrician, haematologist and anaesthetist in order to minimize or prevent the risks associated with anaesthesia and major surgery in cases such as Deborah's. Due to coagulopathy, Deborah is at risk of bruising at injection sites which would preclude the use of spinal anaesthetic techniques (Addo et al. 2008; Kakar and O'Sullivan 2010). If a haematoma was to occur at the site of insertion of a spinal needle, then one or more of the nerve roots of the cauda equina could be compressed which may cause lower back pain, sciatica, perineal numbness, or bladder/bowel dysfunction. These serious complications known as the *cauda equina syndrome* are recognized as a medical emergency as there may be permanent neurological damage (Yatis et al. 2007). Thus, a general anaesthetic would be advised in the presence of coagulopathy.

The particular risks to Deborah of surgery are that it will be difficult to achieve haemostasis at every stage of the operation. Furthermore, accumulated blood loss may be considerable and as the uterus is particularly prone to atony following placental abruption as a consequence of FDP interfering with myometrial contraction, Deborah would also be at risk of experiencing a postpartum haemorrhage (PPH) (McDonald 2009; RCOG 2011b) (see *Case 8*).

Think

The 'Four Ts' are potential causes of PPH, and Deborah presents with all four:

- *Tone* (distended uterus due to placental abruption)
- *Tissue* (retained clots)
- *Trauma* (lower segment caesareen section (LSCS))
- *Thrombin* (APS/DIC).

---

13 **What preventative measures could be taken to avoid a PPH?**

A In anticipation of uterine atony, the surgeon would need to work efficiently once the baby is born to remove the placenta, check that the uterine cavity is empty and then repair the uterus. Agents to promote sustained uterine contraction should be given routinely, such as Syntocinon infusion. If the uterus remains poorly contracted once closed, or there is heavy vaginal bleeding or heavy bleeding from the uterine incision, then the anaesthetist could be asked to administer other agents such as IV ergometrine, carboprost, misoprostol (RCOG 2011b). In certain circumstances, uterine brace sutures or additional compression sutures might need to be used as an adjunct, to promote continued uterine contraction and reduce the risk of hysterectomy, following the birth of Deborah's stillborn baby and placenta and membranes (B-Lynch et al. 1997; RCOG 2011b).

14 **Describe the appearance of a couvelaire uterus and its significance in childbirth.**

A A *couvelaire uterus* is also known as *uterine apoplexy* and is more commonly seen in cases of placental abruption where blood is retained behind the placenta rather than draining through the vagina. This blood is forced into the myometrium, infiltrating between the muscle fibres of the uterus, causing marked damage. At operation, the uterus will appear bruised and oedematous. Deborah would have all the symptoms of hypovolaemic shock caused by *concealed* bleeding into the uterine muscle as there will be no vaginal bleeding. Due to the bleeding causing uterine enlargement, Deborah would also experience extreme pain. According to Konje and Taylor (2006) concealed haemorrhage is said to account for 20–35 per cent of placental abruptions.

The assessment of Deborah's physiological status is vital in such a situation. The midwife would be expected to monitor the vital signs by use of a MEOWS system and promptly communicate any concerns to experienced obstetricians, bearing in mind that in a concealed haemorrhage, the extent of visible blood loss cannot be taken as a guide to the severity of the haemorrhage (see Case 2 and Case 8). Deborah is at risk of experiencing DIC and PPH as complications of a moderate to severe antepartum haemorrhage (APH). Renal failure may also occur as a result of hypovolaemia leading to poor perfusion of the kidneys, as may Sheehan's syndrome (pituitary necrosis) due to prolonged and severe hypotension. Maternal mortality due to APH, however, continues to decline; Norman (2011) reports that during 2006–2008, there were only two deaths from placental abruption, but continues to advocate the use of regular drills and skills exercises, guidelines and closer multidisciplinary working regarding management of obstetric haemorrhage to continue making improvements.

15 **What is the purpose of a CVP line in cases such as Deborah's?**

A A central venous pressure (CVP) line measures the filling pressure on the right side of the heart, the right atrium or superior vena cava, and provides an indication of the degree to which the vascular space is filled, reflecting the competence of the heart as a pump and the peripheral vascular resistance (Coates 2009). CEMACH (2004) recommended that CVP and direct arterial pressure monitoring should be implemented when a woman's cardiovascular system (CVS) is compromised by either haemorrhage or maternal disease to reduce significant maternal morbidity. In Deborah's case, it helps to establish that she has been given sufficient volume replacement for all the blood she has lost both before and during surgery. As the normal pressure varies between +5 and +10 cmH$_2$0, a CVP of +7 cmH$_2$0 indicates that her vascular space is well filled and that she does not need further red cell transfusion at this point in her management. These readings should then be recorded at frequent intervals on the MEOWS chart that monitors Deborah's overall condition and well-being.

16 **Considering the risks and benefits of different agents and methods of administration, what would be the most appropriate analgesia for Deborah to have post-operatively?**

A The most appropriate post-operative analgesia for Deborah would be paracetamol or opiates, given orally or IV as a bolus or in the form of PCA as recommended by NICE (2004). Due to the risk of bruising within the muscle, IM injections of opiates should be avoided. Non-steroidal anti-inflammatory drugs (NSAIDs), such as aspirin, should be avoided due to the adverse impact they have on renal and platelet function which would increase the bleeding risk at this time (Rutherford 2009).

17 **What do the blood results taken 4 hours post-operatively inform us about the DIC process and subsequent management? (Results Chart 5.3)**

A These results demonstrate that the DIC process has been brought under control. Fibrinogen levels are now higher, APTT and INR measurements are within the normal range. The platelet count remains low, but is fairly stable. Overall, there has been restoration of the ability of blood to clot at an appropriate speed. Renal function remains normal, so efforts to replace intravascular volume have been successful in allowing continued perfusion of the kidneys. In the absence of continued bleeding, there is no need for further transfusion of platelets or cryoprecipitate. Fibrinogen levels are now adequate and do not need further support. This would support the observation by Addo et al. (2008) that the coagulation process usually resolves between 24–48 hours following the birth of the baby, and the low platelet count within a week.

18 **As Deborah has had an operative birth, what thromboprophylactic measures should be taken?**

A The time of greatest risk for VTE associated with pregnancy is the early puerperium for women who have experienced an uncomplicated pregnancy and birth and thus, for someone such as Deborah who has APS, the risk is further increased (Robson and Hodgett 2008). A comprehensive risk assessment and postnatal care plan should be drawn up with the specialist haematologist and obstetrician involved in Deborah's care and these details should be clearly evident in the maternity records for members of the multidisciplinary team to consult. This would involve the midwives closely monitoring Deborah for early signs of VTE and CAPS and encouraging her to mobilize as soon as her recovery allows to minimize the risk of thrombosis.

Although RCOG (2009) specify that women who have undergone an emergency LSCS have a four times higher chance of VTE than women giving birth vaginally and should there-fore be given LMWH for 7 days following surgery, there should be careful consideration of the balance of Deborah's risk of bleeding and clotting due to her developing DIC. As a result, NICE (2010a), DH (2008) and Greer and Nelson-Piercy (2005) advocate that LMWH should be avoided, discontinued or postponed in such cases until the balance is sustained.

The advantages and limitations of graduated compression stockings and other mechanical methods of VTE prevention in the general setting were reviewed by Geerts et al. (2008) on behalf of the American college of Chest Physicions (ACCP). The review concluded that these methods be used primarily for women with a high risk of bleeding and where pharmacological thromboprophylaxis is contraindicated as well as an adjunct to anticoagulant thrombopro-phylaxis where this had been shown to improve efficacy in surgical cases. In addition, Bates et al. (2008) recommended the use of graduated compression stockings for childbearing women such as Deborah who are considered to be at high risk of VTE after LSCS and antenatally/postpartum for all women with a previous DVT.

19 **What advice should Deborah and Robert be given about future pregnancies and the risk of developing DIC in a subsequent pregnancy?**

A As Deborah and Robert's baby was stillborn due to experiencing a placental abruption, they should allow themselves time to reflect on the events and grieve their loss along with other family members. The midwife can help support the couple in this respect or put them in touch with a support group, such as the Stillbirth and Neonatal Death Society (SANDS), a coun-sellor or chaplain as they require (NMC 2004; Thomas 2011).

It is essential that Deborah's health and well-being are closely monitored during the post-natal period and any advice that is given about subsequent pregnancies is determined in consul-tation with the obstetrician, haematologist and immunologist. It is assumed that Deborah and Robert would be well versed with the pregnancy risks of APS (Khare and Nelson-Piercy 2003) but will require advice on the recurrent risk of developing DIC. Addo et al. (2008) specify that this is determined by the precipitating cause of DIC, which in Deborah's case was placental abruption. Although Konje and Taylor (2006) refer to placental abruption occurring in 0.49–1.8 per cent of *all* pregnancies, Deborah's risk will be significantly increased due to the consequential risk of pregnancy complications associated with APS.

Until such a time as another pregnancy is contemplated, appropriate contraception should be used by Deborah and Robert (NICE 2006) in conjunction with anticoagulant therapy. Lakasing and Khamashta (2001) have found there is a high incidence of thromboses in women with APS using the combined oral contraceptive pill containing either second or third generation progestogens and thus suggest that these women should be advised against using this form of contraception. The use of IUCDs in Deborah's case would also be unsuitable as far as those containing oestrogen are concerned as there is a susceptibility to infection and the development of SAPS. As a consequence, barrier methods of contraception with spermi-cides or natural family planning methods may be the only valid options available to Deborah and Robert.

20 **Would you consider any changes in antenatal management for a subsequent pregnancy to prevent a placental abruption?**

A Although most cases of placental abruption cannot be directly prevented, there are factors that can be avoided or treated to reduce the risk of its recurrence in a subsequent pregnancy. To optimize fetal health and development in terms of reducing the risk of neural tube defects, Deborah should take a daily dose of 400 micrograms of folic acid prior to conception and then for up to 12 weeks of pregnancy (DH 2000).

To reduce the risk of developing pre-eclampsia, Deborah should also take 75 mg of aspirin each day from 12 weeks of pregnancy until the baby is born to minimize the risk of any poten-tial complications (NICE 2010a, 2010b). LMWH, such as enoxaparin (Clexane) 1 mg/kg twice daily, would help prevent VTE and also help reduce the risk of platelet-clot formation occurring around the placental site, leading to placental abruption and consequential APH. Robson and Hodgett (2008) recommend an early dating scan and regular serial scans to detect IUGR. In addition, Khare and Nelson-Piercy (2003) advocate that uterine artery waveforms be undertaken at 20 weeks and 24 weeks and if normal, the cessation of LMWH could be considered.

Summary of key points

- The risks of APS to a pregnant woman are vast in terms of fetal and maternal morbidity, especially if left untreated.
- Concealed blood loss with placental abruption can be considerable.
- The first indication of DIC may be quite subtle prolongation of coagulation times; these must be interpreted in the light of normal ranges for pregnancy.
- The full extent of DIC becomes apparent when additional tests (e.g. fibrinogen levels) are ordered and trends followed in serial blood tests.
- Communication between the multidisciplinary team is vital for safe outcomes.
- Careful documentation of observations using MEOWS and serial blood tests is invaluable.
- The balance of risk of bleeding and clotting in women with DIC should be carefully considered before commencing LMWH following emergency caesarean section where there is a four-fold increase of VTE.
- When parents experience a stillbirth/neonatal death, they should be given time to grieve, and be referred to appropriate support agencies.

REFERENCES

Addo, A., Robson, S.E. and Oppenheimer, C. (2008) Haematological disorders, in Robson, S.E. and Waugh, J. (eds) *Medical Disorders in Pregnancy: A Manual for Midwives.* Oxford: Blackwell Publishing, pp.169–184.

American College of Obstetricians and Gynecologists Committee on Practice Bulletins-Obstetrics (2010) ACOG Practice Bulletin No. 111: Inherited thrombophilias in pregnancy, *Obstetrics and Gynecology,* 115(4): 877–87.

Ananth, C.V., Peltier, M.R., Chavez, M.R., Kirby, R.S., Getahun, D. and Vintzileos, A.M. (2007) Recurrence of ischemic placental disease, *Obstetrics and Gynecolology,* 110(1): 128–33.

Bates, S.M., Greer, I.A., Pabinger, I., Sofaer, S. and Hirsh, J. (2008) Venous thromboembolism, thrombophilia, antithrombotic therapy, and pregnancy: American College of Chest Physicians Evidence-Based Clinical Practice Guidelines (8th edn), *Chest,* 6 (Suppl.): 844S–6S.

B-Lynch, C., Coker, A., Lawal, A.H., Abu, J. and Cowen, M.J. (1997) The B-Lynch surgical technique for the control of massive postpartum haemorrhage: an alternative to hysterectomy? Five cases reported, *British Journal of Obstetrics and Gynaecology,* 104(3): 372–5.

Brenner, B. (2004) Clinical management of thrombophilia-related placental vascular complications, *Blood,* 103(11): 4003–9.

Carrington, M. and Down, J. (2009) Recognition and assessment of critical illness, *Anaesthesia and Intensive Care Medicine,* 11(1): 6–8.

Coates, T. (2009) Midwifery and obstetric emergencies, in Fraser, D.M. and Cooper, M.A. (eds) *Myles Textbook for Midwives,* 15th edn. Edinburgh: Churchill Livingstone, Elsevier, pp. 625–47.

Confidential Enquiry into Maternal and Child Health (2004) *Why Mothers Die, 2000–2002: Sixth Report on Confidential Enquiries into Maternal Deaths in the United Kingdom*. London: RCOG Press.

Crafter, H. (2009) Problems of pregnancy, in Fraser, D.M. and Cooper, M.A. (eds) *Myles Textbook for Midwives*, 15th edn. Edinburgh: Churchill Livingstone, Elsevier, pp. 333–59.

Department of Health (2000) *Folic Acid and the Prevention of Disease: Report of the Committee on Medical Aspects of Food and Nutrition Policy*. London: HMSO.

Department of Health (2008) *Venous Thromboembolism (VTE) Risk Assessment*. London: HMSO.

Empson, M.B., Lassere, M., Craig, J.C. and Scott, J.R. (2005) Prevention of recurrent miscarriage for women with antiphospholipid antibody or lupus anticoagulant, *Cochrane Database Systematic Reviews*, (2): CD002859.

Geerts, W.H., Bergqvist, D., Pineo, G.F., Heit, J.A., Samama, C.M. and Lassen, M.R. (2008) Prevention of venous thromboembolism. American College of Chest Physicians Evidence-Based Clinical Practice Guidelines, 8th edn, *Chest*, 133: 381–453.

Greer, I.A. and Nelson-Piercy, C. (2005) Low molecular weight heparins for thromboprophylaxis and treatment of venous thromboembolism in pregnancy: a systematic review of safety and efficacy, *Blood*, 106(2): 401–7.

Hughes, G. (1984) Autoantibodies in lupus and its variants: experience in 1000 patients, *British Medical Journal*, 289(6441): 339–42.

Kaandorp, S., Di Nisio, M., Goddijn, M. and Middeldorp, S. (2009) Aspirin or anticoagulants for treating recurrent miscarriage in women without antiphospholipid syndrome, *Cochrane Database Systematic Review*(1): CD004734.

Kakar, V. and O'Sullivan, G. (2010) Management of obstetric haemorrhage: anesthetic management, in Pavord, S. and Hunt, B. (eds) *The Obstetric Haematology Manual*. Cambridge: Cambridge University Press, pp. 158–65.

Khare, M. and Nelson-Piercy, C. (2003) Acquired thrombophilias and pregnancy, *Best Practice and Research in Obstetrics and Gynaecology*, 17(3): 1333–44.

Konje, J.C. and Taylor, D.J. (2006) Bleeding in late pregnancy, in James, D.K. Steer, P.J. Weiner, C.P. and Gonik, B. (eds) *High Risk Pregnancy Management Options*. London: WB Saunders, pp. 1259–75.

Lakasing, L. and Khamashta, M. (2001) Contraceptive practices in women with systemic lupus erythematosus and/or antiphospholipid syndrome: what advice should we be giving? *Journal of Family Planning and Reproductive Health Care*, 27(1): 7–12.

Lefkou, E. and Hunt, B. (2010) Management of obstetric haemorrhage: hemostatic management, in Pavord, S. and Hunt, B. (eds) *The Obstetric Haematology Manual*. Cambridge: Cambridge University Press, pp. 166–75.

McDonald, S. (2009) Physiology and management of the third stage of labour, in Fraser, D.M. and Cooper, M.A. (eds) *Myles Textbook for Midwives*, 15th edn. Edinburgh: Churchill Livingstone, Elsevier, pp. 531–54.

Mitchell, E. (2010) Specific features of critical care medicine: recognition of critical illness, in Smith, F.G. and Yeung, J. (eds) *Core Topics in Critical Care Medicine*. Cambridge: Cambridge University Press, pp. 1–5.

National Institute for Health and Clinical Excellence (2004) *Caesarean Section*. Clinical Guidance No. 13. London: NICE. Available at: http://www.nice.org.uk/Guidance/CG13

National Institute for Health and Clinical Excellence (2006) *Postnatal Care: Routine Postnatal Care of Women and Their Babies*. Clinical Guideline No. 37. London: NICE. Available at: http://www.nice.org.uk/Guidance/CG37

National Institute for Health and Clinical Excellence (2010a) *Venous Thromboembolism: Reducing the Risk of Venous Thromboembolism (Deep Vein Thrombosis and Pulmonary Embolism) in Patients Admitted to Hospital*. Clinical Guideline No. 92. London: NICE. Available at: http://www.nice.org.uk/Guidance/CG92

National Institute for Health and Clinical Excellence (2010b) *Hypertension in Pregnancy: The Management of Hypertensive Disorders During Pregnancy.* Clinical Guideline No. 107. London: NICE. Available at: http://www.nice.org.uk/Guidance/CG107

Norman, J. (2011) Haemorrhage, in Centre for Maternal and Child Enquiries (CMACE) *Saving Mothers' Lives: Reviewing Maternal Deaths to Make Motherhood Safer: 2006–2008. The Eighth Report on Confidential Enquiries into Maternal Deaths in the United Kingdom.* Ed. Lewis, G . *BJOG:* 118 (Suppl. 1): 71–6.

Nursing and Midwifery Council (2004) *Midwives Rules and Standards.* London: NMC.

Nursing and Midwifery Council (2010) *Record Keeping: Guidance for Nurses and Midwives.* London: NMC.

Ramsay, M.M. (2010) Normal haematological changes during pregnancy and the puerperium, in Pavord, S. and Hunt, B. (eds) *The Obstetric Haematology Manual.* Cambridge: Cambridge University Press, pp. 3–12.

Robson, S.E. and Hodgett, S. (2008) Autoimmune disorders, in Robson, S.E. and Waugh, J. (eds) *Medical Disorders in Pregnancy: A Manual for Midwives.* Oxford: Blackwell Publishing, pp. 137–46.

Royal College of Obstetricians and Gynaecologists (2009) *Thrombosis and Embolism during Pregnancy and the Puerperium: Reducing the Risk.* Green Top Guideline No. 37a. London: RCOG Press.

Royal College of Obstetricians and Gynaecologists (2011a) *The Use of Antithrombotics in the Prevention of Recurrent Pregnancy Loss: Scientific Advisory Committee Opinion Paper 26.* London: RCOG.

Royal College of Obstetricians and Gynaecologists (2011b) *Prevention and Management of Post-partum Haemorrhage.* Green Top Guideline No. 52. London: RCOG.

Rutherford, J.M. (2009) Pharmacology and childbirth, in Fraser, D.M. and Cooper, M.A. (eds) *Myles Textbook for Midwives,* 15th edn. Edinburgh: Churchill Livingstone, Elsevier, pp. 945–58.

Thomas, J. (2011) Grief and bereavement, in McDonald, S. and Magill-Cuerden, J. (eds) *Mayes Midwifery,* 14th edn. Edinburgh: Ballière Tindall, Elsevier, pp. 953–68.

Yatis, S., May, A. and Malhotra, S. (2007) *Analgesia, Anaesthesia and Pregnancy: A Practical Guide.* Cambridge: Cambridge University Press.

ANNOTATED FURTHER READING

Pavord, S. and Hunt, B. (2010) *The Obstetric Haematology Manual.* Cambridge: Cambridge University Press.

This multi-authored text addresses the many haematological conditions that can cause serious problems during childbirth for both mother and baby and includes up-to-date, evidence-based guidelines on best care. An ideal text for all members of the multidisciplinary team: obstetricians, anaesthetists, haematologists and midwives.

Robson, S.E. and Waugh, J. (2008) *Medical Disorders in Pregnancy: A Manual for Midwives.* Oxford: Blackwell Publishing.

This is one of the first texts written for midwives outlining common medical conditions that may be affected by pregnancy or may cause pregnancy complications. The management, treatment and care by both doctors and midwives are included to enable an understanding of each other's roles and responsibilities.

USEFUL WEBSITES

www.bcshguidelines.com	British Committee for Standards in Haematology
www.b-s-h.org.uk	British Society for Haematology
www.dh.gov.uk	Department of Health
www.hqip.org.uk	Healthcare Quality Improvement Partnership
www.nice.org.uk	National Institute for Health and Clinical Excellence
www.npsa.nhs.uk	National Patient Safety Agency
www.rcog.org.uk	Royal College of Obstetricians and Gynaecologists
www.shotuk.org	Serious Hazards of Transfusion
www.uk-sands.org	Stillbirth and Neonatal Death Society

Obstetric cholestasis
Karen Jackson and Jane Rutherford

Pre-requisites for the chapter: the reader should have an understanding of:

- The anatomy and physiology of the liver.
- The altered physiology of the liver during pregnancy.
- The midwife's role and responsibilities within the interprofessional team.
- Knowledge of drugs/medicines used in the management of obstetric cholestasis.
- Clinical governance/risk management procedures.
- The statutory framework and guidelines governing midwifery practice.
- Local NHS Trust medicine code, policies and guidelines.

Pre-reading self-assessment

1 What are the functions of the liver?
2 Describe briefly four of the main functions of the liver.
3 Describe briefly physiological changes that occur to the liver during pregnancy.
4 Identify the causes of common itching/pruritus during pregnancy.
5 What are the signs and symptoms of obstetric cholestasis?
6 What are the possible complications of obstetric cholestasis for mother and fetus/ neonate?
7 Outline the care and management of obstetric cholestasis during pregnancy and for the labour and birth.
8 What specific postnatal care and advice will be offered to women who have developed obstetric cholestasis?

Recommended prior reading

Kenyon, A. and Girling, J. (2005) Liver disease in pregnancy, *Women's Health in Medicine*, 2(2): 26–8.

Lee, R., Kwok, K., Ingles, S., Wilson, M., Mullin, P., Incerpi, M., Pathak, B. and Murphy Goodwin, T. (2008) Pregnancy outcomes during an era of aggressive management for intrahepatic cholestasis of pregnancy, *American Journal of Perinatology*, 25(6): 341–5.

Royal College of Obstetricians and Gynaecologists (RCOG) (2011) *Obstetric Cholestasis*. RCOG Guideline No. 43. London: RCOG.

Saleh, M.M. and Abdo, K.R. (2007) Consensus on the management of obstetric cholestasis: national UK survey, *BJOG*, 114: 99–103.

CASE STUDY

Imogen, a 25-year-old primigravida attends a routine antenatal appointment with her community midwife at 35 weeks gestation. All has been previously well with the pregnancy. The routine observations assessed and recorded by the midwife are P 82 bpm, BP 124/80 mmHg, RR 14 breaths per min. T 36.9°C, urinalysis NAD. On abdominal examination, symphysis pubis fundal height (SPFH) measurement is 35 cm. The lie is longitudinal, cephalic presentation, right occiput anterior (ROA) position and the fetal head 3/5th engaged. At Imogen's request, auscultation of the FHR is performed by the midwife using a Pinard stethoscope for 1 minute. This is not routinely performed in accordance with NICE (2008) antenatal care guidelines. Findings following auscultation are recorded as: FHR 155 bpm and regular, baseline variability > 5 bpm, no accelerations or decelerations are noted during the auscultation. All these findings are recorded in Imogen's hand-held records.

The midwife enquires about Imogen's general health and well-being. Imogen mentions that she is feeling quite tired lately; she also mentions that she has been experiencing itching for a few weeks that has progressively become more problematic. The itching has interfered with her sleep on a number of occasions. The midwife further enquires about the nature of this 'itching'. Imogen states that it started on the palms of her hands, and a little on the soles of her feet, but is now on her arms and on her abdomen. On examining Imogen's arms, the midwife notices that these are quite red through vigorous scratching. However, the presence of a rash is not obvious.

1 **What are your initial thoughts concerning a diagnosis for Imogen's condition?**

A Imogen's history is generally normal, apart from the severe itching (pruritus) that has developed over the preceding few weeks. The nature and timing of the itching would initially lead the health professional to consider obstetric cholestasis (also known as intrahepatic cholestasis of pregnancy (ICP)). This commonly presents in the third trimester of pregnancy (Dixon and Williamson 2008), but can sometimes be in the second trimester (Milkiewicz et al. 2002). The description of itching occurring in the first instance on the palms of the hands and the soles of the feet are classic symptoms (Ambros-Rudolph et al. 2007); this itching can then spread to other areas.

The main systems that are implicated are:

- liver/biliary;
- skin/cutaneous.

2 **What actions should the midwife take regarding Imogen's pruritus?**

A The midwife should make a detailed record of her findings and after discussing her concerns with Imogen, make a referral to a hospital for an immediate review by an experienced obstetrician. This will uphold rules 6 and 9 of the NMC (2004) *Midwives Rules and Standards*.

3 **What other conditions could cause Imogen's signs and symptoms?**

A Itching in pregnancy is not uncommon. Therefore, although all the signs point to obstetric cholestasis, there are other possible explanations for Imogen's condition and it is important to consider and exclude them.

It is imperative to consider a differential diagnosis in this situation as outlined in Box 6.1. Although itching *per se* is not an obstetric emergency, the management of the condition could vary greatly depending on its aetiology. See Box 6.1 for a list of differential diagnoses for maternal pruritus.

Box 6.1 Differential diagnosis to explain maternal pruritus

- Eczema or other dermatological conditions
- Liver disease due to other causes:
  - Hepatitis A
  - Hepatitis B
  - Hepatitis C
  - Cytomegalovirus (CMV)
  - Epstein–Barr virus (EBV)
  - Autoimmune liver disease
  - Liver disease as a result of drug or alcohol misuse
  - Normal physiological itching in pregnancy.

(RCOG 2011)

---

4 **What is the definition of pruritus?**

A The itchiness that gives rise to the medical term pruritus means that it can be defined as an unpleasant sensation that triggers the need to scratch (Bergassa 2005).

Check point

Morbidity in the form of pruritus can be extremely troublesome and debilitating in women with obstetric cholestasis.

---

5 **With reference to relevant pathophysiology, briefly describe the causes of obstetric cholestasis and subsequent pruritus.**

A The cause of obstetric cholestasis is not well understood, and is probably multifactorial with genetic, environmental and hormonal factors all having an influence. It appears that bile acid secretion from the liver into bile is impaired. The intense pruritus (itching) is due to accumulation of bile acids in the bloodstream and subsequent deposition in skin.

A number of theories have been proposed to explain this malfunction of bile secretion. It does appear to have genetic and hormonal associations. A woman with a first-degree relative who has suffered from obstetric cholestasis, e.g. mother or sister, is more likely to develop the disease. Obstetric cholestasis is also more common in women whose children subsequently develop rare types of inherited cholestatic liver disease (Milkiewicz et al. 2002). The presence of oestrogen and progesterone can also have an impact on the secretion of bile from the liver (Brannon 2004).

6 **What are the possible implications for Imogen's pregnancy if it is confirmed as being complicated by obstetric cholestasis?**

A The possible implications for a pregnancy complicated by obstetric cholestasis are outlined in Figure 6.1.

- *Increased risk of stillbirth*: Stillbirth is the most concerning of the risks which have been associated with obstetric cholestasis. However, when considering the evidence on this, it is important to recognize that the data has changed with time. The earliest reported study of cholestasis in 1976 found a perinatal mortality rate of 107/1000 pregnancies (Reid et al. 1976). However, when all later studies are reviewed, the mortality rate is comparable with the background rate. It is not certain whether this is because of general improvements in obstetric care, or specific active management of cholestasis (RCOG 2011).
- *Increased risk of premature birth*: The rate of spontaneous pre-term birth is slightly increased compared to the general population but the rate of iatrogenic prematurity is high with a range of 7–25 per cent (Reid et al. 1976; Fisk and Storey 1988; Rioseco et al. 1994; Alsulyman et al. 1996; Kenyon et al. 2002; RCOG 2011).

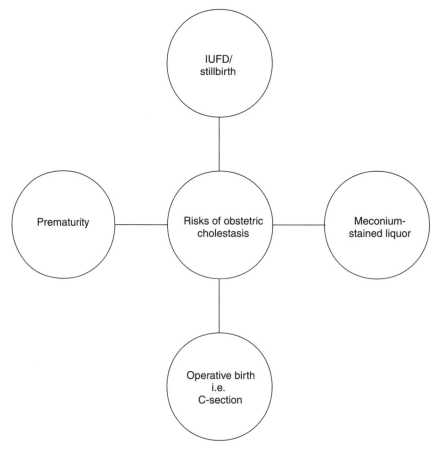

Figure 6.1 Risks of obstetric cholestasis

- *Increased risk of meconium staining of the liquor*: Some studies show an increase in meconium staining of liquor (Kenyon et al. 2002).
- *Increased risk of caesarean section*: Caesarean section rates are high in women with obstetric cholestasis. It is, however, unclear as to whether this is due to an increased intervention rate with early induction, or genuine obstetric indications.

The actual risks of the factors outlined above remain unclear, and more research is required to provide more definitive information regarding obstetric cholestasis and its effects on pregnancy (RCOG 2011).

7 **How can obstetric cholestasis be diagnosed?**

A In addition to a detailed history of the timing and nature of the pruritus outlined earlier, other sources of evidence should be elicited, for example, a family history of cholestasis (usually in a first-degree relative), previous occurrence of obstetric cholestasis, pale stool, dark urine, right upper quadrant pain, malaise, intolerance of fatty foods (Kenyon and Girling 2005; RCOG 2011). Imogen's skin should be inspected to look for rashes. However, care should be taken to avoid mistaking dermatitis artefacta caused by intense scratching for other skin conditions such as eczema.

Serum liver function tests should be checked to enable the diagnosis to be made. Abnormalities of transaminases such as alanine aminotransferase (ALT) and aspartate aminotransferase (AST), gamma glutamyl transferase (gamma GT), bilirubin and bile salts may occur. Bilirubin levels are raised in only 25 per cent of women. Most will have an increased level of one or more of the other liver function tests with 60 per cent having elevated transaminases. Most will have elevated bile salts, but normal levels do not exclude the diagnosis (Milkiewicz et al. 2002; RCOG 2011). When considering liver function tests, pregnancy-specific normal ranges should be used (Ramsay 2011); however, in many cases hospital laboratories will give a non-pregnant normal range.

It is important to recognize that other liver conditions may have the same pattern of abnormalities of liver function, and the diagnosis of obstetric cholestasis can only be confirmed if other liver conditions have been excluded. Other pregnancy-related causes of abnormal liver function should also be considered such as pre-eclampsia, HELLP syndrome (see Case 3) and acute fatty liver of pregnancy. Imogen should have detailed laboratory investigations identified, as shown in Box 6.2, if it is confirmed that her liver function tests are abnormal to exclude other causes of liver dysfunction.

Box 6.2 Laboratory investigations to be performed when LFTs are abnormal

Serum viral screen for:

- hepatitis A, B, C
- Epstein–Barr virus (EBV)
- cytomegalovirus (CMV)

(Continued overleaf)

Autoimmune liver screen:

- anti-smooth muscle antibodies for chronic active hepatitis
- anti-mitochondrial antibodies for primary biliary cirrhosis

Liver ultrasound scan

Many women will have pruritus for days or weeks before abnormalities in the liver function tests occur (Kenyon et al. 2001). Therefore, if pruritus persists, even if the liver function tests are initially normal, they should be repeated regularly, every one to two weeks (RCOG 2011).

As the abnormalities of liver function in obstetric cholestasis are confined to pregnancy, the diagnosis should be finally confirmed by establishing that the serum liver function tests normalize postpartum.

Check point

In women with suspected obstetric cholestasis, it is imperative that other liver conditions are screened for and excluded.

Imogen attends the maternity hospital assessment unit where she is seen by a midwife and then by an obstetric consultant. She has a full history taken and is examined. No additional features are discovered. There are no fetal concerns. She has blood taken for liver function tests which reveal that the bile acid level is 20 micromol/L, and ALT 50 U/L. All her other liver function tests are normal. In view of her liver function tests, she also has blood taken for serum viral screening and liver autoantibodies, and a liver ultrasound scan is performed. All these further investigations are normal.

8 **How is obstetric cholestasis managed/monitored?**

A Imogen should be given information about obstetric cholestasis and informed about the risks. Ideally she should be given written information such as the RCOG information leaflet for pregnant women, *Obstetric Cholestasis (Itching Liver Disorder): Information for You* (RCOG 2007).

Liver function tests should be measured weekly. In cholestasis, transaminases vary from just above the normal range to several hundred. If the levels rise rapidly or, alternatively, return to normal, then the diagnosis should be reviewed as this is not the usual pattern in obstetric cholestasis (RCOG 2011).

There are now a number of studies which suggest that the level of bile salts is related to the fetal complication rate (Laatikainen and Ikonen 1977; Laatikainen and Tulenheimo 1984; Glantz et al. 2004; Lee et al. 2008).

It is not clear from current evidence how to monitor the fetus in women with obstetric cholestasis in order to predict and prevent fetal death. When it occurs, intrauterine fetal death is usually sudden and is probably due to acute hypoxic injury. It does not appear to occur as a result of placental dysfunction and intrauterine growth restriction, oligohydramnios and abnormal umbilical artery Doppler measurements are not a feature of these pregnancies (Zimmerman et al. 1991; Rioseco et al. 1994; Alsulyman et al. 1996; Bacq et al. 1997; RCOG 2011).

Cases have been reported where routine CTG has detected pathological patterns which have led to emergency caesarean section being carried out (Fisk and Storey 1988; Rioseco et al. 1994; Alsulyman et al. 1996). However, CTG is not able to predict future fetal well-being and is therefore limited in its usefulness. Maternal perception of movements is simple and non-invasive, but has not been evaluated formally as a tool for monitoring fetal condition in obstetric cholestasis.

Despite the lack of evidence for any of the monitoring modalities, the difficulties should be discussed with Imogen by the obstetrician with support from the midwife in the hospital and the community. As she is likely to be anxious, an individual plan should be made to monitor her and her fetus, which might include fetal movement monitoring and CTG.

9 **What treatment can be offered?**

A There are currently no therapies available that have, in good quality trials, been shown to improve maternal symptoms or neonatal outcomes. Any treatment which is offered to Imogen should be discussed in advance with the evidence and rationale explained. Treatments that can be offered are identified in Box 6.3.

Box 6.3 Possible pharmacological treatments in obstetric cholestasis

- Topical emollients
- Antihistamines
- Ursodeoxycholic acid
- Dexamethasone
- Other treatments
- Vitamin K

- *Topical emollients*: Simple topical emollients can be useful to provide transient relief from pruritus and soothe areas which have been subjected to intense scratching. Examples include aqueous cream, aqueous cream with menthol, calamine lotion and other proprietary creams and lotions. There are no trial data to support or refute their use, but they are safe to apply topically in pregnancy and it is worth suggesting their use to Imogen. If they prove helpful to her, she can continue to use them. These are all available without prescription at local pharmacies and the midwife and/or GP might recommend their use.
- *Antihistamines*: Antihistamines such as chlorpheniramine can be prescribed to give symptomatic relief for the itch. None of them are licensed for use in pregnancy, but particularly chlorpheniramine has a well-established safety profile in pregnancy. These drugs can cause sedation, which may be useful in order to assist with sleep at night. The usual dose is 4 mg as required up to 6 hourly.

- *Ursodeoxycholic acid*: Ursodeoxycholic acid (UDCA) has been shown in some animal studies to have beneficial effects in clearing bile acids across the placenta from the fetus and in protection of cardiac muscle cells from the effects of bile acids. However, there have been only a few small randomized controlled trials of UDCA in pregnancies complicated by obstetric cholestasis. In the Cochrane Database of Systematic Reviews, three trials including 56 women in total, are identified in which UDCA is compared with placebo (Burrows et al. 2001). Two trials looked at symptomatic relief and showed no difference. One showed a reduction in bile salts and liver function tests with UDCA. A more recent study comparing UDCA, dexamethasone and placebo showed benefit in symptoms and liver function tests in women on UDCA, but not with placebo or dexamethasone (Glantz et al. 2005). There have been no studies which have investigated the effect of UDCA on perinatal outcome (RCOG 2011). In the UK, UDCA is frequently offered to women with obstetric cholestasis as clinicians believe that it has beneficial effects (Saleh and Abdo 2007). There is an urgent need for further large-scale studies. If Imogen is offered UDCA, she should have a full discussion with the obstetrician who should inform her of the data. The usual dose is 500 mg twice daily.
- *Dexamethasone*: One study has shown benefit in alleviating symptoms and improving biochemical markers with high doses of oral dexamethasone (Hirvioja et al. 1992). Subsequent studies have failed to show this effect (Glantz et al. 2005; Diac et al. 2006) and there is concern about the fetal risks of high doses of corticosteroids. Dexamethasone is therefore not a recommended therapy (RCOG 2011).
- *Other treatments*: Other treatments which have been used include cholestyramine, s-adenosylmethionine and guar gum. None of these agents have sufficient evidence to support their use in practice.
- *Vitamin K*: Obstetric cholestasis can adversely affect the absorption of fat from the diet because of the reduced excretion of bile salts into the gastrointestinal tract. This may, therefore affect the absorption of fat soluble vitamins from the diet, such as vitamin K. Vitamin K is required for the production of several clotting factors. Prescription of water-soluble vitamin K (10 mg daily orally) is recommended to optimize both maternal and fetal vitamin K levels to reduce the risk of postpartum haemorrhage and fetal/neonatal bleeding (RCOG 2011). Postnatal vitamin K must also be offered to Imogen's baby in the usual way, and if Imogen does not take vitamin K antenatally, the midwife at the birth should stress the increased risks of neonatal haemorrhagic disease because of Imogen's obstetric cholestasis.

Check point

Further research is needed in the recognition, management and treatment of women who develop obstetric cholestasis.

---

10 **How should birth be planned for women with obstetric cholestasis?**

A Many obstetricians will offer elective birth at 37 weeks gestation in order to reduce the chance of stillbirth (Saleh and Abdo 2007). This practice is not evidence based. In over 1500 pregnancies complicated by obstetric cholestasis, 13 out of 18 stillbirths occurred before 37 weeks and 5 were at 37–38 weeks (RCOG 2011). Clearly, offering Imogen elective induction of labour at 37 weeks will avoid the risk of stillbirth beyond 37 weeks gestation; however, there is insufficient evidence to be able to identify exactly what that risk is. The disadvantages of offering induction of labour at 37 weeks include an increased risk of respiratory morbidity in the neonate and increased risk of admission to neonatal intensive care unit, and an increased risk of failed induction leading to increased risk of caesarean section and thus an impact on future pregnancies. An experienced obstetrician should discuss the plans for birth with Imogen and this discussion should include the balance of risks (RCOG 2011). The agreed plan was for Imogen to be closely monitored, and for the labour to be induced at 39 weeks gestation, provided that mother and fetus remained well.

11 **What postnatal care would be given to Imogen?**

A Postnatally, the pruritus should resolve and liver function should return to normal; this will usually occur in 3 days to 6 weeks (Kenyon and Girling 2005). If this does not happen, then a different diagnosis may be considered. Imogen can be reassured that there are no long-term sequelae for either her or her baby (RCOG 2011). However, Imogen should be informed that obstetric cholestasis has a high recurrence rate, approximately 90 per cent will develop the condition in future pregnancies (Kenyon and Girling 2005). It would be prudent to ensure that Imogen is aware of the possible implications for close female relatives.

In those previously affected by obstetric cholestasis, the advice is that the combined oral contraceptive (COC) pill should not be used for contraception (although this is not an absolute contraindication). This is because there is some evidence that recurrent pruritus and abnormal liver function tests may be associated with taking the COC pill in these women (RCOG 2011). In addition, if Imogen chooses to breastfeed her infant, contraceptives other than COC methods would be recommended, as oestrogen-containing products may interfere with lactation (Guillebaud 2008). Imogen will have a range of options available to her including: natural family planning methods, male and female condoms, the intra-uterine contraceptive device (IUCD) and any of the progesterone only methods, for example, the progesterone only pill (POP), the intra-uterine system (IUS, Mirena), the contraceptive injection (Depo-Provera) and the contraceptive implant (Nexplanon) (Guillebaud 2008; Faculty of Sexual and Reproductive Healthcare 2010).

Psychosocial aspects of care are an important part of the midwives' role, including cultural and spiritual needs. Imogen, her partner or other family members may appreciate discussing the events of her pregnancy and birth with an appropriate member of the interprofessional team.

There are a number of resources that can be given to, or accessed by Imogen. As previously highlighted by the RCOG (2007) information leaflet *Obstetric Cholestasis (Itching Liver Disorder): Information for You*, the British Liver Trust has an information leaflet, which can be accessed at www.britishlivertrust.org.uk. Furthermore, an obstetric cholestasis support group exists which can be contacted by email at: jennychambersoc@aol.com or by phoning 07970 367973.

CASE OUTCOME

Imogen went into spontaneous labour at 38 weeks gestation, had a straightforward normal labour and gave birth to a healthy baby girl, Ellie. They were transferred to the postnatal ward. All aspects of postnatal care related to obstetric cholestasis were given to Imogen and Ellie as highlighted previously. Mother and baby were discharged home two days following the birth.

Summary of key points

- The signs and symptoms of obstetric cholestasis commonly present in the third trimester of pregnancy but can sometimes occur in the second trimester.
- The classic early symptoms of obstetric cholestasis are itching on the palms of the hands and the soles of the feet which may then spread to other areas. A rash is not present in cases of obstetric cholestasis.
- A differential diagnosis should always be considered when a pregnant woman presents with pruritus.
- Although increased risk of stillbirth is a commonly cited complication of obstetric cholestasis, there is little evidence to support this. However, there is evidence of associations with meconium staining of liquor, premature birth, and increased caesarean section rates, although the latter two may be iatrogenic effects.
- In addition to clinical examination, serum liver function tests should be checked to enable the diagnosis of obstetric cholestasis to be made. These should be repeated regularly throughout the pregnancy.
- Surveillance of the fetus is usually by CTG monitoring and by checking fetal movements.

REFERENCES

Alsulyman, O., Ouzounian, J., Ames Castro, M. and Goodwin, T. (1996) Intrahepatic cholestasis of pregnancy: perinatal outcome associated with expectant management, *American Journal of Obstetrics and Gynecology*, 175(4): 957–60.

Ambros-Rudolph, C., Glatz, M., Trauner, M., Kerl, H. and Müllegger, R. (2007) The importance of serum bile acid level analysis and treatment with ursodeoxycholic acid in intrahepatic cholestasis of pregnancy: a case series from Central Europe, *Archives of Dermatology*, 143(6): 757–62.

Bacq, Y., Sapey, T., Brechot, M., Peirre, F., Fignon, A. and Dubois, F. (1997) Intrahepatic cholestasis of pregnancy: a French prospective study, *Hepatology*, 26(2): 358–64.

Bergassa, N. (2005) The pruritus of cholestasis, *Journal of Hepatology*, 43(6): 1078–88.

Brannon, H. (2004) Intrahepatic cholestasis of pregnancy, *Dermatology*. Available at: http://dermatology.about.com/cs/pregnancy/a/icp.htm (accessed 30 August 2011).

Burrows, R., Clavisi, O. and Burrows, E. (2001) Interventions for treating cholestasis in pregnancy, *Cochrane Database of Systematic Reviews* Issue 4. Art. No.: CD000493. DOI: 10.1002/14651858. CD000493.

Davidson, K.M. (1998) Intrahepatic cholestasis of pregnancy, *Seminars in Perinatology*, 22(2):104–11.

Diac, M., Kenyon, A., Nelson-Piercy, C. et al. (2006) Dexamethasone in the treatment of obstetric cholestasis: a case series, *Journal of Obstetrics and Gynaecology*, 26(2): 110–14.

Dixon, P. and Williamson, C. (2008) The molecular genetics of intrahepatic cholestasis of pregnancy, *Obstetric Medicine*, 1(2): 65–71.

Faculty of Sexual and Reproductive Healthcare (FSRH) (2010) *Nexplanon*, FSRH Clinical Effectiveness Unit. London: RCOG.

Fisk, N. and Storey, G. (1988) Fetal outcome in obstetric cholestasis, *British Journal of Obstetrics and Gynaecology*, 95: 1137–43.

Glantz, A., Marschall, H.U., Lammert, F. and Mattsson, L.A. (2005) Intrahepatic cholestasis of pregnancy: a randomised controlled trial comparing dexamethasone and ursodeoxycholic acid, *Hepatology*, 42(6): 1399–405.

Glantz, A., Marschall, H. and Mattsson, L.A. (2004) Intrahepatic cholestasis of pregnancy: relationships between bile acid levels and fetal complication rates, *Hepatology*, 40(2): 467–74.

Guillebaud, J. (2008) *Contraception: Your Questions Answered* (5th edn). London: Churchill Livingstone.

Hirvioja, M.L., Tuimala, R. and Vuori, J. (1992) The treatment of intrahepatic cholestasis of pregnancy by dexamethasone, *British Journal of Obstetrics and Gynaecology*, 99(2): 109–11.

Kenyon, A. and Girling, J. (2005) Liver disease in pregnancy, *Women's Health in Medicine*, 2(2): 26–8.

Kenyon, A., Nelson-Piercy, C., Girling, J., Williamson, C., Tribe, R. and Shennan, A. (2001) Pruritus may precede abnormal liver function tests in pregnant women with obstetric cholestasis: a longitudinal study, *British Journal of Obstetrics and Gynaecology*, 108(11): 1190–2.

Kenyon, A., Nelson-Piercy, C., Girling, J., Williamson, C., Tribe, R. and Shennan, A. (2002) Obstetric cholestasis, outcome with active management: a series of 70 cases, *British Journal of Obstetrics and Gynaecology*, 109(3): 282–8.

Laatikainen, T. and Ikonen, E. (1977) Serum bile acids in cholestasis of pregnancy, *Obstetrics and Gynecology*, 50(3): 313–18.

Laatikainen, T. and Tulenheimo, A. (1984) Maternal serum bile acid levels and fetal distress in cholestasis of pregnancy, *International Journal of Gynaecology and Obstetrics*, 22(2): 91–4.

Lee, R., Kwok, K., Ingles, S., Wilson, M., Mullin, P., Incerpi, M., Pathak, B. and Murphy Goodwin, T. (2008) Pregnancy outcomes during an era of aggressive management for intrahepatic cholestasis of pregnancy, *American Journal of Perinatology*, 25(6): 341–5.

Lewis, G. (ed.) (2007) *The Confidential Enquiry into Maternal and Child Health (CEMACH). Saving Mothers' Lives: Reviewing Maternal Deaths to Make Motherhood Safer, 2003–2005. The Seventh Report on Confidential Enquiries into Maternal Deaths in the United Kingdom.* Available at: http://www.cmace.org.uk (accessed 27 August 2011).

Milkiewicz, E., Williamson, C. and Weaver, J. (2002) Editorials. Obstetric cholestasis may have serious consequences for the fetus and needs to be taken seriously, *British Medical Journal*, 324(7330): 123–4.

National Institute for Health and Clinical Excellence (2008) *Antenatal Care: Routine Care for the Healthy Pregnant Women.* Clinical Guideline No. 62. London: NICE.

Nursing and Midwifery Council (2004) *Midwives Rules and Standards.* London: NMC.

Ramsay, M. (2011) Normal values, in D.K. James, P.J. Steer, C.P. Weiner and B. Gonik (eds) *High Risk Pregnancy.* London: Elsevier.

Reid, R., Ivey, K., Rencoret, R. and Storey, B. (1976) Fetal complications of obstetric cholestasis, *British Medical Journal*, 1(6014): 870–2.

Rioseco, A., Ivankovic, M., Manzur, A., Hamed, F., Kato, S., Parer, J. and Germain, A. (1994) Intrahepatic cholestasis of pregnancy: a retrospective case-control study of perinatal outcome, *American Journal of Obstetrics and Gynecology*, 170(3): 890–5.

Royal College of Obstetricians and Gynaecologists (RCOG) (2007) *Obstetric Cholestasis (Itching Liver Disorder): Information for You.* Available at: http://www.rcog.org.uk/womens-health/clinical-guidance/obstetric-cholestasis-itching-liver-disorder-information-you (accessed 3 July 2011).

Royal College of Obstetricians and Gynaecologists (RCOG) (2011) *Obstetric Cholestasis.* RCOG Guideline No. 43. London: RCOG.

Saleh, M. and Abdo, K. (2007) Consensus on the management of obstetric cholestasis: national UK survey, *British Journal of Obstetrics and Gynaecology*, 114(1): 99–103.

Zimmerman, P., Koshiken, J., Vaalamo, P. and Ranta, T. (1991) Doppler umbilical artery velocimetry in pregnancies complicated by intrahepatic cholestasis, *Journal of Perinatal Medicine*, 19: 155–64.

ANNOTATED FURTHER READING

Chappell, L., Gurung, V., Chambers, J., Seed, P., Williamson, C., and Thornton, J. (2011) Pitch: two randomised controlled trials in obstetric cholestasis: ursodeoxycholic acid versus placebo and early delivery versus expectant management, *Archive of Disease in Childhood: Fetal and Neonatal Edition*, 96: Fa110–Fa111.

Geenes, V. and Williamson, C. (2009) Intrahepatic cholestasis of pregnancy, *World Journal of Gastroenterology*, 15(7): 2049–66.

Reports on RCTs examining two interventions in the treatment and management of obstetric cholestasis.

This is an up-to-date review of all aspects of obstetric cholestasis.

James, D., Steer, P., Weiner, C. and Gonik, B. (eds) (2011) *High Risk Pregnancy*. Oxford: Elsevier.

This text comprehensively explores all major complications and emergencies in childbearing including obstetric cholestasis and other conditions related to the liver.

Powrie, R., Greene, M. and Camann, W. (2010) *De Swiet's Medical Disorders in Obstetric Practice*, 5th edn. Oxford: Wiley-Blackwell.

This textbook comprehensively explores all of the major medical complications of pregnancy and provides the reader with a useful chapter on disorders of the liver and biliary system.

USEFUL ORGANIZATIONS

The British Liver Trust
2 Southampton Road
Ringwood BH24 1HY
Tel: 0870 770 8028
Website: www.britishlivertrust.org.uk
Email: info@britishlivertrust.org.uk

Obstetric Cholestasis Support and Information Line
Website: www.ocsupport.org.uk
Email: JennyChambersOC@aol.com
Tel: 07970 367973.

Provides support and information about Obstetric Cholestasis and promote research into the condition.

Royal College of Obstetricians and Gynaecologists
Obstetric Cholestasis – Green Top Guidelines
Website: www.rcog.org.uk/womens-health/clinical-guidance/obstetric-cholestasis-green-top-43

Guidelines for health professionals.

USEFUL WEBSITES

www.cemace.org.uk	Centre for Maternal and Child Enquiries
www.dh.gov.uk	UK Department of Health
www.institute.nhs.uk	National Health Service Institute for Innovation and Improvement
www.nice.org.uk	National Institute for Health and Clinical Excellence
www.npeu.ox.ac.uk	National Perinatal Epidemiology Unit
www.rcm.org.uk	Royal College of Midwives
www.rcog.org.uk	Royal College of Obstetricians and Gynaecologists (RCOG)

Haemoglobinopathies
Karen Jackson and Jane Rutherford

Pre-requisites for the chapter: the reader should have an understanding of:

- The structure and function of haemoglobin.
- Normal blood serial values/haematological indices including some of the routine laboratory investigations performed during pregnancy.
- The anatomy and physiology of systems (including maternal physiological adaptation during pregnancy), such as the circulatory system especially the structure and function of red blood cells.
- The value of SBAR as a communication tool in the interprofessional team.
- The midwife's role and responsibilities within the interprofessional team.
- Drugs/medicines used in the management of haemoglobinopathies.
- Clinical governance/risk management procedures.
- Statutory framework and guidelines governing midwifery practice.

Pre-reading self-assessment

1 What are the functions of haemoglobin?
2 What happens to haemoglobin in sickle cell disease?
3 What are the implications of sickle cell disease in pregnancy?
4 What happens to haemoglobin in β-thalassaemia major?
5 What are the implications of β-thalassaemia major in pregnancy?

Recommended prior reading

CMACE (2011) *Saving Mothers' Lives: Reviewing Maternal Deaths to Make Motherhood Safer: 2006–2008. The Eighth Report on Confidential Enquiries into Maternal Deaths in the United Kingdom*. Ed. G. Lewis. *BJOG:* 118 (Suppl. 1): 30–56.

Roberts, S. (2008) Sickle cell disease, in J. Queenann (ed.) *Management of High Risk Pregnancy: An Evidence Based Approach*. Chichester: John Wiley & Sons Ltd.

This case study is split into two parts to examine the care of two women, one with sickle cell disease (Case study 7.1: Julia) and one with β-thalassaemia major (Case study 7.2: Anna).

CASE STUDY 7.1: SICKLE CELL DISEASE

Julia, a 23-year-old multigravida (G2 P1), is 30 weeks pregnant. She has been referred to hospital by her community midwife after she reported suffering from a period of vomiting and complains of feeling generally unwell. She also has severe pain in both legs and is known to have sickle cell disease.

The routine observations are as follows: P 120 bpm, BP 110/60 mmHg, RR 16 breaths per min., T37.8°C, urinalysis with nothing abnormal detected (NAD). On abdominal examination symphysis pubis fundal height (SPFH) measures 29 cm, longitudinal lie, cephalic presentation, left occipito anterior (LOA) position with the fetal head 4/5th palpable. Due to the clinical picture, auscultation of the fetal heart rate (FHR) is performed by the midwife using a Pinard stethoscope for 1 minute (NICE 2008). Findings following auscultation are FHR 160 bpm and regular, baseline variability > 5 bpm; no accelerations or decelerations are noted during the auscultation. All these findings are recorded in Julia's notes and hand-held records.

Julia admits that she has had similar pain in her legs when she has had viral infections in the past and that she has previously been admitted to hospital with these symptoms.

1   **What is sickle cell disease?**

A   Sickle cell disease is the most common disorder related to the presence of abnormal haemoglobin in red blood cells. There are over 300 abnormal variant haemoglobins (Strong and Rutherford 2011). Sickle cell disease is caused by haemoglobin S. It is a result of a point mutation in the β-globin gene. This disorder is seen in ethnicities originating from Africa, Mediterranean countries, Asia, the Caribbean and the Far East (Addo et al. 2008; RCOG 2011). Sickled cells are removed from the circulation resulting in haemolytic anaemia, the iron that is released in this process is then stored and reused for new blood cells. The average life span of a normal red blood cell is 120 days, the life span of a sickled cell is 5–30 days (Johnston 2005). Homozygous sickle cell disease (HbSS) is an autosomal recessive disorder in which the individual has inherited the mutated gene from both parents (homozygous). Those with a sickle cell trait (HbAS) have received one defective and one healthy allele (heterozygous). These individuals remain healthy but are known as carriers of the disease. If two carriers have a child, there is a 1-in-4 chance that the child will be affected by the disease and a 1-in-2 chance that they will be a carrier. The risk odds will remain the same for each pregnancy (Johnston 2005; RCOG 2011).

2   **What are the complications of sickle cell disease?**

A   There are a number of complications associated with sickle cell disease as listed in Box 7.1.

Box 7.1 Complications of sickle cell disease

- Chronic haemolytic anaemia
- Hyposplenism
- Increased risk of infection
- Iron overload
- Avascular bone necrosis
- Increased risk of cerebrovascular accident
- Cardiac failure (caused by chronic hypoxaemia)

- Chest syndrome (manifested by cough, severe chest pain, dyspnoea, fever, severe anaemia)
- Pulmonary hypertension
- Pulmonary embolism
- Retinal disease
- Vaso-occlusive or painful crisis (exacerbated by stress, cold, infection, dehydration, exercise).

  (Johnston 2005; Addo et al. 2008; RCOG 2011; Strong and Rutherford 2011)

3 **What are the implications of sickle cell disease during pregnancy?**

A In the latest CMACE report Harper (2011) identified 29 deaths attributed to genital tract sepsis (see Case 11). Two of these women had sickle cell disease and one had sickle cell trait. All of the women were of Black African origin. Two died from coliform sepsis and one died from *Staphylococcus aureus* infection (Harper 2011). It is known that women with sickle cell disease are more susceptible to infection. This is mainly because of damage to the spleen caused by repeated episodes of sequestration of sickle cells. This has a long-term effect on splenic function. Sickle cell disease was also associated with an indirect maternal death where cardiac disease was also present (Nelson-Piercy 2011). Maternal mortality from sickle cell disease is estimated to be 1 in 220 (National Institutes of Health 2002).

Check point

When caring for pregnant women who have sickle cell disease, the maternity interprofessional team should be aware that these women are more susceptible to infection and therefore to the subsequent development of sepsis. Adhering to infection control measures is particularly important for these women.

4 **What are your initial thoughts regarding Julia's current problems?**

A Julia is known to have sickle cell disease. She has presented with vomiting and pain in her legs. Sickle cell crises are precipitated by situations such as cold, infection, dehydration, exercise and stress. Since she may have gastroenteritis and is probably dehydrated due to her vomiting, it is likely that this may have precipitated a sickle cell crisis.

Check point

Every effort should be made for pregnant (and non-pregnant) women to avoid where possible any of the 'triggers' that may induce a sickle cell crisis.

5 **What initial actions should the midwife take?**

A The midwife should make an immediate referral and ask for Julia to be reviewed by an experienced senior obstetrician.

6 **Why does Julia have pain in her legs?**

A A sickle cell crisis is an acutely painful vaso-occlusive event which has an increased incidence in pregnancy. People with sickle cell disease have red blood cells that contain mostly haemoglobin S, an abnormal type of haemoglobin. Because the red blood cells contain abnormal haemoglobin, they are prone to alter their shape and become sickle, or crescent, shaped (Figure 7.1). These cells cannot pass smoothly through blood vessels and therefore can cause the vessel to become obstructed. This blockage causes tissue ischaemia and results in pain (Johnston 2005; Roberts 2008; Strong and Rutherford 2011).

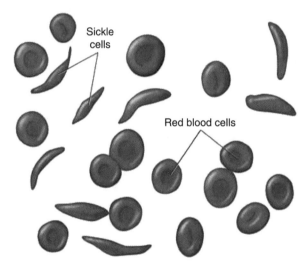

Figure 7.1 Sickle cells and normal red blood cells

7 **Why has Julia developed the pain in her legs?**

A When the oxygen tension within the bloodstream is low, which may occur when there is underlying infection, this promotes more aggregation of the abnormal haemoglobin within the red blood cells and this results in decreased flexibility of the cells and their characteristic change in shape. As Julia appears to have an underlying infection resulting in vomiting, this is likely to have promoted increased sickling of the red blood cells and thus has led to a vaso-occlusive crisis with pain in her legs.

8 **What is the appropriate management of Julia's condition at this time?**

A The mainstay of management of acute vaso-occlusive crisis is analgesia and hydration. Outside pregnancy, non-steroidal anti-inflammatory drugs (NSAIDS) are widely used; however, these should be avoided in the second half of pregnancy because of the risk of premature closure of the ductus arteriosus. In the second half of pregnancy, opiate analgesia should be used together with regular paracetamol. Box 7.2 summarizes the initial management of sickle cell crisis.

Box 7.2 Initial management of sickle cell crisis

- Give opiate analgesia.
- Ensure that Julia is kept warm.
- Monitor oxygen saturation. If < 96 per cent on air, then give inhaled oxygen.
- Ensure adequate hydration. In Julia's case, this will require intravenous fluids in view of her vomiting.
- Monitor fluid balance carefully.
- If Julia is immobile for more than 24 hours, thromboprophylaxis is required with LMWH.
- If the vaso-occlusive crisis does not respond to conservative treatment, then an exchange transfusion may be required.

(Johnston 2005; Roberts 2008; Strong and Rutherford 2011)

---

9 **How might sickle cell disease affect Julia and the fetus/neonate?**

A There are some common maternal and fetal/neonatal complications associated with sickle cell disease as outlined in Table 7.1.

Table 7.1 Sickle cell disease complications

Maternal complications	Fetal/neonatal complications
Anaemia	Increased risk of miscarriage
Increased risk of thromboembolism	Increased risk of pre-term labour
Ischaemic injury	Increased risk of intrauterine growth restriction
Vaso-occlusion (painful crisis)	Increased risk of stillbirth
Organ damage (due to stress of pregnancy)	Increased morbidity and mortality
Infection – chest and urinary tract	Haemolytic disease of the newborn
Hypertensive disorders of pregnancy	

Source: Johnston 2005; Roberts 2008; Strong and Rutherford 2011.

10 **What tests should be offered in pregnancy with regard to sickle cell disease?**

A Table 7.2 outlines the tests and purpose of tests that may be performed in pregnant women with sickle cell disease.

11 **What other antenatal management would Julia receive?**

A • *Early multiprofessional team involvement*: In addition to the tests highlighted in question 10, Julia should have early referral to a multiprofessional team: obstetrician, haematologist, midwife or nurse with expertise in the management of women with haemoglobinopathies.
- *Initial visit in early pregnancy*: A detailed history would be taken from Julia, including obstetric/gynaecological history. The pattern of any previous crises is particularly relevant. The members of the multiprofessional team should have a detailed discussion with Julia regarding the possible complications of sickle cell disease in pregnancy.

Table 7.2 Tests carried out in pregnancy for women with sickle cell disease

Test	Purpose
Full blood count	To assess anaemia
Serum ferritin concentration	To determine whether there is iron deficiency
Serum folate	Because of the rapid turnover of red cells, there is increased utilization of folate
Reticulocyte count	Reticulocytes are immature red blood cells. When there is increased turnover of red cells, the reticulocyte count will be high
Urea and electrolytes	To assess renal function
Lactate dehydrogenase (LDH)	LDH is released when red cells are destroyed, and is an index of haemolysis
Liver function	Raised bilirubin is indicative of haemolysis. Abnormalities of other liver function tests may suggest the presence of gall stones which may occur in sickle cell disease
Blood typing and red cell antibody screen	If transfusion is necessary, it is important to have accurately assessed blood group and the presence of any antibodies which would affect cross-matching
HIV and hepatitis screening	To treat any underlying infection

Source: Johnston 2005; Roberts 2008; Strong and Rutherford 2011.

Julia's partner should be screened for haemoglobinopathies if his sickle cell status is not already known. If the result is positive, Julia and her partner should have counselling and be offered prenatal diagnosis.

Julia should be advised to avoid precipitating factors of crises, e.g. dehydration, infection and cold, and should receive information regarding the signs and symptoms of infection.

- *Management during pregnancy*: The following may be prescribed for Julia:
  - *Analgesia*: Analgesia will be required for pain associated with painful occlusive sickle episodes. Opiate analgesia is the mainstay of therapy. In the first half of pregnancy non-steroidal anti-inflammatory drugs may be used, but these are contra-indicated in the second half of pregnancy because of the risks of premature closure of the ductus arteriosus.
  - *Top–up or exchange transfusion*: Women with sickle cell disease will often have a low haemoglobin level. Typically, the haemoglobin level outside pregnancy will be 6–10 g/dL. However, symptoms of anaemia tend to be less since haemoglobin S has a lower affinity for oxygen and therefore gives up oxygen to the tissues more readily than haemoglobin A. Top-up transfusions may be given if there is symptomatic anaemia, or prior to the birth. There is insufficient evidence to recommend prophylactic transfusions during pregnancy (Mahomed 2000). There is also an increased likelihood of developing red cell antibodies with increased numbers of transfusions (Rosse and Gallagher 1990). Exchange transfusions may be indicated in the event of sickle cell crises.
  - *Folic acid supplementation (5 mg daily)*: Because of the increased red cell turnover, and the requirements of the fetus, folate supplementation is recommended.

- *Iron supplements only if required*: The need for iron supplementation can be assessed based on serum ferritin levels.
- *Penicillin V (250 mg twice a day)*: This is recommended since hyposplenism is common and women are therefore prone to infection with organisms such as *Haemophilus influenzae* and pneumococcus.
- *Maternal and fetal surveillance*: During pregnancy, women should be offered regular antenatal appointments every 2–4 weeks. The majority of these should, where possible, be done in the context of a multidisciplinary clinic. Regular BP monitoring and urinalysis should be performed to screen for hypertensive disorders of pregnancy.

In addition to routine dating and fetal anomaly scans, regular ultrasound scanning should be performed in the third trimester to assess fetal growth, liquor volume and umbilical artery Doppler velocimetry. The ideal is spontaneous labour at term. Induction should be offered for medical or obstetric indications (Johnston 2005; Roberts 2008; Strong and Rutherford 2011).

Julia recovers from the acute vaso-occlusive crisis, following conservative management and is discharged from hospital after two days. The rest of the pregnancy is uneventful until Julia goes into spontaneous labour at 39 + 2 weeks gestation. The routine observations are: P 92 bpm, BP 110/74 mm/Hg, RR 16 breaths per min., T 36.9°C, urinalysis NAD. On abdominal examination the SPFH measures 39 cm, longitudinal lie, cephalic presentation, LOA position with the fetal head 3/5th palpable. Auscultation of the fetal heart rate (FHR) is performed by the midwife using a Pinard stethoscope for 1 minute in accordance with NICE (2007) intrapartum care guidelines. Findings following auscultation are recorded as: FHR 145 bpm and regular, baseline variability > 5 bpm; no accelerations or decelerations are noted during the auscultation. Julia does not wish to have a vaginal examination and requests to stay mobile during the labour, and use Entonox if required for pain relief. All these findings are recorded in Julia's intrapartum notes.

12 **What are the main principles of care/management for Julia's labour?**

A Close monitoring is required during labour. The risk of sickle cell crisis in labour will be higher if Julia becomes dehydrated or has hypoxia, acidosis, or infection. Care should be taken to prevent these complications.

Labour is also a time of increased cardiac output, exacerbated by the pain of uterine contractions. Cardiac function may be reduced by chronic hypoxaemia and anaemia. Pain relief is important in reducing cardiac work, and epidural analgesia is particularly effective (Winder et al. 2011). Prolonged labour should be avoided. The key principles of care/management during labour are identified in Box 7.3.

Box 7.3 The main principles of care/management during Julia's labour

- Keep warm.
- Avoid dehydration (commonly by intravenous fluids).
- Avoid hypoxia (oxygen therapy if required), sepsis and acidosis.
- Continuous fetal monitoring with a cardiotocograph (CTG).
- Take blood for FBC, group and save (G_p & S).

(Continued overleaf)

- Keep mobile for as long as possible.
- Pain relief if required; low threshold for epidural to reduce cardiac demand.
- Thromboprophylaxis is not given routinely but Julia should be assessed for the need for thromboprophylaxis using a standard risk scoring process (RCOG 2009).
- Active management of third stage of labour.
- Cord blood may be sent for haemoglobinopathy screening of the newborn; however, there is a risk of maternal contamination. Since universal neonatal screening for sickle cell disorders has been introduced in England as part of the newborn blood spot test, cord blood screening is no longer advised.

(Strong and Rutherford 2011)

13 **What are the key principles of postnatal care for Julia and her baby?**

- Vigilance is maintained as the risk of vaso-occlusive crisis remains following the birth.
- Maintain oxygenation.
- Maintain hydration.
- Monitor for infection.
- Thromboprophylaxis is considered if risk factors are present, e.g. impaired mobility.
- Consider prophylactic antibiotics if surgical intervention has been required.
- Discussion regarding contraception.

Although there are no absolute contraindications to the type of contraception used, if oral hormonal methods are preferred by Julia, progesterone-only methods are often advised as they are safe, effective and may reduce the risk of sickling. Low-dose combined pills may also be used. The risks of infection with intrauterine contraceptive devices (IUCD/coil) and intra-uterine systems (IUS/Mirena) should be considered, but do not preclude their use (Johnston 2005). There are no contraindications to barrier methods and natural family planning methods.

The newborn baby should have screening for haemoglobinopathies. In England this is done using the blood spot testing (UK National Screening Committee Regional Teams 2011).

Psychosocial aspects of care are an important part of the midwives' role, including cultural and spiritual needs. Julia, her partner or other family member may appreciate discussing the events of her birth with an appropriate member of the interprofessional team.

In terms of pre-conception care for any subsequent pregnancy, it is advisable for Julia to be given the following information:

- the role of dehydration, cold, hypoxia, overexertion and stress in the frequency of sickle cell crises;
- how nausea and vomiting in pregnancy can result in dehydration and the precipitation of crises;
- the risk of worsening anaemia, the increased risk of crises and acute chest syndrome (ACS) and the risk of increased infection (especially urinary tract infection) during pregnancy;
- the increased risk of having a growth-restricted baby, which increases the likelihood of fetal distress, induction of labour and caesarean section;

- the chance of the baby being affected by sickle cell disease;
- an up-to-date assessment for chronic disease complications;
- genetic screening of father, if not already conducted.

(RCOG 2011)

CASE OUTCOME

Julia had a normal vaginal birth after a 9-hour labour. Her baby boy, Alex, was born in good condition. They were transferred to the postnatal ward. She was provided with the postnatal care as outlined previously. Mother and baby were discharged home on day 3.

CASE STUDY 7.2: β-THALASSAEMIA MAJOR

Anna and her husband Tomas would like a baby. Anna is 28 years of age and has β-thalassaemia major. They would like to know what their options are regarding conception.

1 **What is β-thalassaemia major?**

A β-thalassaemia major is an autosomal recessive inherited disorder affecting haemoglobin synthesis. It is caused by a quantitative defect affecting the globin chain production. This leads to haemoglobin being unstable and thus to ineffective blood cell production. Most individuals with β-thalassaemia major are dependent on regular blood transfusions to maintain their haemoglobin levels. The incidence is approximately 1 in 10,000 in the UK (Strong and Rutherford 2011). Similar to sickle cell disease, populations in which β-thalassaemia major is prevalent are those with origins from Africa, the Caribbean, the Mediterranean, South-East Asia and the Middle East (Addo et al. 2008).

2 **What advice would Anna and Tomas be given preconceptionally?**

A Tomas should be offered haemoglobin electrophoresis to determine the risk of major haemoglobinopathy in their children. If he is found to have a haemoglobinopathy, then Tomas and Anna should be offered counselling by a professional with expertise in haemoglobinopathies.

One of the effects of thalassaemia is iron overload which may result in organ damage, particularly hepatic, endocrine and cardiac. Any pre-existing organ damage should be assessed using thyroid function tests, tests of parathyroid function and blood glucose. Anna should be reviewed by a cardiologist. Significant cardiomyopathy secondary to iron deposition in the myocardium would be associated with a high risk of maternal mortality, and Anna should be informed of this (Johnston 2005).

Because of the risks of iron overload, Anna is likely to be on iron chelation therapy. This treatment needs to be reviewed. Outside pregnancy, iron chelation is usually carried out using desferrioxamine mesylate which is given as a subcutaneous infusion over 12 hours, 5–7 days per week. The safety of this drug in pregnancy has not been established, and therefore, ideally, iron status should be optimized pre-pregnancy and chelation discontinued periconceptually, at least for the first trimester, and if possible, throughout pregnancy. A risk–benefit assessment of continuing iron chelation in pregnancy is required, and the results will depend on the degree of iron overload at the start of pregnancy (Strong and Rutherford 2011).

Bone problems with osteopenia and osteoporosis often occur in transfusion-dependent thalassemics, and these can worsen during pregnancy. Anna's bone density should be assessed and vitamin D and calcium supplements are advisable if bone density is reduced.

Anna should be informed that fertility is reduced in women with transfusion-dependent thalassaemia and she is likely to require assisted conception to become pregnant. Fertility treatment will not be considered until her iron levels are as low as possible. If there is a risk of an affected child, then it may be possible to perform pre-implantation diagnosis. Otherwise, Anna and Tomas could opt for prenatal diagnosis with chorionic villus sampling (CVS) or amniocentesis (Addo et al. 2008; Strong and Rutherford 2011).

Anna subsequently becomes pregnant through IVF, the embryo was screened prior to implantation and is unaffected. Anna is now 8 weeks pregnant.

3   **What would Anna's antenatal management consist of?**

A   Anna should have early referral to a multiprofessional team including an obstetrician with expertise in the management of haemoglobinopathies, a haematologist and a midwife or nurse with experience of haemoglobinopathies. A detailed history would be taken from Anna, including obstetric/gynaecological history.

Folate supplementation 5 mg daily is recommended throughout pregnancy. Her iron status should be assessed and iron chelation treatment stopped if she is still taking it. Iron supplementation should be avoided as this will not improve anaemia and will exacerbate iron overload. If Anna becomes anaemic, then this should be treated with blood transfusions. Because of multiple transfusions, it is common for women with thalassaemia major to have multiple red cell alloantibodies and cross-matching may be challenging. It may also increase the risk of haemolytic disease in the fetus and neonate.

Maternal blood should be tested for red cell antibodies and, if present, the fetus should be carefully monitored for signs of anaemia if indicated, using middle cerebral artery peak systolic velocities.

There should be ongoing assessment of the degree of organ damage.

As there is a high incidence of gestational diabetes, glucose tolerance testing should be carried out.

There should be regular assessment of the fetal growth by ultrasound scanning.

There is limited data regarding pregnancy outcome in women with β-thalassaemia major since pregnancy itself is rare in these women (Johnston 2005; Strong and Rutherford 2011).

4   **How might β-thalassaemia major affect Anna and the fetus/neonate?**

A   There are a number of common maternal and fetal/neonatal complications of β-thalassaemia major as summarized in Table 7.3.

At 38 + 5 weeks pregnant, Anna goes into spontaneous labour. She has been having regular, painful uterine contractions for 6 hours. She has a history of spontaneous rupture of membranes (SROM) an hour ago. The baby is moving well.

The routine observations are as follows: P 76 bpm, BP 125/70 mmHg, RR 15 breaths per min., T 37.3°C, urinalysis NAD. On abdominal examination SPFH measures 37 cm, longitudinal lie, cephalic presentation, LOA position with the fetal head 4/5th palpable. Auscultation of the FHR is performed by the midwife using a Pinard stethoscope for 1 minute in accordance with NICE (2007) intrapartum care guidelines. Findings following auscultation are recorded as:

Table 7.3 Complications with β-thalassaemia major

Maternal complications	*Fetus/neonate*
Anaemia	Haemolytic disease of the newborn
Increased transfusion needs	
Increased iron accumulation	
Infection	
Increased risk of gestational diabetes	
Thromboembolic disorders	
Possible cephalopelvic disproportion	

Source: Johnston 2005; Addo et al. 2008; Strong and Rutherford 2011.

FHR 145 bpm and regular, baseline variability > 5 bpm; two accelerations and no decelerations are noted during the auscultation.

Following discussion with the couple, Anna decides that she would like to have a vaginal examination to assess if her labour is established. This is conducted and Anna's cervix is assessed as being 5 cm dilated.

All these findings are recorded in Anna's notes and hand-held records.

5 **What would be Anna's care during labour?**

A Anna would already have a provisional plan for labour made in conjunction with the team caring for her during pregnancy. An individualized plan would be made dependent on her cardiac condition and taking into account her stature. Women with β-thalassaemia major are often of small stature and may therefore be more likely to have cephalopelvic disproportion.

- Her vital signs should be monitored regularly, including BP, TPR and oxygen saturation.
- There should be continuous monitoring of FHR via cardiotocograph.
- Maintain her mobility as long as possible.
- As with all women Anna should have one-to-one support in labour and be offered analgesia as required.
- Active management of the third stage.
- Cord blood should be sent for determination of the haemoglobinopathy status of the fetus.

Check point

With the development of reproductive technologies, more women with β-thalassaemia major are having the opportunity to become mothers. The maternity interprofessional team should be knowledgeable in the care and management of women with this condition.

---

6 **What are the key principles of Anna's care postnatally?**

A Postnatally Anna would have an individualized plan of care involving the obstetricians, haematologists, midwives and neonatal paediatricians. She should be observed in hospital for

24–48 hours and a plan should be made to recommence iron chelation as necessary. Desferrioxamine is safe in breast feeding (Strong and Rutherford 2011). The baby should be observed.

Psychosocial aspects of care are an important part of the midwives' role, including cultural and spiritual needs. Anna, her partner or other family member may appreciate discussing the events of her pregnancy and birth with an appropriate member of the interprofessional team.

CASE OUTCOME

Anna had a Neville-Barnes forceps delivery, following a long labour. A baby girl, Catrina, was born in good condition. They were transferred to the postnatal ward where they received postnatal care as previously described. Mother and baby were discharged home on day 3.

Summary of key points

Sickle cell disease

- Joint care with consultant obstetrician and haematologist.
- All immunizations should be up to date.
- Prompt treatment of any infection.
- Prophylactic antibiotics with penicillin is recommended.
- A clear plan of care should be documented in women's notes in early pregnancy (Harper 2011).

Thalassaemia

- Multiprofessional team involvement.
- Folate supplementation.
- Individualized plan of care for labour and birth (Strong and Rutherford 2011).

The future

Sickle cell disease in pregnancy is being researched by the UK Obstetric Surveillance System (UKOSS) which was due for completion in February 2011 (Harper 2011). The results of this study are due to be published late in 2011.

REFERENCES

Addo, A., Robson, E. and Oppenheimer, C. (2008) Haematological disorders, in E. Robson and J. Waugh (eds) *Medical Disorders in Pregnancy*. Oxford: Blackwell.

Harper, A. (2011) Sepsis, in G. Lewis (ed.) for the Centre for Maternal and Child Enquiries (CMACE) *Saving Mothers' Lives: Reviewing Maternal Deaths to Make Motherhood Safer: 2006–2008. The Eighth Report on Confidential Enquiries into Maternal Deaths in the United Kingdom*. Available at: http://www.cmace.org.uk (accessed 29 March 2011).

Johnston, T. (2005) Haemoglobinopathies in pregnancy, *The Obstetrician and Gynaecologist*, 7(3): 149–57. Available at: http://www.rcog.org.uk/togonline (accessed 15 February 2011).

Mahomed, K. (2000) *Prophylactic Versus Selective Blood Transfusion for Sickle Cell Anaemia During Pregnancy*. Cochrane Database Syst. Rev. 2:CD000040.

National Institute for Health and Clinical Excellence (NICE) (2007) *Intrapartum Care: Care of Healthy Women and Their Babies during Labour*. Clinical Guidance No. 55. London: NICE.

National Institute for Health and Clinical Excellence (NICE) (2008) *Antenatal Care: Routine Care for the Healthy Pregnant Women*. Clinical Guidance No. 62. London: NICE.

National Institutes of Health (NIH) (2002) *The Management of Sickle Cell Disease*. NIH. National Heart, Lung and Blood Institute, Division of Blood Diseases and Resources, 4th edn. NIH publication number 02-2117. London: NIH.

Nelson-Piercy, C. (2011) Cardiac disease, in Centre for Maternal and Child Enquiries (CMACE) *Saving Mothers' Lives: Reviewing Maternal Deaths to Make Motherhood Safer: 2006–2008. The Eighth Report on Confidential Enquiries into Maternal Deaths in the United Kingdom*. Ed. G. Lewis. Available at: http://www.cmace.org.uk (accessed 4 March 2011).

Roberts, S. (2008) Sickle cell disease, in J. Queenann (ed.) *Management of High Risk Pregnancy: An Evidence Based Approach*. Chichester: John Wiley & Sons Ltd.

Rosse, W. and Gallagher, D. (1990) Transfusion and alloimmunisation in sickle cell disease: the Co-operative Study of Sickle Cell Disease, *Blood*, 76: 1431–7.

Royal College of Obstetricians and Gynaecologists (RCOG) (2009) *Reducing the Risk of Thrombosis and Embolism During Pregnancy and the Puerperium*. RCOG Green Top Guideline No. 37a. London: RCOG.

Royal College of Obstetricians and Gynaecologists (RCOG) (2011) *Management of Sickle Cell Disease in Pregnancy*. RCOG Green Top Guideline No. 61. London: RCOG.

Strong, J. and Rutherford, J. (2011) Anaemia and white blood cell disorders, in D. James, P. Steer, C. Weiner, and B. Gonik (eds) *High Risk Pregnancy: Management Options*, 4th edn. Philadelphia, PA: Elsevier Saunders.

UK National Screening Committee Regional Teams (2011) *NHS Antenatal and Newborn Screening Programmes: Key Messages*. Available at: http://www.screening.nhs.uk (accessed 9 May 2011).

Winder, A., Johnson, S., Murphy, J. and Ehsanipoor, R. (2011) Epidural analgesia for treatment of a sickle cell crisis during pregnancy, *Obstetrics & Gynecology*, 118(2): 495–7.

ANNOTATED FURTHER READING

Pavord, S. and Hunt, B. (2010) *The Obstetric Haematology Manual*. Cambridge: Cambridge University Press.

A useful chapter on the management of haemoglobinopathies in pregnancy.

Powrie, R.O., Greene, M.F. and Camann, W. (2010) *De Swiet's Medical Disorders in Obstetric Practice*, 5th edn. Chichester: Wiley-Blackwell.

A comprehensive and up-to-date text on medical conditions that may affect pregnancy, including a chapter on haematologic disease in pregnancy.

USEFUL ORGANIZATIONS

Centers for Disease Control and Prevention: Hemoglobin S Allele and Sickle Cell Disease
http://www.cdc.gov/genomics/hugenet/reviews/sickle.htm

An informative website about a range of disorders and diseases including sickle cell genetics and epidemiology.

Genetic Alliance

http://www.geneticalliance.org

A support organization for different genetic problems. The site is American but has some resources that would be useful to health professionals working in the UK.

Harvard Sickle Cell Program

http://sickle.bwh.harvard.edu

A comprehensive source of information for patients and health care providers concerning both sickle cell disease and thalassaemia.

National Newborn Screening and Genetics Resource Center (NNSGRC)

http://genes-r-us.uthscsa.edu

Information and resources for health professionals, the public health community, consumers and government officials. The site is American but has some resources that would be useful to health professionals working in the UK.

National Sickle Cell/Thalassaemia Centres

http://www.sickle-thal.nwlh.nhs.uk/Information/NationalSickleCellThalassaemiaCentres.aspx

A website including regional contacts for sickle cell and thalassaemia specialists.

Sickle Cell Disease Association of America (SCDAA)

http://www.sicklecelldisease.org

A US patient advocacy site with information for the public.

Sickle Cell Society

http://www.sicklecellsociety.org/

A UK-based support website for sickle cell disease.

UK National Screening Committee

http://www.screening.nhs.uk/index.php

Information about screening programmes in the United Kingdom including haemoglobinopathy screening.

CASE STUDY 8
Antepartum and postpartum haemorrhage
Karen Jackson

Pre-requisites for the chapter: the reader should have an understanding of:

- The anatomy and physiology of the pregnant uterus.
- Placental implantation during pregnancy.
- The predisposing factors for antepartum and postpartum haemorrhage.
- The MEOWs assessment chart.
- The signs and symptoms of placental abruption.
- The signs and symptoms of placenta praevia.
- The midwife's role and responsibilities within the interprofessional team.
- The value of SBAR as a communication tool in the interprofessional team.
- Drugs/medicines used in the management of antepartum and postpartum haemorrhage.

Pre-reading self-assessment

1 What are the possible causes of antepartum haemorrhage (APH)?
2 Discuss four main differences between the presentation of placental abruption and placenta praevia.
3 Describe the classifications of placenta praevia.
4 Define placental abruption.
5 List six predisposing factors for postpartum haemorrhage (PPH).

Recommended prior reading

Norman, J. (2011) Haemorrhage, in Centre for Maternal and Child Enquiries (CMACE) *Saving Mothers' Lives: Reviewing Maternal Deaths to Make Motherhood Safer: 2006–2008. The Eighth Report on Confidential Enquiries into Maternal Deaths in the United Kingdom*. Ed. G. Lewis. *BJOG*. 118 (Suppl. 1): 1–203.

Royal College of Obstetricians and Gynaecologists (RCOG) (2009) *Prevention and Management of Postpartum Haemorrhage*. Green Top Guidelines, No. 52. London: RCOG.

Royal College of Obstetricians and Gynaecologists (RCOG) (2011) *Placenta Praevia, Placenta Praevia Accreta and Vasa Praevia: Diagnosis and Management*. Green Top Guideline, No. 27. London: RCOG.

This case is split into two parts to examine the care of two women, one with an APH caused by placental abruption, followed by a PPH (Case study 8.1: Cathy) and one with an APH caused by placenta praevia (Case study 8.2: Andrea).

CASE STUDY 8.1: APH AND PPH

Cathy, a 26-year-old gravida 2, para 1, is 36 weeks pregnant. She is admitted to labour suite via an emergency ambulance, with a history of abdominal pain which is constant and has become increasingly worse over the past 4 hours. She reported a small amount of blood loss per vaginum (PV). Her history revealed a normal pregnancy until 34 weeks when she was admitted to the labour suite after experiencing a small blood loss per vaginum with no other signs or symptoms reported. All observations and investigations during this previous admission were normal and Cathy was discharged home on this occasion. The routine observations were: P 125 bpm, BP 110/60 mmHg, RR 16 breaths per min., T 37°C, urinalysis NAD. On abdominal examination the uterus felt rigid and tender, a lie and presentation were therefore not ascertained but the fetus felt large for gestation, SPFH measured 38 cm. Attempts at auscultating the fetal heart with a Pinard stethoscope were unsuccessful and monitoring the fetal heart electronically was also difficult. An ultrasound scan revealed a live fetus with a heart rate of 160 bpm. The 20-week scan and current scan showed the placenta to be normally situated, not low lying.

1   **What are your initial thoughts concerning a diagnosis for Cathy's condition?**

A   Cathy presents with constant abdominal pain, rigid and tender uterus, PV blood loss, difficulty with auscultating fetal heart, uterus palpated as large for dates, and normally-sited placenta. The signs and symptoms present in this scenario are consistent with a placental abruption.

2   **What other conditions could be causing Cathy's signs and symptoms?**

A   It is important to consider differential diagnosis to ensure other underlying conditions are not missed. To aid diagnosis and early recognition, Table 8.1 accounts for differences between the presentations of placenta praevia and placental abruption. Box 8.1 lists other conditions as a differential diagnosis for placental abruption.

Box 8.1 Differential diagnosis for placental abruption

In addition to placenta praevia, differential diagnosis for placental abruption may also include:

Acute polyhydramnios
Chorioamnionitis
Peritonitis
Vasa praevia
Incidental causes of bleeding from the genital tract.

(Beckman et al. 2009; Cunningham et al. 2010)

Table 8.1 Differential diagnosis that compares the differences between placenta praevia and placental abruption

Clinical sign	Placenta praevia	Placental abruption
Warning haemorrhages	Yes	No
Abdominal pain	Usually none	Can be severe
Colour of blood loss	Bright red, fresh	May be dark red
Onset of bleeding	At rest, sometimes post-coital	Following exertion or trauma
Degree of shock	In proportion to the visible vaginal blood loss	May be more severe than visible vaginal blood loss
Consistency of uterus	Soft, not tender	Hard, tense, painful, 'woody'
Palpation	Fetus usually easy to palpate	Fetus difficult to palpate
Presentation	Malpresentation	Usually cephalic
Engagement	Not engaged	May be engaged
FHR pattern via CTG	Usually normal	May show fetal compromise, may be absent
Coagulation defects	Rare	Can be present but infrequent. DIC can develop
Abdominal girth	Equal to gestation	May be increased due to concealed haemorrhage

Source: Beckman et al. 2010; Hutcherson 2011.

3 **How is placental abruption defined?**

A A placental abruption is the premature separation of a normally-sited placenta (Lala and Rutherford 2002).

4 **What are the predisposing factors associated with placental abruption?**

A Predisposing factors include: advanced maternal age, previous abruption, smoking, cocaine use, multiple pregnancy, trauma, hypertension, pre-eclampsia, thrombophilias, pre-term pre-labour rupture of membranes, intrauterine infections and polyhydramnios (Oyelese and Ananth 2006).

5 **With reference to relevant pathophysiology, how would you account for the signs and symptoms associated with a placental abruption?**

A In most cases bleeding is slight with no obvious cause. Placental abruption may be mild, moderate or severe. It may also be referred to as: (a) concealed; (b) revealed; or (c) concealed and revealed.

Abruptio placentae arises due to haemorrhage into the decidua basalis of the placenta (Ngeh and Bhide 2006). In mild placental abruption, blood loss may be minimal; the woman will complain of mild abdominal pain, the uterus is not normally tender, the fetal heart is normally present and maternal observations are within normal limits.

In moderate placental abruption, blood loss is heavier, the woman may be hypotensive, tachycardic, and will complain of more severe abdominal pain. The uterus is more tender and firm, and there will usually be signs of fetal compromise.

In severe placental abruption, blood loss can be heavier but this is variable as blood can be concealed within the uterus. Visible assessment of blood loss is therefore unreliable. The woman complains of severe abdominal pain. The uterus is hard and painful on palpation, there are likely to be signs of hypovolaemic shock (despite apparent minimal vaginal blood loss). The fundus is often higher than gestation of pregnancy, fetal parts are difficult to palpate and the fetal heart may not be heard; fetal death is common in severe placental abruption. Severe placental abruption can lead to coagulation disorders, e.g. DIC (see Case 5). Intrauterine tension rises, blood infiltrates into the uterine muscle sometimes as far as the myometrium; this is known as a couvelaire uterus. The woman will suffer from pain and shock due to blood loss, causing gross distension of the uterus (Oyelese and Ananth 2006).

6   **How would the interprofessional team manage Cathy's case?**

A   It is important to call for help early. In cases where a potentially serious APH has occurred, the following interprofessional team would be required and must be alerted, using the SBAR tool (see Case 2) to maximize good communication (NHS Institute for Innovation and Improvement 2008): senior obstetrician, anaesthetist, midwives (to assist with running and to document actions), paediatrician, haematologist and blood bank, theatre team, hospital porters and ICU/HDU team to ensure high level of care. The subsequent management of a suspected placental abruption is summarized in Box 8.2.

Box 8.2 Key management principles of APH: suspected placental abruption

- Ensure good communication with woman, family members and all members of the multidisciplinary team are maintained throughout.
- It is recommended that with appropriate help, many of these procedures can be executed simultaneously.
- Documentation of events should take place as contemporaneously as possible.
- Cathy's condition is reasonably stable at present; however, she is tachycardic which is a sign of hypovolaemia. All other observations appear to be within normal limits but this could be due to effective compensatory mechanisms working well initially within young healthy women.
- Continue with ¼-hourly observations of BP, P, T and RR. Commence MEOWS chart.
- Gentle palpation of the uterus.
- Estimate blood loss.
- Assess likely cause of APH.
- Intravenous access must be gained, using two wide-bore (14G or 16G) cannulae.
- Send blood samples for full blood count, clotting screen, urea and electrolytes and cross-match for 4 units of blood.
- Resuscitation in the first instance is with crystalloids until cross-matched blood is available.
- Assess for ABC resuscitation (see Case 12).
- Monitor oxygen saturation.
- Oxygen therapy.
- Monitor level of consciousness using AVPU or Glasgow Coma Scale (see Case 10).

- Urinary catheterization will be performed and strict fluid balance should be observed.
- Cathy is likely to be in pain, therefore appropriate analgesia should be offered, such as an opiate in accordance with local guidelines.
- The fetus should be monitored continuously with a CTG if possible.

(Lala and Rutherford 2002; NMC 2004;
Beckman et al. 2009; Cunningham et al. 2010)

After the above measures have been taken, it is advisable that the obstetrician assesses the most appropriate mode of birth. Speculum examination may be performed. With the exclusion of a placenta praevia, a gentle vaginal examination can be conducted; in Cathy's case, the cervix was 9 cm dilated with the fetal head well descended in the pelvis. A careful assessment of the overall clinical picture by a senior obstetrician must be made. If birth is not likely to be imminent, it is probable that an urgent or emergency caesarean section will be conducted. However, in Cathy's case, she had given birth vaginally before and this labour was well advanced. Provided that both maternal and fetal conditions are stable, Cathy may be able to progress to a vaginal birth.

7 **What are the possible implications for a pregnancy complicated by placental abruption?**

A Haemorrhage is a complication affecting 3 per cent of pregnancies, one-third caused by placental abruption, one-third caused by placenta praevia and one-third by other causes (Harrington and Black 2005). In the 2003–2005 triennial report into maternal deaths, haemorrhage accounted for 17 maternal deaths (Liston 2007). Two deaths were due to placental abruption, three to placenta praevia, nine to postpartum haemorrhage and three to genital tract trauma. While there has been an impressive decline in haemorrhage during the past 50 years, suboptimal care has been highlighted in many of these maternal deaths (Liston 2007).

In the Confidential Enquiry into Maternal Deaths for the triennium 2006–2008, there were a total of nine deaths caused by haemorrhage: two from placental abruption, two from placenta praevia and five from postpartum haemorrhage (PPH) (Norman 2011). Complications such as PPH, DIC, acute renal failure, infection, anaemia, or psychological disorders can also occur following placental abruption.

Check point

All cases of APH of unknown origin should be treated as a placenta praevia until this has been excluded.

Cathy's labour progresses rapidly and she has a normal vaginal birth of a live male infant weighing 3.100 kg with apgars of 9/10 at 1 min. and 10/10 at 5 mins; the baby's condition was good. However, following the birth, there is a constant trickle of blood that appears to be coming from the uterus, blood loss to this point is estimated to be 650 mL. Cathy looks pale and sweaty.

8 **How is primary postpartum haemorrhage defined?**

A Primary PPH is defined as a blood loss of over 500 mL in a vaginal birth (sometimes defined as 1000 mL blood loss in a caesarean delivery) (Thami 2007). It is recognized that most women in the UK could cope well with a blood loss of 500 mL, therefore blood loss over 1000 mL would be referred to as a major PPH (RCOG 2009). Because of the arbitrary nature of the amounts of blood loss and the acknowledgement that blood loss is notoriously under-assessed, the definition often incorporates 'or any amount of blood loss that adversely affects the woman's condition'. PPH is categorized into two groups: (1) primary, occurring within the first 24 hours of birth; and (2) secondary, occurring after 24 hours and within 6–12 weeks following the birth (Mukherjee and Arulkumaran 2009).

9 **What are the predisposing factors for postpartum haemorrhage?**

A PPH is often due to one or a combination of what is commonly regarded as the 4Ts. These are:

1 *Tone* (poor uterine tone);
2 *Tissue* (blood clots, placental tissue or any retained products of conception);
3 *Trauma* (to the genital tract);
4 *Thrombin* (coagulopathies).

Predisposing factors for PPH are listed in Box 8.3.

Box 8.3 Predisposing factors for PPH

- Over-distended uterus, e.g. multiple pregnancy, polyhydramnios, macrosomic fetus.
- Antepartum haemorrhage.
- Previous PPH.
- Coagulation disorders.
- Chorioamnionitis.
- Uterine fibroid.
- Induction of labour.
- Instrumental delivery.
- Previous caesarean delivery (high risk associated with placenta accreta and percreta; site of placenta should be determined in current pregnancy).
- Prolonged labour.
- Obesity.
- Pre-eclampsia.
- It is important to note that in most cases of PPH, no risk factor is identified.

(Mousa and Alfirevic 2007; Mukherjee and Arulkumaran 2009;
RCOG 2009)

10 **How would a primary postpartum haemorrhage be managed?**

A The actions taken are dependent on the severity of the blood loss, the woman's clinical condition and whether the different stages of management have any effect. The following management is suggested but should not be considered as being a linear progression. Indeed, it is recommended that with appropriate help many of these procedures can be executed simultaneously.

Postpartum haemorrhage is an obstetric emergency, therefore the midwife should seek immediate help from appropriate members of the interprofessional team, using the SBAR tool to maximize good communication (NHS Institute of Innovation and Improvement 2008). In this case, most of the appropriate interprofessional team would already be in attendance or would have been alerted to Cathy's condition: senior obstetrician, anaesthetist, midwives (to assist with co-ordination of the team and documentation of actions), haematologist/ blood bank, theatre team, hospital porters and ICU/HDU nurses and physicians. Subsequent management of PPH is summarized in Box 8.4.

Box 8.4 Management of postpartum haemorrhage

- Ensure good communication with woman, family members and all members of the multidisciplinary team are maintained throughout.
- Documentation of events should take place as contemporaneously as possible and in a systematic way.
- If placenta is *in situ*, this needs to be removed to enable uterine contraction and haemostasis, by controlled cord traction (CCT) or by manual removal if necessary.
- Accurate assessment and estimation of blood loss.
- Establish aetiology (systematically reviewing the 4Ts). If the uterus is contracted, there may be genital tract trauma; if blood lost is not clotting, consider coagulopathy:
  - Are placenta and membranes complete (*Tissue*)?
  - Is uterus boggy (*Tone*)?
  - Is there trauma to the genital tract (*Trauma*)?
  - Clotting disorder (*Thrombin*)?
  - Could there be a combination of the above?
  - Find cause of bleeding promptly.
- Massage uterus to stimulate contractions.
- Assess for ABC resuscitation (see Case 12).
- Assess BP, P, T and RR and monitor at regular intervals e.g. ¼ hourly. Commence MEOWS chart.
- Monitor oxygen saturation.
- Oxygen therapy.
- Monitor level of consciousness using AVPU or Glasgow Coma Scale (see Case 10).
- Insert two wide-bore cannulae (14G or 16G) for resuscitation with crystalloids or colloids.
- Ongoing assessment of uterine tone is necessary because uterine atony is the most common cause of PPH; massage the uterus, repeat oxtocic injection, e.g. 10 units

(Continued overleaf)

Syntocinon IM, Syntometrine 1 ml IM (if not contraindicated) or therapeutic dose of 5 units of Syntocinon by slow intravenous injection or ergometrine 0.5 mg slow intravenous or IM injection, providing the woman is normotensive, then may proceed to administer Syntocinon IV (e.g. 40 units in 500 mL normal saline).
- Consider a CVP line.
- Strict fluid balance.
- Take blood for FBC, Gp & S, and cross-match 6 units, coagulation screen, and LFTs.
- Ensure bladder is empty, consider urinary catheterization.

In most cases the initial stages of management are all that is required to stem bleeding and achieve haemostasis. And, indeed, in Cathy's case, this is what happened; however, for some women, if bleeding persists further measures will be taken as follows:

- A prostaglandin such as carboprost may be administered intramuscularly or intramyometrically (0.25 mg every 15–20 minutes up to a maximum dose of 2 mg, contraindicated in women with asthma).
- Misoprostol 1000 micrograms rectally (some units may not use this drug due to the unwelcome and debilitating side effects of nausea and vomiting).
- Attempt bimanual compression of uterus (see Figure 8.1).

If these measures fail, then surgical procedures should be effected by the obstetrician sooner rather than later. These include:

- Ligation of vessels:
  - Bilateral uterine artery ligation
  - B-Lynch suture (see Figure 8.2)
  - Hypogastic artery ligation
- Interventional radiology:
  - Balloon tamponade
  - Selective arterial embolization
- Uterine packing
- Hysterectomy
- Consider transfer to ITU

(NMC 2004; Rogers and Chang 2005; Beckman et al. 2009; RCOG 2009; Cunningham et al. 2010)

---

11 **What are the implications of a primary PPH?**

A In the 2003–2005 Confidential Enquiry into Maternal Deaths, nine deaths were attributed to PPH. Many of these deaths were said to involve sub-standard care. There were also implications of severe morbidity such as hysterectomy (Liston 2007).

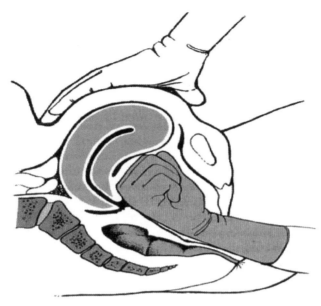

Figure 8.1 Internal bimanual compression

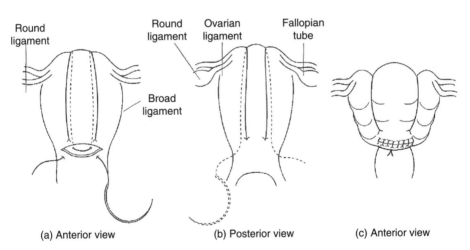

(a) Anterior view   (b) Posterior view   (c) Anterior view

Figure 8.2 The B-Lynch suture

In the confidential enquiry report for the triennium 2006–2008, there were five deaths related to PPH. Although this reduction in deaths is commendable, Norman (2011) reports that these deaths could be further reduced by improving the most elementary aspects of care. These include early referral to senior multidisciplinary team members, vigilant post-operative monitoring, and acting on signs and symptoms that women are seriously unwell, i.e. from recordings on the MEOWS chart (Norman 2011).

CASE OUTCOME

The P P H that Cathy experienced was brought under control by the interprofessional team using repeat doses of 10 units Syntocinon I M, followed by 40 units Syntocinon in 500 mL of normal saline IV and by massaging the uterus and emptying the bladder. Cathy's total blood loss was estimated to be 1,200 mL. Cathy had 2 units of cross-matched blood following the birth. She was kept in the high dependency unit on the labour suite for 24 hours. She was then transferred to the postnatal ward. Psychosocial aspects of care, including cultural and spiritual needs, are an important part of the midwives' role. Cathy, her partner, and/or other family members may appreciate discussing the events of her birth with an appropriate member of the interprofessional team. The consultant obstetrician discussed the possible risks for a subsequent pregnancy.

Cathy made a full recovery and mother and baby were discharged home on day 4. She was informed that it would be advisable to have consultant care for her next pregnancy and to have her baby in hospital.

CASE STUDY 8.2: APH

Andrea, a 32-year-old gravida 3, para 1 (1 miscarriage), is 20 weeks pregnant. Her last baby was born by LSCS for breech presentation. She attends for her routine ultrasound (US) scan that reveals a low-lying placenta.

1 | **What are your initial thoughts concerning a diagnosis for Andrea's condition?**

A | A low-lying placenta will be found in approximately 5 per cent of pregnancies. At term this will reduce to 0.5 per cent. This is because of the apparent migration of the placenta following the development of the upper and lower uterine segment. This is usually complete at around 34 weeks gestation (Lala and Rutherford 2002).

2 | **What would be the subsequent management for Andrea's pregnancy?**

A | The US scan would be repeated at around 32–34 weeks gestation, to assess if the placenta has remained low lying and Andrea would be informed of the importance of any bleeding during her pregnancy, and to contact the hospital immediately if this happens.

3 | **How is placenta praevia defined?**

A | Placenta praevia is when the placenta is situated partially or wholly in the lower uterine segment (RCOG 2011). It is caused by the blastocyst being implanted low in the uterine cavity (Ngeh and Bhide 2006).

4 | **What are the classifications of placenta praevia?**

A | In order to plan the management of a pregnancy complicated by placenta praevia, it is categorized into four types. See Table 8.2 for classifications. Figure 8.3 illustrates the differences in the classification of placenta praevia.

5 | **What are the predisposing factors for placenta praevia?**

A | A number of factors are associated with developing the complication of placenta praevia during pregnancy, as identified in Box 8.5.

Table 8.2 Types of placenta praevia

Type	Definition
Type 1	Placenta is lying in the lower uterine segment but the lower edge does not reach the internal cervical os. Sometimes called low lying or minor placenta praevia.
Type 2	The edge of the placenta reaches the internal cervical os but does not cover it. Sometimes called marginal or minor placenta praevia.
Type 3	The placenta covers the internal cervical os, but not when it is dilated. Sometimes called partial or major placenta praevia.
Type 4	The placenta covers the cervical os at full dilatation. Sometimes called complete or major placenta praevia.

Source: Lala and Rutherford 2002; Oyelese 2008.

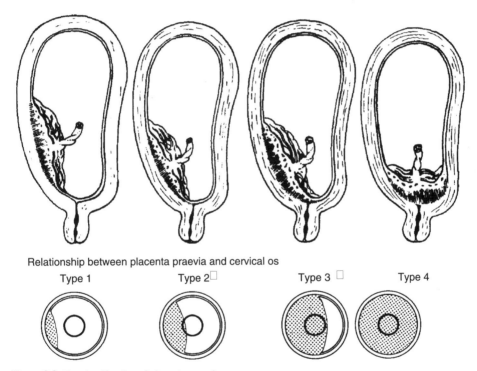

Figure 8.3 The classification of placenta praevia

Box 8.5 Predisposing factors for placenta praevia

- Prior caesarean section
- Smoking
- Multiple pregnancy
- Prior uterine surgery

(Continued overleaf)

- Endometrial damage
- Increasing parity
- Increasing maternal age
- Previous placenta praevia
- Cocaine use

(Ngeh and Bhide 2006; Oyelese 2008; Cunningham et al. 2010)

6 **How can placenta praevia be diagnosed?**

A This is usually achieved via careful history taking and ultrasonography for placental localization. The main features to consider are well documented (Ngeh and Bhide 2006; Oyelese 2008; Cunningham et al. 2010).

Think

Is there a presence of any of the following?

- Painless haemorrhage.
- Fresh bright red bleed.
- Haemorrhage at rest or following sexual intercourse.
- Bleeding more common from 28–30 weeks onwards with formation of lower uterine segment, and cervical effacement, causing detachment of inelastic placenta.
- Recurrent 'spotting'.
- On abdominal palpation fundus usually = dates.
- Fetal head not engaged.
- Fetal activity and F H R usually normal (unless bleeding is severe).
- Fetal malpresentation/unstable lie.

If there is anterior placenta praevia, then palpation of fetus may be difficult, loud maternal pulse may be found below the umbilicus, the fetal H R may be more difficult to auscultate and fetal movements may be felt by woman above the umbilicus. This is usually diagnosed via ultrasonography (preferably transvaginal). Use magnetic resonance imaging (M RI) in suspected cases of placenta accreta.

7 **What are the implications of Andrea possibly having a placenta praevia during pregnancy?**

A In the 2007 Confidential Enquiry into Maternal Deaths, three women died following a placenta praevia. In the most recent enquiry there were two deaths and one late death of women with placenta praevia. Two of these three women also had placenta accreta, one of whom also had a uterine rupture (Norman 2011). This indicates that placenta praevia is still a potentially serious complication of pregnancy. In addition to this, Andrea has had a previous caesarean section, and this is a risk factor for having an abnormally adherent placenta such as accreta, increta or percreta.

8 **What are the maternal and fetal complications associated with placenta praevia?**

A There are a number of maternal and fetal/neonatal morbidities that may arise as a consequence of placenta praevia, as identified in Table 8.3.

Table 8.3 Placenta praevia: maternal and fetal/neonatal complications

Maternal complications	Fetus/neonate
APH	Prematurity
Anaemia especially with repeated bleeds	Congenital malformations
Caesarean delivery	Fetal hypoxia/compromise
Thromboembolic disease	IUGR
Placenta accreta	Respiratory distrus syndrome
PPH	↑ Perinatal mortality
Hysterectomy	↑ Neonatal deaths
Psychological sequelae	
Maternal death	

Source: Beckman et al. 2009; Cunningham et al. 2010.

At 32 weeks gestation Andrea attends for a follow-up scan for placental localization. This shows that she has placenta praevia grade 3. Up until this point, her pregnancy has been uneventful. However, she reveals that she has experienced a small blood loss PV this morning. She is transferred to the labour suite. The routine observations were: P 92 bpm, BP 125/70 mmHg, RR 15 breaths per min., T 36.8°C, urinalysis NAD. She currently has spots of blood on her sanitary towel. As a scan had been conducted and confirmed a normally-grown live fetus equal to 34 weeks gestation, an abdominal palpation was not attempted.

9 **What would be the recommended management for the remainder of Andrea's pregnancy?**

A Management depends on the condition of mother and fetus, the amount of bleeding and the gestation of the pregnancy. It would be advisable for Andrea to stay in hospital for the remainder of her pregnancy, due to her having significant placenta praevia that is currently symptomatic (Norman 2011; RCOG 2011). Blood will be taken for cross-matching, at least 4–6 units of blood should be readily available, and full blood count; rhesus status will need to be established (Kleihauer test and anti-D if rhesus negative). Correction of anaemia if present. An USS, preferably transvaginal as this provides a more accurate assessment (Oyelese 2008), will be conducted at regular intervals. As Andrea has had a previous caesarean, she is at increased risk of an abnormally adherent placenta, therefore an MRI scan is recommended to diagnose this condition. If Andrea's pregnancy gestation was between 24–32 weeks, corticosteroids such as dexamethasone or betamethasone would be given to stimulate production of surfactant; however, at 34 weeks the benefits of steroid administration are unproven. Daily or twice daily cardiotocography (CTG). Serial USS for fetal growth. If bleeding subsides for at least 24–48 hours, Andrea may be managed as an outpatient. In well-informed, motivated women, who have a companion and transport readily available to them at all times, there appears to be no benefit in managing women with asymptomatic placenta praevia in hospital; indeed; there are no differences in maternal or fetal morbidity in inpatient or outpatient managed cases, according to Mouer (1994) and Wing et al. (1996). The RCOG (2011) suggest that more research is required in this area. The aim is to conservatively manage cases of placenta praevia, where appropriate, until the fetus is deemed to be mature. This decision has to be carefully balanced to avoid iatrogenic prematurity of the baby but also to ensure maternal condition is not compromised (Oyelese 2008; Beckman et al. 2009).

Andrea is hospitalized and assessed by twice daily observations of BP, P, T, RR, with close observation for vaginal blood loss; the fetus is monitored by CTG daily, weekly USS to assess fetal growth, weekly transvaginal scan (TVS) to assess degree of placenta praevia, and weekly bloods. An MRI scan was conducted at 34 weeks gestation and confirmed the presence of a grade 3 anterior placenta praevia and placenta accreta. Possible interventions and outcomes were explained to Andrea such as hysterectomy, the placenta being left *in situ*, and interventional radiology (cell salvage is not applicable in Andrea's case). A planned caesarean section was due at 38 weeks gestation, with consultant obstetrician and anaesthetist involvement. A level 2 critical bed (HDU bed) was available for Andrea following the caesarean section. However, on the morning that the operation is due, Andrea wakes to find her bed soaked with fresh red blood; she presses the buzzer for assistance and the midwife arrives to find Andrea pale and clammy.

10   **What would be the recommended management of a significant haemorrhage with known placenta praevia?**

A   Haemorrhage with a placenta praevia is a potentially serious obstetric emergency. The midwife would need to call for help from the appropriate members of the interprofessional team using the SBAR tool to maximize good communication (NHS Institute for Innovation and Improvement 2008). The multidisciplinary team would consist of a senior obstetrician, anaesthetist, midwives (to assist with running and to document actions), haematologist and blood bank, theatre team, hospital porters, and ICU/HDU team alerted. The subsequent management of haemorrhage from placenta praevia is summarized in Box 8.6.

Box 8.6 Management of haemorrhage with known placenta praevia

- Ensure good communication with woman, family members and all members of the multidisciplinary team is maintained throughout.
- It is recommended that with appropriate help many of these procedures can be executed simultaneously.
- Documentation of events should take place as contemporaneously as possible.
- Andrea's condition needs to be stabilized, prior to emergency caesarean section. In addition to the management below, Andrea will be prepared for theatre, using local guidelines/checklists for this purpose.
- Palpation of the uterus not necessary as the cause of APH is highly likely to be placenta praevia.
- Accurate assessment and estimation of blood loss.

- Assess for ABC resuscitation (see Case 12).
- Assess BP, T, P, RR and monitor at regular intervals e.g. ¼ hourly. Commence MEOWS chart.
- Monitor fetus with CTG.
- Monitor oxygen saturation.
- Oxygen therapy.
- Monitor level of consciousness using AVPU or Glasgow Coma Scale.
- Insert two wide-bore cannulae (14G or 16G) for resuscitation with crystalloids or colloids.
- Blood for FBC, Gp & S, cross-match, coagulation screen, and LFTs should already have been taken. At least 4–6 units of cross-matched blood should be ready for use.
- Consider a CVP line.
- Strict fluid balance.
- Ensure bladder is empty via urinary catheterization.
- Mode of birth – LSCS as grade 3 placenta praevia.
- A consultant obstetrician should perform or directly supervise the caesarean section.
- A consultant anaesthetist should administer or directly supervise the administration of the anaesthetic. In emergency situations, a general anaesthetic is usually administered.
- In Andrea's case, where the placenta is anterior, a vertical incision of the uterus is performed, preferably avoiding the placenta to reduce fetal bleeding. However, if the placenta is not anterior, a transverse incision of the uterus may be performed.
- In Andrea's case, placenta accreta has already been confirmed. The presence of placenta accreta should be borne in mind with all cases of placenta praevia.
- Early recourse to further experienced obstetric help if required.
- Anticipate PPH; if this occurs, management would be as described in Box 8.4 (following CS).

        (NMC 2004; Beckman et al. 2009; Cunningham et al. 2010; RCOG 2011)

11 **What are placenta accreta, placenta increta, and placenta percreta and what is the significance of these conditions?**

A Figure 8.4 illustrates types of placental implantation.

1 *Placenta accreta* is when the placental villi diffusely penetrate into the myometrium. This is the most common form of abnormally adherent placenta; the incidence is 78 per cent.
2 *Placenta increta* is when the placental villi invade the myometrium more deeply; the incidence is 17 per cent.
3 *Placenta percreta* is when the placental villi invade through the myometrium and into the peritoneum. This is the rarest form of abnormally adherent placenta; the incidence is 5 per cent.

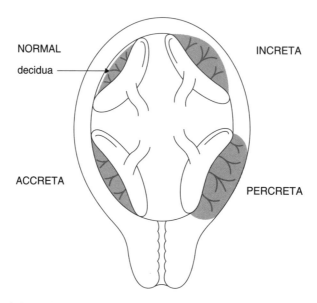

NORMAL

decidua

INCRETA

ACCRETA

PERCRETA

Figure 8.4 Types of placental implantation

Risk factors include previous caesarean sections, and risk increases with the number of c-sections (see Table 8.4), placenta praevia and increasing maternal age.

There is a considerable risk of maternal morbidity and mortality associated with an abnormally adherent placenta. There is a high risk of excessive haemorrhage; this can lead to hysterectomy, increased risk of blood transfusion, and maternal death. If the placenta is morbidly attached, it may be left *in situ* but this can lead to secondary PPH and/or infection. Then it may be left attached and a hysterectomy performed (RCOG 2011).

CASE OUTCOME

Andrea had an emergency caesarean section, and gave birth to a live healthy boy, Harry. The placenta, though difficult to deliver, did separate from the uterine wall, bleeding continued and a B-Lynch suture was applied, which arrested the bleeding. Total blood loss was estimated to be 2.5 L. Andrea was given 4 units of cross-matched blood and kept on the high dependency unit on the labour suite for 24 hours. She and the baby were transferred to the postnatal ward and Andrea recovered well from the surgery. Psychosocial aspects of care are an important part of the midwives' role, including cultural and spiritual needs. Andrea, her partner or other family member may appreciate discussing the events of her birth with an appropriate member of the interprofessional team. Andrea was informed of the risks of placenta praevia and accreta occurring in a subsequent pregnancy. Mother and baby were discharged home on day 5.

Table 8.4 Relationship between number of caesarean sections and incidence of placenta accreta if placenta praevia is present

Number of previous caesarean sections	Chances of placenta accreta if placenta praevia (%)
0	3
1	11
2	40
3	61
4	67
5	67

Source: Silver et al. 2006.

Check point

With the advent of an increased CS rate, and a trend in increasing maternal age, placenta praevia and abnormally adherent placenta will continue to present a challenge to maternity care and resources. The interprofessional team must be well prepared for the advent of these complications.

Following clinical incidents of obstetric haemorrhage, the management and treatment of each case should be audited to ensure that specific recommendations from CMACE have been followed.

Summary of key points
Specific recommendations

- Although there has been a decline in numbers in the triennium 2006–2008, obstetric haemorrhage remains an important cause of maternal death.
- All units should have evidence-based guidelines in place for the identification and management of obstetric haemorrhage, and all clinicians responsible for the care of pregnant women, antenatally, postnatally and intrapartum, including those practising in the community, should carry out regular skills /drills training for such scenarios.
- All clinicians should be aware of the guidelines for management of women who refuse blood transfusion.
- There was an absence of deaths in relation to elective caesarean section for placenta praevia in the most recent CMACE report. This supports the recommendations in earlier reports that senior staff should be involved when there are complications and emergencies.

(Continued overleaf)

- All women who have had a previous caesarean section must have their placental site determined. If there is any doubt, magnetic resonance imaging (MRI) can be used along with ultrasound scanning to determine if the placenta is accreta, increta or percreta. This must be re-emphasized, as scans for placental localization site in women with previous caesarean sections are sometimes still not being performed.
- Women who have delivered by caesarean section should have regular observations of pulse and blood pressure for the first 24 hours after delivery recorded on a Modified Early Obstetric Warning Score (MEOWS) chart. Abnormal scores on MEOWS should be investigated and acted upon immediately. The SBAR chart can help facilitate efficient and timely communication between members of the interprofessional team.
- The RCOG (2011) recommend that women with major placenta praevia who have previously bled should be admitted and managed as inpatients from 34 weeks of gestation. Those with major placenta praevia who remain asymptomatic, having never bled, require careful counselling before contemplating outpatient care. Women with major placenta praevia who elect to remain at home should have the risks explained to them and ideally require close proximity to the hospital.

REFERENCES

Beckman, C., Ling, F., Smith, R., Barzansky, B., Herbert, W. and Laube, D. (eds) (2009) *Obstetrics and Gynaecology*. Philadelphia, PA: Lippincott Williams and Wilkins.

Cunningham, F., Leveno, K., Bloom, S., Hauth, J., Rouse, D. and Spong, C. (2010) *Williams Obstetrics*, 23rd edn. New York: McGraw-Hill.

Harrington, D. and Black, R. (2005) Massive or recurrent ante-partum haemorrhage. *Current Obstetrics and Gynaecology*, 15(4): 267–71.

Hutcherson, A. (2011) Bleeding in pregnancy, in S. Macdonald and J. Magill-Cuerdon (eds) *Mayes Midwifery*. London: Ballière Tindall.

Lala, A. and Rutherford, J. (2002) Massive or recurrent ante-partum haemorrhage, *Current Obstetrics and Gynaecology*, 12(4): 226–30.

Lewis, G. (ed.) (2007) *The Confidential Enquiry into Maternal and Child Health (CEMACH). Saving Mothers' Lives: Reviewing Maternal Deaths to Make Motherhood safer, 2003–2005. The Seventh Report on Confidential Enquiries into Maternal Deaths in the United Kingdom*. Available at: http://cemach.interface-test.com/getattachment/927cf18a-735a-47a0-9200-cdea103781c7/ Saving-Mothers—Lives-2003-2005_full.aspx (accessed 30 August 2011).

Liston, W. (2007) Haemorrhage, in G. Lewis (ed.) *The Confidential Enquiry into Maternal and Child Health (CEMACH). Saving Mothers' Lives: Reviewing Maternal Deaths to Make Motherhood Safer, 2003–2005. The Seventh Report on Confidential Enquiries into Maternal Deaths in the United Kingdom*. Available at: http://cemach.interface-test.com/getattachment/927cf18a-735a-47a0-9200-cdea103781c7/Saving-Mothers—Lives-2003-2005_full.aspx (accessed 30 August 2011).

Mouer, J. (1994) Placenta praevia: ante-partum conservative management, inpatient versus outpatient, *American Journal of Obstetrics and Gynaecology*, 170(6): 1683–5.

Mousa, H. and Alfirevic, Z. (2007) Treatment for primary postpartum haemorrhage (Review), *The Cochrane Collaboration*. The Cochrane Library. Issue 4.

Mukherjee, S. and Arulkumaran, S. (2009) Post-partum haemorrhage, *Obstetrics, Gynaecology, and Reproductive Medicine*, 19(5): 121–6.

Ngeh, N. and Bhide, A. (2006) Ante-partum haemorrhage, *Current Obstetrics and Gynaecology*, 16(2): 79–83.

NHS Institute for Innovation and Improvement (2008) *SBAR: Situation, Background, Assessment, Recommendation*. Available at: http://www.institute.nhs.uk (accessed 8 August 2011).

Norman, J. (2011) Haemorrhage, in Centre for Maternal and Child Enquiries (CMACE) *Saving Mothers' Lives: Reviewing Maternal Deaths to Make Motherhood Safer: 2006–2008. The Eighth Report on Confidential Enquiries into Maternal Deaths in the United Kingdom*. Ed. G. Lewis. *BJOG*: 118 (Suppl. 1): 1–203.

Nursing and Midwifery Council (NMC) (2004) *Midwives Rules and Standards*. London: NMC.

Oyelese, Y. (2008) Placenta praevia and related placental disorders, in J. Queenan (ed.) *Management of High Risk Pregnancy: An Evidence Based Approach*. Chichester: John Wiley & Sons Ltd.

Oyelese, Y. and Ananth, C. (2006) Placental abruption, *Obstetrics and Gynaecology*, 108(4): 1005–16.

Rogers, M. and Chang, A. (2005) Postpartum haemorrhage and other problems of the third stage, in D. James, P. Steer, C. Weiner and B. Gonik (eds) *High Risk Pregnancy*. Philadelphia, PA: Elsevier Saunders.

Royal College of Obstetricians and Gynaecologists (RCOG) (2009) *Prevention and Management of Postpartum Haemorrhage*. Green Top Guideline No. 52. London: RCOG.

Royal College of Obstetricians and Gynaecologists (RCOG) (2011) *Placenta Praevia, Placenta Praevia Accreta and Vasa Praevia: Diagnosis and Management*. Green Top Guideline No. 27. London: RCOG.

Silver, R., Landon, M., Rouse, D., Leveno, K., Spong, C. and Thom, E. et al. (2006) National Institute of Child Health and Human Development Maternal-Fetal Medicine Units Network. Maternal morbidity associated with multiple repeat cesarean deliveries, *Obstetrics and Gynecology* 107: 1226–32.

Thami, M. (2007) Post-partum haemorrhage. *Journal of Postgraduate Medical Education, Training and Research*, 2(3): 34–9.

Wing, D., Paul, R. and Millar, L. (1996) Management of the symptomatic placenta praevia; a randomised controlled trial of inpatient versus outpatient expectant management, *American Journal of Obstetrics and Gynaecology*, 175(4): 806–11.

ANNOTATED FURTHER READING

Khan, K.S., Wojdyla, D., Say, L., Gulmezoglu, A.M. and Van Look, P.F. (2006) WHO analysis of causes of maternal death: a systematic review, *The Lancet*. 367:1066–74.

A useful review of major causes of maternal death including haemorrhage.

Knight, M., Callaghan, W., Berg, C., Alexander, S., Bouvier-Colle, M., Ford, J.B. et al. (2005) Trends in postpartum hemorrhage in high resource countries: a review and recommendations from the International Postpartum Hemorrhage Collaborative Group, *BMC Pregnancy Childbirth*, 9: 55.

An interesting review of PPH in developed countries including recommendations for management.

Neilson, J. (2010) Interventions for suspected placenta praevia. *The Cochrane Library*. Issue 4. John Wiley and Sons Ltd. Available at: http://onlinelibrary.wiley.com/doi/10.1002/14651858.CD001998/full (accessed 9 August 2011).

This is the most up-to-date review of trials that assesses interventions in cases of suspected placenta praevia, such as hospital versus home management, and cervical cerclage versus no cervical cerclage.

Sheiner, E. (ed.) (2011) *Bleeding during Pregnancy: A Comprehensive Guide.* New York: Springer Verlag.

This textbook takes a comprehensive view of all aspects of bleeding in pregnancy, including placental abruption, placenta praevia, placenta accreta and postpartum haemorrhage.

USEFUL WEBSITES

http://www.aagbi.org	The Association of Anaesthetists of Great Britain and Ireland
http://www.cemace.org.uk	Centre for Maternal and Child Enquiries
http://www.dh.gov.uk	UK Department of Health
http://www.institute.nhs.uk	National Health Service Institute for Innovation and Improvement
http://www.nice.org.uk	National Institute for Health and Clinical Excellence
http://www.npeu.ox.ac.uk	National Perinatal Epidemiology Unit
http://www.rcm.org.uk	Royal College of Midwives
http://www.rcoa.ac.uk	Royal College of Anaesthetists
http://www.rcog.org.uk	Royal College of Obstetricians and Gynaecologists (RCOG)

CASE STUDY 9
Uterine inversion and ruptured uterus
Karen Jackson

Pre-requisites for the chapter: the reader should have an understanding of:

- Anatomy and physiology of the uterus.
- The physiology of the third stage of labour.
- The MEOWS assessment chart.
- The value of SBAR as a communication tool in the interprofessional team.
- The midwife's role and responsibilities within the interprofessional team.
- Drugs/medicines used in the management of uterine inversion and uterine rupture.

Pre-reading self-assessment

1 What are the functions of the uterus?
2 Describe briefly the physiology of the third stage of labour.
3 Describe briefly active management of the third stage of labour.
4 What is a uterine inversion?
5 List six predisposing factors for uterine inversion.
6 What is uterine rupture?
7 List six predisposing factors for uterine rupture.

Recommended prior reading

Beringer, R. and Patteril, M. (2004) Puerperal uterine inversion and shock, *British Journal of Anaesthesia*, 92(3): 439–41.

Grady, K., Howell, K. and Cox, C. (eds) (2007) *Managing Obstetric Emergencies and Trauma: The MOET Course Manual*, 2nd edn. London: RCOG Press.

NHS Institute for Innovation and Improvement (2008) *SBAR: Situation, Background, Assessment, Recommendation*. Available at: http://www.institute.nhs.uk (accessed 8 August 2011).

This case study is split into two parts to examine the care of two women, one with uterine inversion (Case study 9.1: Cindy) and one with a uterine rupture (Case study 9.2: Althea).

CASE STUDY 9.1: UTERINE INVERSION

Cindy, a 34-year-old gravida 3 para 2 is 40 weeks pregnant. Previous births were straightforward. She has had a normal labour and has given birth to a live male infant. Her last recorded observations on the partogram were: P 80 bpm, BP 128/78 mmHg, RR 15 breaths per min., T 37.4°C, urinalysis NAD. Cindy has been previously fit and well but currently has a heavy cold and a chesty cough. Cindy opted to have active management of the third stage of labour. Following IM administration of Syntocinon 10 units, as per hospital guidelines, Cindy has a violent coughing fit; following this, the midwife notices that there is 'something visible at the vulva' and Cindy immediately looks pale and clammy and is complaining of severe pain.

1 **What are your initial thoughts concerning a diagnosis for Cindy's condition?**

A Cindy had a violent coughing fit, which will mean that there is increased intra-abdominal pressure; she looks pale and clammy which is indicative of shock, something is 'visible' at the vulva and she is complaining of severe pain. This history is consistent with an initial likely diagnosis of uterine inversion.

2 **What other conditions could cause Cindy's signs and symptoms?**

A If the uterus is clearly seen at the vulva, then the diagnosis is uterine inversion. If the uterus is not visible, then uterine rupture, gestational trophoblastic disease, occult genital tract disease, undiagnosed second twin, neurogenic collapse and retained placenta without inversion could be suspected as a differential diagnosis (Bhalla et al. 2009).

3 **How would you define uterine inversion?**

A Uterine inversion is a rare but potentially life-threatening occurrence. The incidence of uterine inversion varies according to geographical location, from 1 in 2500 to 1 in 20,000 (You and Zahn 2006). It usually occurs during the third stage of labour and is associated with significant blood loss. Shock is also present but may not be reflective of the degree of haemorrhage (Beringer and Patteril 2004). The uterus may be partially or completely turned inside out. In incomplete (first or second degree) uterine inversion, the inner surface of the fundus is drawn down into the uterine cavity. In complete (third degree) uterine inversion, the inside of the fundus protrudes through the cervix into the vagina. If the uterus is fully inverted, it may be visible outside of the vulva (Stables and Rankin 2010). In a total (fourth degree) inversion, the vagina may also be prolapsed (Bhalla et al. 2009). See Figure 9.1 for an illustration of uterine inversion and Box 9.1 for classifications of uterine inversion.

Box 9.1 Classification of uterine inversion

Uterine inversion is often classified in degrees of severity as follows:

First (incomplete): the fundus lies within the endometrial cavity, not beyond the cervical os.

Second (incomplete): the fundus protrudes through the external cervical os but remains within the vagina.
Third (complete or prolapsed): the fundus extends to or through the introitus.
Fourth (total): the vagina is also inverted.

Uterine inversion is also classified in relation to the timing of the inversion:

1 *Acute inversion*: occurs within the first 24 hours.
2 *Subacute inversion*: occurs after the first 24 hours and within 4 weeks.
3 *Chronic inversion*: occurs after 4 weeks (very rare).

(Beringer and Patteril 2004; Bhalla et al. 2009; Stables and Rankin 2010)

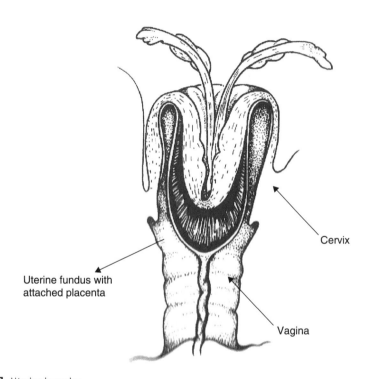

Cervix

Uterine fundus with
attached placenta

Vagina

Figure 9.1 Uterine inversion

4 **What are the predisposing causes of uterine inversion?**

A A variety of risk factors have been highlighted as being associated with uterine inversion. These are listed in Box 9.2.

Box 9.2 Predisposing factors for uterine inversion

- Manual removal of placenta.
- Mismanagement of the third stage of labour, e.g. fundal pressure or inappropriate controlled cord traction.
- Pathologically adherent placenta, e.g. placenta accreta particularly if involving the uterine fundus.
- Short cord.
- Primiparity.
- Fetal macrosomia.
- Sudden emptying of a distended uterus.
- Raised intra-abdominal pressure, e.g. caused by coughing, sneezing or vomiting.
- Spontaneous inversion.

(Stables and Rankin 2010; Uzoma and Ola 2010)

Check point

It is well established and documented that mismanagement of the third stage of labour is the commonest cause of uterine inversion. This is an avoidable cause of a potentially catastrophic event. Midwives should be skilled in the active management of the third stage of labour and, when caring for women, choosing the physiological third stage of labour.

---

5   **How is uterine inversion diagnosed?**

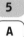 Diagnosis of uterine inversion is usually based on clinical features. However, the use of MRI scans has been reported in rare cases when faced with uncertainty and the woman's condition is stabilized to ensure that it is safe to move her to specialized departments for such investigations.

There may be a number of signs and symptoms as reported by Beringer and Patteril (2004), and You and Zahn (2006) such as:

- Severe abdominal pain.
- Shock (neurogenic) – thought to be due to the parasympathetic effect caused by traction of the ligaments supporting the uterus, and hypotension with inadequate tissue perfusion; this may be disproportionate to the amount of blood loss.
- Collapse may suddenly occur.
- On palpation of the uterus, the fundus may be difficult to locate. A hollow in the fundus may be felt.
- There is often a complaint of feeling 'something in the vagina'.
- Haemorrhage is present in most cases.

6 **What is the management of uterine inversion?**

A In cases where a uterine inversion has occurred, the following interprofessional team would be required, using the SBAR tool to maximize good communication (NHS Institute for Innovation and Improvement 2008): senior obstetrician, anaesthetist, midwives (to assist with co-ordination and documentation of actions), paediatrician, haematologist and blood bank, theatre team, hospital porters, and ICU/HDU team alerted. Subsequent management principles are summarized in Box 9.3.

Box 9.3 Management of uterine inversion

- Ensure good communication with woman, family members and all members of the multidisciplinary team is maintained throughout.
- It is recommended that with appropriate help many of these procedures can be executed simultaneously.
- Documentation of events should take place as contemporaneously as possible.
- The midwife should attempt to replace the uterus to relieve neurogenic shock. The uterine fundus is pushed backwards with the palm of the hand, along the vagina towards the posterior fornix. Steady pressure is used to push the uterus towards the umbilicus and returned to its original position.
- If the uterus cannot be completely repositioned, it should be replaced into the vagina. Prompt action will reduce risks to the mother. However, avoid rough or prolonged manipulation as this may induce vaso-vagal shock.
- A uterine muscle relaxant may be used, e.g. terbutaline 0.25 mg by slow IV bolus or magnesium sulphate 2–4 g given I.U. over 5 minutes, to facilitate repositioning of the uterus.
- Elevate foot of bed, to relieve traction on uterine ligaments.
- Pain relief such as opiates that are used locally.
- Maternal vital signs: BP, P, RR taken at regular intervals, usually ¼ hourly.
- Estimate blood loss.
- Commence MEOWS chart.
- Assess for ABC resuscitation (see Case 12).
- Wide-bore cannulae should be inserted (14G or 16G).
- Bloods taken for FBC, cross-matching, clotting studies.
- Commence intravenous infusion of fluids, colloids and/or crystalloids.
- Urinary catheterization.
- Accurate fluid balance chart.
- Monitor oxygen saturation.
- Oxygen therapy.
- Monitor level of consciousness. If applicable, using AVPU or Glasgow Coma Scale (see Case 10).
- If the placenta remains *in situ* at this stage, then no attempt should be made to remove it, as this may result in serious haemorrhage.

(NMC 2004; Vijayaraghavan and Sujatha 2006; Soleymani et al. 2009; Uzoma and Ola 2010; Keriakos and Chaudri 2011)

Once the uterus has been repositioned, the midwife's hand should remain *in situ* until a firm contraction has been achieved. Oxytocics such as Syntometrine (if not contraindicated) or Syntocinon 10 units followed by 40 units in 500 mL of normal saline are given to maintain a contraction. Carboprost and misoprostol may also be administered.

If manual replacement fails, then the hydrostatic method may be employed (Figure 9.2). This involves the infusion of 2–3 litres of warm saline, given via a tube set into the vagina. The woman lies in the lithotomy position and the fluid is held about 1 m above the level of the uterus. The fluid rapidly fills and distends the uterus which then repositions itself.

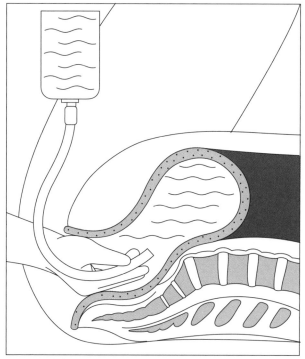

Figure 9.2 Hydrotatic method of uterine replacement in uterine inversion
Note position of hand at vaginal orifice, acting as a plug in order to prevent the warm saline seeping out as the fluid pressure is needed to help the uterus revert back into place.

Once the uterus has been repositioned, the placenta can be removed. More recently there have been reports of using the insertion of a Rusch balloon, filled with approximately 700 mL of saline, to arrest bleeding. A vaginal pack is often used and IV antibiotics administered. The Rusch balloon can be removed 12–24 hours following the birth.

If all the above fail, then surgical intervention may be required as follows:

- The Huntington technique involves laporotomy, the cup of the uterus is located and Allis forceps are used to apply gentle upward traction to correct the inversion.
- The Haultain procedure involves making a posterior incision in the cervical ring and manually reducing the inversion. Repair the incision after giving oxytocin and manually remove the placenta.

- A modified laparoscopic reduction has also been reported but this procedure requires further evaluation (Vijayaraghavan and Sujatha 2006; Soleymani et al. 2009; Uzoma and Ola 2010; Keriakos and Chaudri 2011).
- Hysterectomy is the last resort.

Think

All these procedures should be covered by IV antibiotics.

Check points

- Moderate to excessive traction on the cord prior to placental separation should be avoided.
- Prompt recognition and treatment of a uterine inversion increase the chances of a successful outcome.
- Attempted replacement is the appropriate first–line management of uterine inversion.

CASE OUTCOME

With effective communication between the interprofessional team and prompt recognition, diagnosis and treatment, Cindy's case was successfully managed with the hydrostatic method of reversing uterine inversion. Blood loss was 750 mL, clear intravenous fluids were maintained for 24 hours. Psychosocial aspects of care are an important part of the midwives' role, including cultural and spiritual needs. Cindy, her partner and/or other family members may appreciate discussing the events of her birth with an appropriate member of the interprofessional team. Cindy made a good recovery, and mother and baby were transferred home 3 days postnatally.

CASE STUDY 9.2: UTERINE RUPTURE

Althea is a 32-year-old gravida 3, para 1 + 1 miscarriage who is 39 weeks pregnant. She had a ventouse delivery 18 months ago, and surgery to remove a fibroid 6 years ago. She had an in-depth discussion with the consultant obstetrician who informed her of the advantages and disadvantages of having a vaginal birth versus a caesarean birth. She decided that she wanted to have a normal vaginal birth this time as there had been no complications during her pregnancy. She is in established labour contracting 3–4 in ten minutes; contractions are moderate to strong. She is using Entonox with good effect. Findings on abdominal examination: uterine fundus is equal to gestational date, i.e. 39 weeks, lie is longitudinal, presentation cephalic, head 2/5ths palpable. The last vaginal examination found her cervix to be 6 cm dilated, central, well applied to the presenting part, membranes intact, cephalic presentation at 1 cm above the ischial spines. FHR is being continuously monitored, the rate is 145 bpm, good variability, accelerations are present, no decelerations noted, and the CTG trace is classified as 'normal'. The admission routine observations were: P 85 bpm, BP 125/20 mmHg, RR 15 breaths per min., T 36.8°C, urinalysis showed a small trace of blood.

Althea informs the midwife that she feels a little 'strange', and that she is experiencing 'a different type of pain in her abdomen which is quite unlike the contractions and is continuous'. The CTG trace has started to show variable decelerations. Althea looks pale and there is approximately 400 mL of fresh red blood loss from her vagina.

1 **What are your initial thoughts concerning a diagnosis for Althea's condition?**

A The combination of signs and symptoms, i.e. Althea saying she feels 'strange', and reporting a 'different' type of continuous abdominal pain, with early signs of shock and a CTG tracing showing variable decelerations, are consistent with uterine rupture.

2 **What other conditions could cause Althea's signs and symptoms?**

A There are a number of factors that might explain the clinical features that have manifested as well as the sudden unexpected change in Althea's condition. These are outlined in Box 9.4.

Box 9.4 Differential diagnosis for uterine rupture

- Placenta praevia
- Vasa praevia
- Placental abruption
- Uterine inversion
- Incidental causes of bleeding from the genital tract
- Coagulopathy
- Uterine atony
- Uterine artery rupture.

(Mazzone and Woolever 2006)

---

3 **How would you define uterine rupture?**

A Uterine rupture is a full thickness tear through the myometrium and serosa; this can extend to the bladder or broad ligament (Rogers and Chang 2005; RCOG 2007). Kroll and Lyne (2002) define it as the separation of the uterine wall, with or without expulsion of the fetus. They classify uterine rupture as follows: a complete rupture involves a full thickness tear of uterine wall and peritoneum (see Figure 9.3). The fetus is normally partially or wholly expelled into the peritoneal cavity. An incomplete rupture involves a tear to the myometrium but does not involve the peritoneum (Kroll and Lynne 2002). The rate of uterine rupture is 2–8 per 10,000 births, incidence 0.05 per cent (Belfort and Dildy 2011).

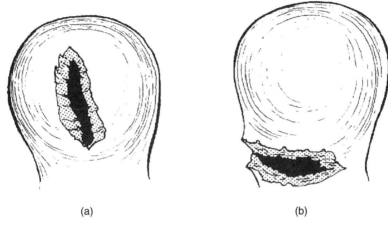

(a) (b)

Figure 9.3 Rupture through classical CS scar (a) and transverse rupture through lower uterine segment (b)

4 **What are the predisposing factors associated with uterine rupture?**

A These are manifold as identified by Lydon-Rochelle et al. (2001), Kroll and Lyne (2002), Johanson et al. (2001), Rogers and Chang (2005), Seracchioli et al. (2006) and RCOG (2007). They are listed in Box 9.5.

Box 9.5 Predisposing factors to uterine rupture

Traumatic or iatrogenic

- Misuse of oxytocic drugs and prostaglandins.
- Instrumental delivery – particularly associated with mid– or high–cavity forceps. (Cervical tears can extend into lower uterine segment causing severe haemorrhage.)
- Intra-uterine manipulations during pregnancy or labour, e.g. external cephalic version or internal podalic version.
- Manual removal of placenta.
- Shoulder dystocia.
- Fundal pressure in second stage of labour.

Spontaneous rupture

- Often the reasons for spontaneous rupture are unknown.
- Previous uterine surgery, particularly classical caesarean section.
- Very strong naturally occurring contractions.
- Unrecognized earlier trauma.
- Unrecognized obstructed labour resulting in tonic contractions.
- Abruptio placentae because of distension and disruption of uterine wall.
- Occurrence in primigravidae is rare but has been reported.

---

5 **With reference to relevant pathophysiology, how would you account for the signs and symptoms associated with uterine rupture?**

A This will depend on the severity of the rupture but according to the RCOG (2007) may include:

- Acute onset scar tenderness.
- Continuous severe abdominal pain.
- Abnormal CTG tracing, e.g. variable or late decelerations, fetal tachycardia. May lead to fetal compromise or death.
- Reduction or cessation of uterine contractions.
- Maternal tachycardia, hypotension or shock, may lead to maternal collapse or death.
- Fresh red blood loss PV.
- Easily palpable fetal parts.
- Haematuria.
- Loss of station of the presenting part.

6 **What are the implications of a labour complicated by uterine rupture?**

A This is an extremely serious emergency, requiring prompt recognition and treatment. In the last confidential enquiry into maternal deaths, one parous woman died as a result of uterine rupture which was not recognized until after maternal collapse and cardiac arrest (Liston 2007). In the 2006–2008 CMACE triennial report, 111 cases of uterine rupture were reported as causing morbidity in women. This translates as 17.4 cases per 100,000 maternities. Some 86 per cent of the incidences of uterine rupture occurred in women who had had a previous caesarean delivery (Norman 2011). Intra-uterine death is common with a uterine rupture (Nahum and Chelmow 2010). Lydon-Rochelle et al. (2001) report the perinatal mortality rate with uterine rupture as being 5.5 per cent.

7 **What is the management of uterine rupture?**

A Uterine rupture is an obstetric emergency and the following interprofessional team would be required, using the SBAR tool to maximize good communication (NHS Institute for Innovation and Improvement 2008): senior obstetrician; anaesthetist; midwives (to assist with running and to document actions); paediatrician; haematologist and blood bank; theatre team; hospital porters; ICU/HDU team alerted. The subsequent management of uterine rupture is summarized in Box 9.6.

Box 9.6 Key management principles of uterine rupture

- Ensure good communication with woman, family members and all members of the multidisciplinary team is maintained throughout.
- It is recommended that with appropriate help many of these procedures can be executed simultaneously.
- Documentation of events should take place as contemporaneously as possible.

- Prepare for theatre immediately.
- Continue with ¼–hourly observations of BP, P, T and RR. Commence MEOWS chart.
- Estimate blood loss.
- Intravenous access must be gained, using two wide-bore (14G or 16G) cannulae.
- Blood will have been sent for full blood count, clotting screen, urea and electrolytes and cross-matched for 4 units of blood.
- Resuscitation with intravenous fluids.
- Assess for ABC resuscitation (see Case 12).
- If fetus is alive, attempt to continuously monitor FHR.
- Nahum and Chelmlow (2010) state that the time available for a successful intervention following a uterine rupture and before the onset of major fetal morbidity is 10–37 minutes.
- Emergency laparotomy is the only treatment if a uterine rupture is suspected.
- The fetus must be delivered promptly.

Following this, the types of surgical management depend on the type of uterine rupture, the extent of the rupture, the amount of haemorrhage, the condition of the mother, and the mother's future childbearing wishes.
Surgical options are:

- Repair of rupture to preserve uterus if possible.
- Uterine and hypogastric artery ligation to control haemorrhage.
- Hysterectomy.

Following the laparotomy, the following management is recommended:

- Continue with MEOWS chart.
- Observe for blood loss.
- Monitor oxygen saturation.
- Oxygen therapy.
- Monitor level of consciousness using AVPU or Glasgow Coma Scale (see Case 10).
                                        (NMC 2004; Nahum and Chelmlow 2010)

Check points

- Diagnosis and prompt treatment of uterine rupture is essential as any delay may seriously affect the woman's chances of survival.
- In women who have had a previous CS, induction and acceleration of labour are associated with a higher incidence of uterine rupture.

(Continued overleaf)

- The decision to use prostaglandins and/or oxytocin in women who have a scarred uterus from a previous CS (or other uterine surgery) must be carefully made between a senior obstetrician and the childbearing woman.

CASE OUTCOME

The midwife caring for Althea and the rest of the interprofessional team correctly diagnosed a uterine rupture. She was prepared for theatre and the baby was delivered via an emergency CS, under general anaesthetic (GA) within 20 minutes of the diagnosis. The baby was mildly asphyxiated at birth, due to the acute insult as a result of the uterine rupture, but recovered well without resuscitation. The uterine rupture was found and repaired by a consultant obstetrician. The total blood loss was estimated to be 1,800 mL. Althea agreed to have 2 units of blood transfused following the operation. Althea and her baby were admitted to the high dependency unit on the labour suite for 24 hours and were then transferred to the postnatal ward. Psychosocial aspects of care are an important aspect of the midwives' role, including cultural and spiritual needs. Althea, her partner and/or other family members may appreciate discussing the events of her birth with an appropriate member of the interprofessional team. The consultant obstetrician discussed the possible risks for a subsequent pregnancy. Althea made a good recovery and mother and baby were discharged home on day 6.

Summary of key points

- Uterine inversion and rupture are potentially catastrophic life-threatening conditions. Their prompt diagnosis, management and treatment are imperative to reduce the incidence of maternal and perinatal morbidity and mortality.
- Use of the SBAR tool and MEOWS chart facilitate efficient and timely communication with obstetricians, anaesthetists, paediatricians and other key members of the interprofessional team.
- Hyper-vigilant record keeping in all aspects of care including documentation of vital signs, with no omissions is essential. The midwife has a professional responsibility to report any deviations in the vital signs to the medical team.
- The midwife has a professional responsibility to ensure the woman's holistic needs are met. This includes psychosocial support for the woman's partner and/or relatives to help to ameliorate the stress and anxiety associated with medical and technological interventions.
- Good team working and collaboration between the interprofessional team are recognized as being vital to a successful outcome when obstetric emergencies arise.
- Regular skills drills and training in obstetric emergencies including uterine inversion and rupture, are recommended as good practice for the interprofessional team.

(Norman 2011; RCOG 2011)

REFERENCES

Belfort, M. and Dildy, G. (2011) Postpartum haemorrhage and other problems of the third state of labour, in D. James, P. Steer, C. Weiner, B. Gonik, C. Crowther and S. Robson (eds) *High Risk Pregnancy, Management Options*, 4th edn. St Louis, MO: Elsevier.

Beringer, R. and Patteril, M. (2004) Puerperal uterine inversion and shock, *British Journal of Anaesthesia*, 92(3): 439–41.

Bhalla, R., Wuntakal, R., Odejinmi, F. and Khan, R. (2009) Acute inversion of the uterus, *The Obstetrician and Gynaecologist*, 11(1): 13–18.

Cunningham, F., Leveno, K., Bloom, S., Hauth, J., Rouse, D. and Spong, C. (2010) *Williams Obstetrics*, 23rd edn. New York: McGraw-Hill.

Grady, K., Howell, K. and Cox, C. (eds) (2007) *Managing Obstetric Emergencies and Trauma: The MOET Course Manual*, 2nd edn. London: RCOG.

Johanson, R., Kumar, M., Obhrai, M. and Young, P. (2001) Management of massive postpartum haemorrhage: use of a hydrostatic balloon catheter to avoid laparotomy, *British Journal of Obstetrics and Gynaecology*, 108(4): 420–2.

Keriakos, R. and Chaudri, S. (2011) Managing post-partum haemorrhage following acute inversion with Rusch balloon catheter, *Case Reports in Critical Care*. Article ID 541479 (accessed 31 July 2011).

Kroll, D. and Lyne, M. (2002) Uterine inversion and uterine rupture, in M. Boyle (ed.) *Emergencies around Childbirth*, Abingdon: Radcliffe Medical Press.

Liston, W. (2007) Haemorrhage, in G. Lewis (ed.) *The Confidential Enquiry into Maternal and Child Health (CEMACH). Saving Mothers' Lives: Reviewing Maternal Deaths to Make Motherhood Safer, 2003–2005. The Seventh Report on Confidential Enquiries into Maternal Deaths in the United Kingdom*. Available at: http://cemach.interface-test.com/getattachment/927cf18a-735a-47a0-9200-cdea103781c7/Saving-Mothers—Lives-2003-2005_full.aspx (accessed 27 August 2011).

Lydon-Rochelle, M., Holt, V., Easterling, T. and Martin, D. (2001) Risk of uterine rupture during labor among women with a prior Cesarean delivery, *The New England Journal of Medicine*, 345(1): 3–8.

Mazzone, M. and Woolever, J. (2006) Uterine rupture in a patient with an unscarred uterus: a case study, *Wisconsin Medical Journal*, 105(2): 64–6. Available at: http://www.wisconsinmedicalsociety.org/_WMS/publications/wmj/issues/wmj_v105n2/Mazzone.pdf (accessed 17 August 2011).

Nahum, G. and Chelmow, D. (2010) Uterine rupture in pregnancy, *Medscape Drugs, Diseases and Procedures*. Available at: http://emedicine.medscape.com/article/275854-overview (accessed 5 August 2011).

NHS Institute for Innovation and Improvement (2008) *SBAR: Situation, Background, Assessment, Recommendation*. Available at: http://www.institute.nhs.uk (accessed 8 August 2011).

Norman, J. (2011) Haemorrhage, in Centre for Maternal and Child Enquiries (CMACE) *Saving Mothers' Lives: Reviewing Maternal Deaths to Make Motherhood Safer: 2006–2008. The Eighth Report on Confidential Enquiries into Maternal Deaths in the United Kingdom*. Ed. G. Lewis. *BJOG*. 118 (Suppl. 1): 1–203.

Nursing and Midwifery Council (NMC) (2004) *Midwives Rules and Standards*. London: NMC.

Rogers, M. and Chang, A. (2005) Postpartum haemorrhage and other problems of the third stage,, in D. James, P. Steer, C. Weiner, B. Gonik, C. Crowther and S. Robson (eds) *High Risk Pregnancy, Management Options*, 4th edn. St Louis, MO: Elsevier.

Royal College of Obstetricians and Gynaecologists (RCOG) (2007) *Birth after Previous Caesarean Birth*. Green Top Guideline No. 45. Available at: http://www.rcog.org.uk/files/rcog-corp/uploaded-files/GT45BirthAfterPreviousCeasarean.pdf (accessed 17 August 2011).

Royal College of Obstetricians and Gynaecologists (RCOG) (2011) *Prevention and Management of Postpartum Haemorrhage*. Green Top Guideline No. 52. London: RCOG.

Seracchioli, R., Manuzzi, L., Vianello, F., Gualerzi, B., Savelli, L., Paradisi, R. and Venturoli, S. (2006) Obstetric and delivery outcome of pregnancies achieved after laparoscopic myomectomy, *Fertility and Sterility*, 86(1): 159–65.

Shiers, C. and Coates, T. (2009) Midwifery and obstetric emergencies, in D.F. Fraser and M.A. Cooper (eds) *Myles Textbook for Midwives*, 15th edn. London: Churchill Livingstone.

Soleymani Majid, H., Pilsniask, A. and Reginald, P. (2009) Recurrent uterine inversion: a novel treatment using SOS Bakri balloon, *British Journal of Obstetrics and Gynaecology*, 116 (7): 999–1001.

Stables, D. and Rankin, J. (eds) (2010) *Physiology in Childbearing*, 3rd edn. London: Elsevier.

Uzoma, A. and Ola, B. (2010) Complete uterine inversion managed with a Rusch balloon catheter, *Journal of Medical Cases*, 1(1): 8–9.

Vijayaraghavan, R. and Sujatha, Y. (2006) Acute postpartum uterine inversion with haemorrhagic shock: laparoscopic reduction: a new method of management, *British Journal of Obstetrics and Gynaecology*, 113(9): 1100–2.

You, W. and Zahn, C. (2006) Postpartum hemorrhage: abnormally adherent placenta, uterine inversion, and puerperal hematomas, *Clinical Obstetrics and Gynecology*, 49(1): 184–97.

ANNOTATED FURTHER READING

Baskett, T. (2002) Acute uterine inversion: a review of 40 cases, *Journal of Obstetrics and Gynaecology Canada*, 24(12): 953–6.

A review of 40 cases of inversion of the uterus including learning points for future management.

Kieser, K. and Baskett, T. (2002) A 10-year population-based study of uterine rupture, *Obstetrics and Gynaecology*, 100(4): 749–53.

This 10-year review explores the outcomes of pregnancies complicated by uterine rupture. It examines the types and extent of maternal and neonatal morbidity and mortality.

Milenkovic, M. and Kahn, J. (2005) Inversion of the uterus: a serious complication at childbirth, *Acta Obstetrics Gynaecology Scandanavia*, 84(1): 95–6.

A useful review and overview of all aspects of inversion of the uterus.

Turner, M. (2002) Uterine rupture, *Best Practice in Research and Clinical Obstetrics and Gynaecology*, 16(1): 69–79.

A comprehensive review of the risk factors, diagnosis and management of uterine rupture.

Yap, O., Kim, E. and Laros, R. (2001) Maternal and neonatal outcomes after uterine rupture in labor, *American Journal of Obstetrics and Gynaecology*, 184(7): 1576–81.

This research article explores the outcomes of pregnancies complicated by uterine rupture. It examines the types and extent of maternal and neonatal morbidity and mortality.

USEFUL WEBSITES

http://www.aagbi.org	The Association of Anaesthetists of Great Britain and Ireland
http://www.cemace.org.uk	Centre for Maternal and Child Enquiries
http://www.dh.gov.uk	U K Department of Health
http://www.institute.nhs.uk	National Health Service Institute for Innovation and Improvement
http://www.nice.org.uk	National Institute for Health and Clinical Excellence
http://www.npeu.ox.ac.uk	National Perinatal Epidemiology Unit
http://www.rcm.org.uk	Royal College of Midwives
http://www.rcoa.ac.uk	The Royal College of Anaesthetists
http://www.rcog.org.uk	Royal College of Obstetricians and Gynaecologists (RCOG)

Anaphylaxis
Maureen D. Raynor and Sam Bharmal

Pre-requisites for the chapter: the reader should have an understanding of:

- Immune response.
- Resuscitation: knowledge and skills of basic and advance life support (adult and neonate).
- Relevant pharmacology.
- Modified Early Obstetrics Warning Scoring System (MEOWS).
- The midwife's role and responsibilities within the interprofessional team.
- Local NHS Trust medicine code and clinical governance/risk management procedures relating to the reporting of critical untoward incidents.

Pre-reading self-assessment

1 What are antigens?
2 In what ways can antigens enter the body?
3 What are antibodies?
4 What are immunoglobulins?
5 The major groups of immunoglobulins reflect an alphabetical chronology; what are they?
6 What is the role of mast cells?
7 What is the role of basophils?
8 What is the role of oesinophils?

Recommended prior reading

CMACE (2011) *Saving Mothers' Lives: Reviewing Maternal Deaths to Make Motherhood Safer: 2006–2008. The Eighth Report of the Confidential Enquiries into Maternal Deaths in the United Kingdom.* Ed. G. Lewis. *BJOG: An International British Journal of Obstetrics and Gynaecology*, 118 (Suppl. 1): Chapters 8, 13, 16.

NHS Institute for Innovation and Improvement (2008) *SBAR: Situation, Background, Assessment, Recommendation.* Available at: http://www.institute.nhs.uk (accessed 12 January 2011).

CASE STUDY

Laura is a 33-year-old primigravida who is admitted at term to her local maternity unit in spontaneous labour. She is accompanied by her partner Sam. Assessment of maternal and fetal well-being on admission is used to establish normal parameters. Laura's vital signs are recorded as pulse 78 bpm, BP 110/68 mmHg, RR 13 breaths per min., T36°C, urinalysis NAD. Slight ankle oedema is noted by the midwife but nothing else of significance is gleaned from history taking on speaking to Laura, and reading her hand-held and hospital records. Findings on abdominal examination reveal SPFH measurement of 38 cm, longitudinal lie, cephalic presentation in a LOA position with the fetal head 3/5th engaged. Auscultation of the FHR is performed by the midwife using a Pinard stethoscope for 1 minute in accordance with NICE (2007a) intrapartum care guidelines. Findings following auscultation are recorded as FHR 140 bpm and regular, baseline variability > 5 bpm, the FH increased transiently from the baseline of 140 bpm by 20 bpm lasting for 20–25 seconds on two consecutive occasions during the 1-minute auscultation period. No audible decrease in the FHR noted.

Several minutes after admission, Laura's midwife recommends a VE to assess cervical status. Donning a pair of sterile powdered latex gloves for the VE, the midwife gains consent and proceeds with the assessment but fails to determine whether Laura has any known allergies.

Within a couple of minutes Laura states that she feels unwell, complains of shortness of breath, difficulty swallowing and a tightness in her chest. She develops a wheeze, feels itchy and has a noticeable urticarial rash over her arms, abdomen and face. Following this, she becomes unrousable.

It is possible that latex allergy is the culprit here. More stringent control measures should have been taken by the midwife to exclude such an allergy by simply asking the question and meticulously reading through the maternity records.

The midwife's assessment of Laura's vital signs when she initially collapsed revealed the following:

BP 60/30 mmHg, Pulse 120 bpm, RR 20 breaths per min., T 36°C.

1   **What is anaphylaxis?**

A   Anaphylaxis has no universally agreed definition; nonetheless it is recognized as an acute, life-threatening multi-system or multi-organ allergic reaction mediated by immunoglobin E (IgE) and non-IgE events. The separate term anaphylactoid (non-IgE dependent reaction) distinct from anaphylaxis (IgE dependent reaction) is unhelpful and should not be used, as both events are indistinguishable critical occurrences that will not change the approach to management (Lieberman 2005; RCUK 2008; AAGBI 2009a; WAO 2009; EAAI 2010).

Both the AAGBI (2009a) and EAAI (2010) offer two sub-categories to anaphylaxis; these are 'allergic anaphylaxis' and 'non-allergic anaphylaxis', which WAO (2009) refers to as 'immunological' and 'non-immunological' in origin. Although the presentation of both these sub-categories of anaphylaxis may be undifferentiated, the term 'allergic anaphylaxis' tends to be applicable when the hypersensitivity reaction is precipitated by an immune response such as IgE mediated antibodies (EAAI 2010).

> **Check point**
>
> Whatever the cause, the diagnosis and treatment of the hypersensitivity reaction known as anaphylaxis are identical (WAO 2009).

Even in cases where the clinical features of anaphylaxis appear mild initially, there is no room for complacency as the potential for progression to a severe outcome that might be intractable and interminable is real and must be recognized.

The main systems that are implicated are:

- cardiovascular
- respiratory
- gastro-intestinal
- skin/cutaneous.

2 **Although all the signs point to anaphylaxis, what are the possible explanations for Laura's collapse?**

A It is important to consider a differential diagnosis in the event of any maternal collapse. There may be several explanations for such an acute occurrence.

The cause of any sudden maternal collapse should be thoroughly investigated as there might be underlying life-threatening conditions or co-morbidities such as thromboembolic disorder and cardiomyopathy, which may disrupt normal organ function. The differential diagnoses that should be considered are listed in Box 10.1.

Box 10.1 Differential diagnoses to explain maternal collapse in the context of the given scenario

Neurological/seizure

Epilepsy

Eclampsia

Cerebrovascular accident

Hypoglycaemia

Circulatory/hypovolaemic shock

Cardiac arrest/myocardial infarction

Vaso-vagal attack/hypotension

Cardiomyopathy

Hypovolaemia

Respiratory distress/arrest

Aspiration syndrome

Pulmonary embolism

Other embolus (air, amniotic fluid)

Haemorrhage

Placental abruption

Uterine rupture

Disseminated intravascular

coagulation

Any pregnancy-related mortality is one death too many with a catastrophic impact on the baby who is left motherless, the relatives left behind and health care professionals involved in the woman's care. Unfortunately, the Anaesthetic chapter of the eighth report of the Confidential Enquiries into Maternal Deaths in the UK (McClure and Cooper 2011) documents one maternal death relating to an unexpected acute anaphylaxis reaction following the administration of antibiotics during the intrapartum period in a woman with no previous history of such allergy. The relative rarity of critical illness in maternity care, combined with the inherent physiological changes during a woman's adaptation to pregnancy, only serve to highlight the challenges and complexities involved in recognition and management of acute critical illness in the maternity context. There were no reported deaths in the previous report (Lewis 2007) from anaphylaxis, proving that maternal demise from this emergency is a very rare event. It is for these reasons that it is strongly recommended that midwives and doctors should be regularly updated on how to recognize and treat such an uncommon occurrence in pregnant women. With this goal in mind, the AAGBI (2009b) Safety Drill and RCUK (2008) anaphylaxis management guideline (Figure 10.1) should be familiar to the interprofessional team and regularly revisited via the interdisciplinary maternity emergencies 'skills and drills' annual updates.

That said, in England and Wales the Department of Health (2006) states the incidence of anaphylaxis is on the increase, and in the context of pregnancy it poses a serious threat to both Laura and her unborn baby. It also suggests that a latex-safe environment is required to prevent inadvertent exposure to latex allergens in latex-sensitive women. This is reflective of the guidance issued in England by the NPSA (2005).

In considering the differential diagnosis, Laura presented with no co-existing morbidity. The presence of a wheeze may not just relate to asthma, it could be a feature of cardiac failure. There is no history of either cardiac disease or any known respiratory disorder. Hence, the presence of a wheeze excludes these conditions. However, the report by the former CEMACH (Lewis 2007) suggests that breathlessness, dyspnoea, tachypnoea and tachycardia can be features of peripartum cardiomyopathy.

As a result of a robust thromboprophylaxis programme, maternal deaths from VTE disorders have slipped to third place, signifying that such fatality is no longer the leading cause of direct deaths in the UK (CMACE 2011). Pulmonary embolism resulting in sudden maternal demise in pregnancy is uncommon. Furthermore, although there might be no accompanying symptomatology in many cases of documented pulmonary embolism, rapid onset of unexplained dyspnoea, tachypnoea, cough, apprehension and chest pain are common features.

Amniotic fluid embolism (AFE) is rare but is reported as the fourth leading cause of direct maternal mortality in the UK (CMACE 2011). There are striking similarities between anaphylactic shock and AFE in the literature (Box 10.2). They both are acute and serious events that can present with sudden unexplained restlessness, acute hypotension, acute hypoxia including features of respiratory distress such as wheezing, stridor, dyspnoea and cyanosis during labour, resulting in respiratory and haemodynamic collapse (Tuffnell and Hamilton 2008). Although a high index of clinical suspicion for AFE is necessary to arrest and avert its catastrophic sequelae, the presenting features are more indicative of anaphylaxis than any of the other critical events listed in Box 10.1. Clark et al. (1995) suggest that AFE tends to mimic anaphylaxis in its immunological response, proposing that AFE should be replaced by the term 'anaphylactoid syndrome of pregnancy'.

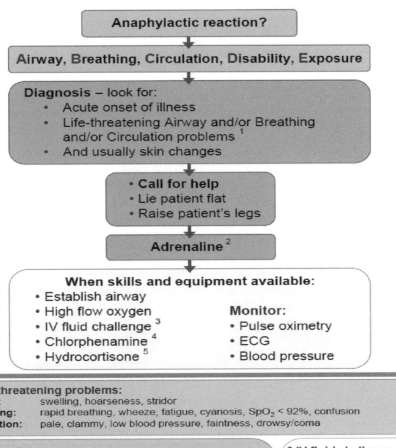

Figure 10.1 Management of anaphylaxis algorithm

Source: Resuscitation Council UK (2008:20) *Emergency treatment of anaphylactic reactions and guidelines for health care providers.* http://www.resus.org.uk Reproduced with kind permission.

Note: Adrenaline has been identified on the list of *Midwives Exemptions for the Administration of Prescription Only Medicines* (NMC 2011). This means midwives within their legal framework are authorized to administer adrenaline via the parenteral route in the first-line management of anaphylaxis in the absence of a doctor.

Box 10.2 Features of AFE vs anaphylaxis

AFE	Anaphylaxis
Acute life-threatening condition with a high incidence of mortality without early recognition, and prompt and skilful management;	Acute life-threatening condition with a high incidence of mortality without early recognition, and prompt and skilful management;
Acute hypoxia (respiratory distress/ arrest, cyanosis, dyspnoea and tachypnoea);	Acute hypoxia (respiratory distress/ arrest, cyanosis, dyspnoea and tachypnoea);
Bronchospasm and angioedema;	Bronchospasm and angioedema;
Nausea and vomiting may feature;	Nausea and vomiting may feature;
Neurological sequelae leading to restlessness, apprehension, confusion and loss of consciousness;	Neurological sequelae leading to restlessness, apprehension, confusion and loss of consciousness;
Unexpected cardiovascular and haemodynamic collapse;	Unexpected cardiovascular and haemodynamic collapse;
Hypotension/hypovolaemic shock;	Hypotension/hypovolaemic shock;
Possibility of seizures;	Possibility of seizures;
Coagulopathy (EARLY FEATURE).	Coagulopathy;
	Urticarial rash/itching.

(Clark et al. 1995; Tufnell and Hamilton 2008)

3   How would you differentiate between AFE and anaphylaxis?

A   In order to treat speedily and accurately it is important to differentiate between anaphylaxis and AFE even though the features of both conditions are almost indistinguishable, as demonstrated in Box 10.2.

Hypersensitivity to latex and anaphylaxis are not a homogenous process (AAGBI 2009a). Anaphylactic reactions are unpredictable as the onset and severity will vary immensely, ranging from mild symptoms to potentially life-threatening complications (EAACI 2010). These reactions may affect any system of the body, varying in severity from mild pruritus at one end of the spectrum, to systemic anaphylaxis.

Check point

It is imperative to recognize the clinical features of anaphylaxis early in order to prevent, arrest and limit any ensuing complication as well as mobilize prompt and appropriate help via the interdisciplinary team, skilled in the management of maternity emergencies.

According to Lieberman (2005), anaphylaxis is diagnosed when *any* of the following criteria present, either immediately or within minutes to hours of exposure to the antigen:

acute clinical manifestation involving the skin, mucosal surface or both, leading to urticaria, itching or oedema of the airways;

hypotension, i.e. a decline in systolic BP > 30 per cent compared to baseline readings, which make the individual symptomatic;

respiratory collapse;

any haemodynamic collapse causing dysfunction of major organs, namely the GI tract, respiratory, skin and CVS compromise.

Laura's history is the most important tool to determine the cause of the hypersensitivity reaction. This takes precedence over other diagnostic tests. She has not had any form of regional analgesia (epidural or spinal). There has been no administration of any pharmacological agents that might contribute to marked maternal compromise, e.g. drugs causing vasodilatation leading to hypotension. There is no history of hypertensive disorder, sudden and acute abdominal pain or vaginal bleeding that often accompanies antepartum haemorrhage (placental abruption). Therefore, the close timing of the introduction of the allergen in relation to Laura's collapse is indicative of a hypersensitivity reaction to latex. This will be known retrospectively from detailed examination of her records.

4 **What are the common causes of anaphylaxis?**

A Antigens are present in diverse forms resulting in many different triggers for anaphylaxis as detailed in Box 10.3.

Box 10.3 Common triggers/allergens or antigens for anaphylaxis

Food	Especially nuts (more commonly peanuts); certain type of fruits, e.g. kiwi fruit, banana, tomatoes, avocados, figs or other; fish, more commonly shellfish/crustaceans.
Environmental factors	Mainly pollen.
Medicines	Commonly antibiotics, anaesthetic drugs, non-steroidal anti-inflammatory drugs (NSAIDs), colloids such as blood or blood products, e.g. anti-D immunoglobulin injections.
Contrast medium	E.g. dyes used mainly for exploratory investigations such as MRI.
Insects	Bee/wasp (yellow jacket) stings.

(Continued overleaf)

Latex	Rubber latex gloves tend to be the main culprit; however, the midwife must be aware that latex can be present in everyday products/medical devices such as catheters and BP cuffs as well as other goods encountered in daily life.
Exercise	In some individuals exercise may trigger anaphylaxis on its own or when combined with other factors such as food or medicines. Drugs such as NSAIDs and beta-blockers, used to control hypertension or other cardiac related problems, can alter mild reactions from another cause into severe anaphylaxis because the body's main defence mechanism against anaphylaxis is impeded. This is why individuals on steroids and beta-blockers are told to seek urgent medical attention in the event of a bee/wasp sting.
Other	Some individuals are allergic to hair dye while in others there is no discernible cause to explain the anaphylactic response.
	(RCUK 2008)

5 **With reference to relevant pathophysiology, how would you account for the common signs and symptoms of anaphylaxis?**

A Anaphylaxis, as stated previously, is very rare indeed. The exact prevalence during pregnancy is unknown (Powrie 2010). It is a rapid systemic hypersensitivity reaction in a sensitized individual to the presence of a foreign substance, i.e. an antigen or allergen, usually introduced into the body by:

- ingestion
- injection
- inhalation
- absorption.

On entering the body of a sensitized individual, antigens cause the systemic release of mediators from the antibodies attached to the surface of mast cells (present in subcutaneous/submucosal tissues, e.g. conjunctival, GI and respiratory tract) and basophils, found in blood plasma. This process is mediated by immunoglobulin E (see p. 164) in the majority of cases, and is classified as type 1 hypersensitivity reaction. The IgE antibodies are produced by T cells as a result of the sensitization. However, complex genetic mechanisms within the body coupled with environmental factors may also have a contributory role. This is less well understood and accounted for (WAO 2009).

The hypersensitivity reaction is triggered by the release of inflammatory mediators from the granulation of mast cells and basophils. The degranulation of mast cells frees the release of histamine in the tissues as part of the inflammatory response to IgE antibodies and a precipitating antigen. Not only histamine as an initial mediator is released; prostaglandins, leukotrienes and platelet-activating factors are also liberated before other secondary mediators. These mediators are responsible for the increased vascular permeability, urticaria, itching, peripheral vasodilatation, heightened mucus secretion as well as contraction of the smooth muscles of the bronchial tree. A large proportion of the chemical features of anaphylaxis are thought to be attributable to histamine (AAGBI 2009a). There are notably three histamine receptors:

H1: the action of histamine causes smooth muscle contraction, increased vascular permeability and prostaglandin generation.
H2: the action of histamine not only leads to increased vascular permeability, but also enhanced gastric acid secretion and further release of histamine from mast cells and basophils.
H3: the action of histamine disrupts nervous system (central and peripheral) activity by inhibiting neurotransmitter release. Further release and formation of histamine are also inhibited.

Further systemic changes may arise, such as autonomic nervous system stimulation, increased GI motility, inflammatory response and platelet aggregation. These reactions account for the variable clinical features of anaphylaxis (Mattson Porth 2007; Powrie 2010).

It is important to remember that the nature in which the antigen or allergen is introduced into Laura's body determines the time of onset of the main clinical features of anaphylaxis. The pathophysiology of this acute emergency is detailed in Box 10.4.

Box 10.4 Pathophysiology: systems approach

Immune system	The introduction of an allergen/antigen causes mast cells to degranulate. Mast cells can be found in connective tissue around blood vessels, bronchi and gastrointestinal mucosa. These cells contain important mediators that are released, namely:

- Histamine, inflammatory activators, spasmogens, platelet activating factor, newly generated leukotrienes, prostaglandins and other factors such as *slow-reacting powerful broncho-constrictors*.

The body responds physiologically to the above mediators. Antigens in the presence of B-lymphocytes lead to proliferation of these cells; some of the lymphocytes then

(Continued overleaf)

	differentiate into memory cells and others produce antibodies. Antibodies are glycoprotein found in all tissue fluids and bodily secretions. Blood has the greatest concentration. *Antibodies are also known as immunoglobulins (Ig)*, the major groups being IgA, IgG, IgM, IgD and IgE. IgE, as mentioned previously, is mobilized as a normal defence mechanism when allergens are introduced into the body. The presence of antibodies on mast cells and basophils in the company of antigens forms antibodies. This leads to the degranulation of cells.
	An exaggerated response leads to symptoms ranging from urticarial rash to the life-threatening condition of anaphylactic shock. This is brought about by the attraction of oesinophils that causes phagocytosis to rid the body of the trouble-seeking antigen.
Cardiovascular	The combination of a fall in circulatory blood volume and marked vasodilatation causes hypotension and shock. If not reversed quickly this may have grave consequences for Laura and her unborn fetus – dependent on adequate placental perfusion to sustain its life.
	There is an increase in vascular permeability leading to oedema, resulting in facial swelling and more importantly, swelling of soft tissue around the airway.
	This increase in vascular permeability can result in more than a third of the circulating volume shifting from the intravascular to extra vascular space within minutes.
	It is the powerful mediators released by mast cells (histamine) that lead to vasodilatation peripherally, thus reducing blood flow back to the heart and resultant low BP.
	Hypoxia may affect the myocardium leading to cardiac arrhythmias noted on ECG.
Respiratory	Marked bronchospasm and laryngeal oedema may make breathing extremely difficult resulting in acute respiratory distress/arrest. Tachypnoea, wheezing or asthma-like features develop due to oedema of the smaller airways.
	Stridor occurs when there is narrowing of the upper airway (larynx).
GI tract	Ingestion of the antigen may cause marked muscle spasms and tissue oedema within the GI tract resulting in abdominal cramps, nausea/vomiting and diarrhoea.

Skin/cutaneous	Vasodilatation and leakage of fluid into the dermis, lead to flushing and urticaria.
	An isolated pruritic urticarial rash or hives may signify local skin irritation where the antigen enters the body via the skin.
	Cyanosis may result from hypoxia if there is associated respiratory or cardiovascular compromise.
Musculoskeletal	Muscle rigidity may occur.
Nervous system	Cerebral hypoxia can lead to neurological sequelae that range from apprehension and confusion to loss of consciousness.
	Seizures may occur, as may nausea and vomiting.
Renal system	Poor circulatory volume and hypotension mean that the kidneys are also compromised due to reduced renal blood flow. This and associated hypoxia result in oliguria.
Reproductive system	Hypoxia will affect the quality of uterine contractions and placental perfusion leading to fetal compromise reflected by abnormal F H R patterns.

6 **What is the significance of latex allergy in the context of maternity care?**

A Although the definitive incidence of latex allergy in the UK is unknown, studies undertaken in other countries with demographics similar to the UK, reveal an incidence of 1 per cent (Charous et al. 2002). This concurs with figures from the RCUK (2008). The AAGBI (2009a) estimates an incidence of approximately 8 per cent of the population being sensitized, which corresponds with the DH (2006) assessment that the problem is under-recognized and is on the increase nationally. Latex allergy is perhaps the most common allergic reaction reported and encountered in maternity care. A survey by the NPSA (2005) highlights 40 per cent of NHS organizations in England and Wales having no discernible latex policy in place to protect those with known sensitivity. Non-latex equipment should be readily available for use when caring for women with known allergy, e.g. BP cuffs, gloves, catheters and other medical devices.

Latex is a milky sap produced by the rubber tree, *Hevea Brasiliensis* (WAO 2009). The known risk factors as identified by AAGBI (2009a) are namely for the following:

- Repeated exposure to latex rubber, e.g. those in occupations requiring frequent use of rubber gloves.
- Individuals with severe dermatitis of the hands.

- Individuals working in industries requiring the use of protective latex gear.
- Individuals allergic to tropical fruits such as kiwi, bananas, avocado and nuts, e.g. peanuts.

The AAGBI (2009a) outlines three distinct categories of latex reactions; these are:

1 *Systemic reaction*: this allergy is life-long and is the most severe but least frequently encountered reaction, occurring in those individuals with a genetic predisposition. This hypersensitivity reaction involves specific IgE to the latex proteins. Clinical features consist of pruritus, asthma-like reaction, oedema, rhinitis and anaphylaxis. Some sensitized individuals will also react to certain fruits/food items previously outlined. It is important for the midwife to record such items at the first contact with the pregnant woman during the antenatal history taking as this will be instrumental in informing care planning and delivery as well as communicating with the other members of the interprofessional team.

2 *Contact dermatitis*: this is a T cell-mediated self-limiting reaction that does not pose a threat to the life of the individual but may act as the precursor to more severe systemic reactions. This hypersensitivity response often culminates in an eczema-type effect commencing 24–48 hours following repeated skin or mucosal contact with the additives used during latex manufacture.

3 *Clinical non-immune-mediated reaction*: this is the most frequently encountered reaction, where irritant dermatitis develops due to the effect of mild irritants, e.g. dust particulates from the presence of powder in latex gloves. The reaction is limited to the site of contact and its main features are irritation, itching and localized blistering of the skin.

7 **What is the first-line management of anaphylaxis in pregnancy?**

A   The RCUK (2008) algorithm is a helpful guideline and a useful *aide-mémoire* in the management of anaphylaxis (Figure 10.1). Key points from this algorithm in conjunction with guidance by Greater Manchester Critical Care Skills Institute (2002, 2009) and ALERT (1999) on the ABCDE skills of haemodynamic assessment in the management of any acute critical illness have been adapted as reflected in Table 10.1 (see also Case 12).

Check point

Epinephrine (adrenaline) is the drug of choice in the management of anaphylaxis in pregnant and non-pregnant adults. It is the most efficacious first-line intervention in the management of this rare life-threatening condition (RCUK 2008).

Midwives now have the legal authority to administer adrenaline via the parenteral route (intramuscular only) in the first-line management of anaphylaxis in the absence of a doctor (NMC 2011).

There are a number of useful assessment tools for measuring levels of consciousness. As identified in Table 10.1, the ABCDE approach is widely recognized as a structured and

Table 10.1 ABCDE assessment tool

	Step	*Assessment*	*Management*	
I F	Step 1 Use ABCDE approach			A S S
U N S U R E C A L L	A Airway	○ Is the airway patent/ maintained? ○ Can Laura speak? ○ Are there added noises e.g. wheezing? ○ Is there a see-sawing movement of the chest and abdomen?	○ Ensure airway is patent/maintained ○ Simple airway manoeuvres ○ Suction ○ Consider using adjuncts to airway management and positioning of Laura (minimize hypotension + fetal compromise by using wedge or left lateral tilt for airway management (Case 12), venous return and to avoid aorto-caval compression by the gravid uterus)	E S S / E V A L U A T E
F O R H E L P	B Breathing	○ Observe rate and pattern ○ Depth of respiratory breaths ○ Symmetry of chest movements ○ Use of accessory muscles ○ Laura's colour ○ Oxygen saturation	○ Oxygen via high concentration mask ○ Positioning of Laura ○ Bag-valve mask	R E S P O N S E S
F R O M M A T E R	C Circulation	○ Manual pulse/BP ○ Capillary refill time ○ Urine output/fluid balance ○ Temperature	○ IV access x 2 using wide-bore (14 gauge) cannulae ○ Obtain appropriate blood specimens (including blood glucose and mast cell tryptase) (AAGBI 2009b) ○ Blood cultures ○ IV fluids – use crystalloids and only administer colloids on instructions of anaesthetist ○ Titrate all IV fluids	A S S E S S A F T
N I T Y	D Disability	○ Conscious level using AVPU or GCS ○ Blood glucose level ○ Pupil reaction and size	○ Optimal positioning of Laura ○ Maintain homeostasis by correcting blood glucose ○ Assess for pain and palpate abdomen to distinguish between uterine contractions from other sources of abdominal pain	E R E A C H

(*Continued overleaf*)

Table 10.1 Continued

	Step	*Assessment*	*Management*	
EMERGENCY TEAM AND RECORD TIME TEAM SUMMONED	E Exposure	○ Do a head-to-toe physical examination, front/back	○ Manage abnormal findings appropriately	INTERVENTION AND LEARN LESSONS FROM THE INCIDENT
	Step 2	Perform a thorough systematic review of records, results of investigation, efficacy of management, i.e. continuously evaluate/reassess to establish whether Laura's condition is improving and whether additional members of the multidisciplinary team need to be summoned, including senior obstetrician, anaesthetist, haematologist, anaesthetists and critical care team. Regular evaluation to determine the efficacy of treatment interventions is important. Successive triennial reports on maternal deaths in the UK (Lewis and Drife 2004; Lewis 2007; CMACE 2011) recommend the use of MEOWS in monitoring and recording vital signs. This should be an integral part of critical care/high dependency care charts used in maternity care.		
	Step 3	The interprofessional team will try to establish firm diagnosis of anaphylaxis but may need to consider additional investigations to exclude other possibilities. This may include ECG, microbiology screen and other specific screening tests.		
	Step 4	It is important for the interprofessional team to debrief, review progress, complete documentation, communicate with senior colleagues, ensure psychosocial support for Laura's partner, follow infection control, health and safety and other risk management procedures including completing an untoward incident form to notify the clinical governance team. This review process is crucial if lessons are to be learnt from such critical incidents and learners should be included in these meetings. Midwives can obtain wider support from their named supervisor of midwives, a statutory requirement in the UK. Student midwives can seek additional support from their midwife mentor(s) and personal teacher. Some midwives and lecturers encourage students to access a supervisor of midwives to discuss critical incidents arising in practice to aid personal reflection on actions and continuing professional development.		
	Step 5 Follow-up	Following initial treatment, if Laura had not been previously assessed at a specialist centre, she should be referred to a specialist Allergy/Immunology centre for further investigation (AAGBI 2009a, 2009b). It is imperative that anyone presenting with suspected anaphylaxis has follow-up investigation and care determined by an agreed referral pathway by the appropriate specialist centre previously identified. Laura's General Practitioner and community-based midwife should be notified.		

Source: Adapted from ALERT (1999); Greater Manchester Critical Care Skills Institute (2002); RCUK (2008).

logical step to undertaking assessment in a systematic way (Alert 1999; Greater Manchester Critical Care Skills Institute 2002; RCUK 2008). Ongoing assessment is important to prevent further deterioration (see Case 1).

Brown et al. (2001) highlight a number of population-based studies that have reported a mortality rate of less than 1 per cent, a figure reflected by RCUK (2008). However, fatality is more common where there are co-morbidities such as asthma (WAO 2009), which might already restrict normal organ function such as lung function, that could further deteriorate as a consequence of anaphylaxis. Fetal outcome is dependent on the well-being of the mother. Laura's condition will need to be stabilized before a decision can be made on the best mode of birth; until such time, continuous electronic fetal monitoring (EFM) should be commenced as soon as possible. Following initial management, reversal of the anaphylaxis and subsequent stabilization, the safe birth of Laura's baby should be the next goal of care. Subsequent care and management should be guided by senior obstetricians and the anaesthetist and maintained by midwives skilled in high dependency care, supported by members of the interprofessional team including those specializing in critical care.

Additional assessment tools in the form of the Glasgow Coma Scale (GCS) and the AVPU method may also be used in conjunction with the initial ABCDE system.

The Glasgow Coma Scale

The Glasgow Coma Scale (Table 10.2) is a validated neurological scale that can be used to achieve objectivity and reliability when assessing Laura's level of consciousness; the scale consists of three main responses:

- eyes
- verbal
- motor.

Table 10.2 The Glasgow Coma Scale

Focus	Response					
	1	*2*	*3*	*4*	*5*	*6*
Eyes	Does not open eyes	Opens eyes in response to painful stimuli	Opens eyes in response to voice	Opens eyes spontaneously	N/A	N/A
Verbal	Makes no sounds	Incomprehensible sounds	Utters inappro- priate words	Confused, disorientated	Oriented, converses normally	N/A
Motor	Makes no movements	Extension to painful stimuli	Abnormal flexion to painful stimuli	Flexion/ withdrawal to painful stimuli	Localizes painful stimuli	Obeys commands

Source: Adapted from Kelly et al. (2005).

The three main responses relating to eyes, verbal command and motor movements are assessed separately and their total considered (see Table 10.2). A score of 3 is the lowest possible GCS sum which signifies at best a deep level of unconsciousness/coma or worse, death (Kelly et al. 2005). The maximum score is 15, indicating full levels of awareness, consciousness and alertness, i.e. the individual is fully awake.

The AVPU Scale

The AVPU Scale (Greater Manchester Critical Care Skills Institute 2002) can be used to determine whether Laura is **A**lert and responsive to both **V**erbal and **P**ainful stimuli, and whether she is **U**nresponsive. This scale is easier to use than the GCS and produces similarly accurate results (Kelly et al. 2005). Hence the AVPU neurological assessment scale is favoured by many maternity units and critical care teams.

Check points

- All health care professionals involved in maternity care should be familiar with an algorithm for managing anaphylaxis, by having their knowledge and skills regularly updated via skills and drills training (Lewis and Drife 2004; Lewis 2007; CMACE 2011).
- The management of anaphylaxis during pregnancy is the same as in non-parturient women. It calls for prompt recognition, and swift, intelligent, aggressive management, to obviate any chance of maternal and fetal demise.

CASE REVIEW

Laura's care was effective due to the management being premised on the following:

- Early recognition and reporting of risk factors coupled with the onset of serious illness followed by thorough assessment, prompt referral and timely intervention/resuscitative measures/first-line treatment of anaphylaxis.
- Good communication within the multidisciplinary team to ensure early mobilization of the maternity emergency team in order to realize prompt involvement of senior staff, e.g. midwives, obstetrician, anaesthetist, neonatologist and haemotologist. This determined clear referral pathways and ensured treatment plans were mobilized.
- Contemporaneous and thorough record keeping.
- Use of the MEOWS chart to record all observations and to report deviation from normality (NICE 2007b).

Summary of key points

- Preparedness: anaphylaxis is a rare but acute, severe, multi-system, life-threatening hypersensitivity reaction that culminates in a maternity emergency.
- Efforts to identify the causative factor of anaphylaxis are crucial to prevent further occurrences.
- Immediate/prompt call for help must be mobilized.
- Epinephrine (adrenaline) therapy is the first-line drug in the management of maternal collapse due to anaphylaxis and is the most efficacious intervention.
- Use of the ABCDE approach to initial assessment and treatment with regular evaluation of the efficacy of each intervention is vital (Greater Manchester Critical Care Skills Institute 2002).
- Record keeping should include systematic documentation of all actions taken, outcome and health care professionals involved in the management of the emergency including their designation.
- Latex-free gloves and other medical devices should be considered as an important risk management priority in an effort to minimize exposure to latex-sensitive women and health care workers (NPSA 2005).
- Follow-up and further investigation by a specialist allergy clinic where there is no previous referral/history of severe allergic reaction are necessary.
- To avoid further episodes of anaphylaxis, individuals with a known allergy should be educated to carry an epinephrine injector pen at all times, with family and friends of the affected individual also educated in its use (WAO 2009).

(RCUK 2008; AAGBI 2009b)

REFERENCES

ALERT (1999) *ABCDE Method of Assessment*. Available at: http://www.alert-course.com/course-information/the-alert-system-of-assessment (accessed 20 November 2010).

Association of Anaesthetists of Great Britain and Ireland (AAGBI) (2009a) *Suspected Anaphylactic Reactions Associated with Anaesthesia*. London: AAGBI. Available at: http://www.aagbi.org (accessed 20 November 2010).

Association of Anaesthetists of Great Britain and Ireland (AAGBI) (2009b) *Management of a Patient with Suspected Anaphylaxis during Anaesthesia: Safety Drill*. London: AAGBI.

Brown, A.F., McKinnon, D. and Chu, K. (2001) Emergency department anaphylaxis: review of 142 patients in a single year, *Journal of Allergy and Clinical Immunology*, 108(5): 861–6.

Charous, B.L., Blanco, C., Tarlo, S., Hamilton, R.G., Baur, X., Beezhold, D., Sussman, G. and Yunginger, J.W. (2002) Natural rubber latex allergy after 12 years: recommendations and perspectives, *Journal of Allergy and Clinical Immunology*, 109(1): 31–4.

Clark, S.L., Hankins, D.A., Dudley, D.A., Dildy, G.A. and Porter, T.F. (1995) Amniotic fluid embolism: analysis of the national registry, *American Journal of Obstetrics and Gynecology*, 172: 1158–67.

CMACE (2011) *Saving Mothers' Lives: Reviewing Maternal Deaths to Make Motherhood Safer: 2006–2008. The Eighth Report of the Confidential Enquiries into Maternal Deaths in the*

United Kingdom. Ed. G. Lewis. *BJOG: An International British Journal of Obstetrics and Gynaecology,* 118 (Suppl. 1): 1–203.

Department of Health (2006) *A Review of Services for Allergy: The Epidemiology, Demand for and Provision of Treatment and Effectiveness of Clinical Interventions.* Available at: http://www.dh.gov. uk (accessed 27 August 2010).

European Academy of Allergology and Clinical Immunology (EAAI) (2010) *Drug Allergy (2010).* Available at: http://www.eaaci.net (accessed 20 November 2010).

Greater Manchester Critical Care Skills Institute (2002) *Acute Illness Management. AIM Course Manual,* 3rd edn. Manchester: Greater Manchester Critical Care Skills Institute.

Greater Manchester Critical Care Skills Institute (2009) *Critical Care Institute Annual Report.* Available at: http://www.gmcriticalcareskillsinstitute.org.uk (accessed 20 November 2010).

Kelly, C.A., Upex, A. and Bateman, D.N. (2005) Comparison of consciousness level assessment in the poisoned patient using the alert, verbal, painful, unresponsive scale and the Glasgow Coma Scale, *Annals of Emergency medicine,* 45(2). Available at: http://www.medscape.com/medline/ abstract/15278081 (accessed 24 September 2010).

Lewis, G. (ed.) (2007) *The Confidential Enquiry into Maternal and Child Health (CEMACH). Saving Mothers' Lives: Reviewing Maternal Deaths to Make Motherhood Safer, 2003–2005. The Seventh Report on Confidential Enquiries into Maternal Deaths in the United Kingdom.* London: CEMACH. Available at: http://www.cmace.org.uk (accessed 27 August 2010).

Lewis, G. and Drife, J. (eds) (2004) *Why Mothers Die, 2000–2002: The Sixth Report of the Confidential Enquiries into Maternal Deaths in the United Kingdom.* Available at: http://www.cmace.org.uk (accessed 27 August 2010).

Lieberman, P. (2005) Biphasic anaphylactic reactions, *Annals of Allergy, Asthma and Immunology,* 95(3): 21–6.

Mattson Porth, C. (2007) *Essentials of Pathophysiology: Concepts of Altered Health States,* 2nd edn. Philadelphia, PA: Lippincott Williams & Wilkins.

McClure, J. and Cooper, G. (2011) Anaesthesia, in CMACE *Saving Mothers' Lives: Reviewing Maternal Deaths to Make Motherhood Safer: 2006–2008. The Eighth Report of the Confidential Enquiries into Maternal Deaths in the United Kingdom.* Ed. G. Lewis. *BJOG: An International British Journal of Obstetrics and Gynaecology,* 118 (Suppl. 1): 102–8.

National Institute for Health and Clinical Excellence (2007a) *Intrapartum Care: Care of Healthy Women and Their Babies.* Clinical Guidance No. 55. London: NICE.

National Institute for Health and Clinical Excellence (2007b) *Acutely Ill Patients in Hospitals: Recognition of and Response to Acute Illness in Adults in Hospital.* Clinical Guidance No. 50. London: NICE.

National Patient Safety Agency (NPSA) (2005) *Protecting People with Allergy Associated with Latex.* Available at: http://www.npsa.nhs.uk (accessed November 2010).

Nursing and Midwifery Council (NMC) (2011) *Changes to Midwives Exemptions,* NMC Circular 07/2011. Available at: http://www.nmc-uk.org (accessed August 2011).

Powrie, R.O. (2010) Anaphylactic shock in pregnancy, in M.A. Belfort, G.R. Saade, M.R. Foley, J.P. Phelan and G.A. Dildy (eds) *Critical Care Obstetrics,* 5th edn. Chichester: Wiley-Blackwell.

Resuscitation Council (RCUK) (2008) *Emergency Treatment of Anaphylactic Reactions and Guidelines for Health Care Providers.* Available at: http://www.resus.org.uk (accessed 20 May 2010).

Tuffnell, D.J. and Hamilton, S. (2008) Amniotic fluid embolism, *Obstetrics, Gynaecology and Reproductive Medicine,* 18(8): 213–16.

World Allergy Organization (WAO) (2009) *Allergic Reactions to Latex.* Available at: http://worldallergy.org (accessed 10 October 2010).

ANNOTATED FURTHER READING

Chaudhuri, K., Gonzales, J., Jesrun, C.A. and Ambat, M.T. (2008) Anaphylactic shock in pregnancy; a case study and review of the literature, *International Journal of Obstetric Anaesthesia*, 17(4): 350–7.

A helpful review.

Lieberman, P., Kemp, S.F., Oppenheimer, J., Lang, D.M., Bernstein, L. and Nicklas, R.A. (2005) The diagnosis and management of anaphylaxis: an updated practice parameter, *Journal of Clinical Immunology*, 115(3): S483–S523.

A comprehensive guide to the management of anaphylaxis.

McNarry, A.F. and Bateman, D.N. (2004) Simple bedside assessment of level of consciousness: comparison of two simple assessment scales with the Glasgow Coma Scale, *Anaesthesia*, 59(1): 34. DOI:10.1111/j.1365-2044.2004.03526.x. Available at: http://www.medscape.com/medline/abstract/14687096 (accessed 24 March 2010).

Provides useful explanation for basis of neurological assessment scales.

USEFUL WEBSITES

http://www.aagbi.org	The Association of Anaesthetists of Great Britain and Ireland
http://www.alert-course.com	ALERT system of assessment
http://www.allergyfoundation.com	British Allergy Foundation
http://www.anaphylaxis.org.uk	The Anaphylaxis Campaign
http://www.bsaci.org	The British Society for Allergy and Clinical Immunology
http://www.dh.gov.uk	UK Department of Health, England
http://www.eaaci.net	The European Academy of Allergology and Clinical Immunology
http://www.gmcriticalcareskillsinstitute.org.uk	Greater Manchester Critical Care Skills Institute
http://www.institute.nhs.uk	NHS Institute for Innovation and Improvement
http://www.npeu.ox.ac.uk/mbrrace-uk	National Perinatal Epidemiology Unit (former CMACE [Confidential Enquiries into Maternal and Child Enquiries] reports can be accessed from this website)
http://www.resus.org.uk	Resuscitation Council UK
http://www.worldallergy.org	The World Allergy Organization

CASE STUDY 11
Sepsis
Maureen D. Raynor

Pre-requisites for the chapter: the reader should have an understanding of:

- Immunology/the inflammatory response including the body's natural defence against infection.
- Normal haematological indices including the rationale for the routine blood investigations performed during pregnancy.
- The physiological changes in the major bodily systems during pregnancy and maternal physiological adaptation.
- Resuscitation – basic/advanced life support of adult and neonate.
- The differences between crystalloids and colloids as intravenous fluids.
- The MEOWS assessment chart.
- Value of SBAR as a communication tool in the interprofessional team.
- The public health role of the midwife in health education/promotion, especially the prevention of infection.

Pre-reading self-assessment

1 Define cardiac output and stroke volume.
2 What is meant by shock?
3 List the different types/causes of shock and compare and contrast their clinical features and management.
4 What is the inflammatory response?
5 Identify the different types of white blood cells (WBCs) and discuss their role in fighting infection.
6 Refer to the recognized international definition and classification relating to maternal deaths and define direct, indirect, coincidental and late death.

Recommended prior reading

Baldwin, K.M., Cheek, D.J. and Morris, S.E. (2006) Shock, multiple organ dysfunction syndrome, and burns in adults, in K.L. McCance and S.E. Huether (eds) *Pathophysiology: The Biologic Basis for Disease in Adults and Children,* 5th edn. Philadelphia: Elsevier/Mosby, pp. 1625–49.

Department of Health (DH) (2009) *Competencies for Recognising and Responding to Acutely Ill Patients in Hospital.* London: DH. Available at: http://www.institute.nhs.uk

(Continued overleaf)

175

Ferns, T. (2007) Shock and the critically ill woman, in M. Billington and M. Stevenson (eds) *Critical Care in Childbearing for Midwives*. Chichester: Wiley-Blackwell, pp. 140–66.

National Institute for Health and Clinical Excellence (NICE) (2007) *Acutely Ill Patients in Hospitals: Recognition of and Response to Acute Illness in Adults in Hospital*. Clinical Guidance No. 50. London: NICE. Available at: http://www.nice.org.uk

NHS Institute for Innovation and Improvement (2008) *SBAR: Situation, Background, Assessment, Recommendation*. Available at: http://www.institute.nhs.uk (accessed 12 January 2011).

CASE STUDY

Fiona is a 27-year-old primigravida and nursery school teacher. At 34 weeks gestation she contacted her community midwife complaining of a sore throat, feeling shivery and achy akin to 'flu-like' symptoms. She also reported nausea, vomiting, abdominal pain and generally feeling unwell. The midwife suspected sepsis on account of the symptoms Fiona described, and contacted the hospital. She arranged for Fiona to be transported via ambulance to be assessed and reviewed at the local consultant-led maternity unit. Fiona's vital signs assessed by the midwife and paramedics prior to her admission to hospital were: pulse 90 bpm, BP 100/60, RR 16 breaths per min., T 35°C; no urine specimen was obtained for urinalysis as she was unable to void.

Having been alerted in advance of Fiona's admission (by the labour suite coordinating midwife) about the community midwife's suspicion of sepsis, an experienced midwife, senior obstetrician and an anaesthetist were on stand-by. The neonatal team, theatre team and haematology department were also notified of Fiona's imminent arrival.

Prior to arrival at hospital, Fiona's condition quickly deteriorated as reflected by her vital signs recorded by the paramedics en route to hospital: BP 70/40 mmHg, pulse 116 bpm, RR 22 breaths per min., T 36.4°C. Fearing haemodynamic instability, the paramedics commenced O_2 therapy, sited a peripheral IV cannula and commenced an infusion of crystalloids.

On arrival at hospital, a second IV cannula was sited; blood cultures and other swabs were taken for microbiology investigations. After excluding any known allergies from Fiona's history, she received a stat dose of a broad spectrum IV antibiotic. A diagnosis of severe sepsis was later confirmed via laboratory investigations.

1   **What is the meaning of sepsis, severe sepsis and septic shock?**

A   Although imprecise, a universal definition of *sepsis, severe sepsis* and *septic shock* was established in 1991 and subsequently revised, having achieved international attention as a direct result of the evidence-based practice guidelines of the Surviving Sepsis Campaign (SSC: available at http://www.survivingsepsis.org) and discussed by Levy et al. (2010). Having an understanding of the classification of sepsis helps in the comprehension of its underlying pathophysiology, determining the severity of the condition and mobilizing standardized evidence-based treatment (Daniels and Nutbeam 2010). It is important to note, however, that due to ongoing research into sepsis, an international definition of the term continues to develop, just like the illness, which is best construed as a dynamic process representing a broad spectrum of an illness along a defined continuum.

Sepsis

Sepsis is a cunning, insidious and non-specific illness, best defined, according to Daniels and Nutbeam (2010), as a systemic inflammatory response syndrome (SIRS) precipitated by the presence of a new infection or if two or more clinical features of SIRS criteria exist. This definition is supported by Clutton-Brock (2011) who, writing on behalf of CMACE, states that sepsis simply means the presence of SIRS alongside an identifiable pathogenic microbial organism. The term is also used to describe an individual with or without organ dysfunction who presents with signs and symptoms suggestive of bacteraemia. Despite intensive efforts at prevention, early recognition and management, this rare, severe and complex clinical syndrome remains a challenge. Sepsis is still a life-threatening critical illness resulting in many fatalities within both maternity and critical care departments globally (Remick 2007; Clutton-Brock 2011).

Severe sepsis

This phase is a continuum of sepsis and the term used when there is major organ dysfunction (Galvagno 2003). There may be dysfunction of one organ or multiple organ dysfunction syndrome (MODS). This clinical state may be precipitated by several causes, namely:

- Tissue hypoperfusion or hypotension leading to serious consequences such as renal dysfunction (oliguria/anuria), metabolic acidosis and noticeable encephalopathy such as the acute alteration in mental state.
- Adult respiratory distress syndrome (ARDS) resulting in respiratory insufficiency and poor tissue oxygenation leading to hypoxia, ischaemia and metabolic acidosis.
- DIC as outlined previously in Case 5.

Septic shock

This is the most severe stage in the sepsis cascade; it arises from marked arterial hypotension that fails to respond to fluid resuscitation, necessitating the use of vasopressors. There is usually underlying organ dysfunction and clinical features of hypoperfusion and hypotension, as outlined in the definition for severe sepsis detailed by Galvagno (2003) who provides a simplified definition of the sepsis cascade (Figure 11.1).

To aid in the recognition of sepsis, Garrod et al. (2011) devised the following mnemonic:

> *SIRS = 3 Ts white with sugar*
> *Temperature (> 38 or < 36°C)*
> *Tachycardia (> 90 bpm)*
> *Tachypnoea (> 20 breaths per min.)*
> *White* blood cell count (< 4 × 10^9 cells/L or > 12 × 10^9 cells/L)
> *Sugar* – blood glucose (> 7.7 mmol in the absence of diabetes mellitus)

Although sepsis is considered to represent three distinct stages as outlined above, the literature presents a conflicting view at times such as Nelson et al. (2009) who identify four main

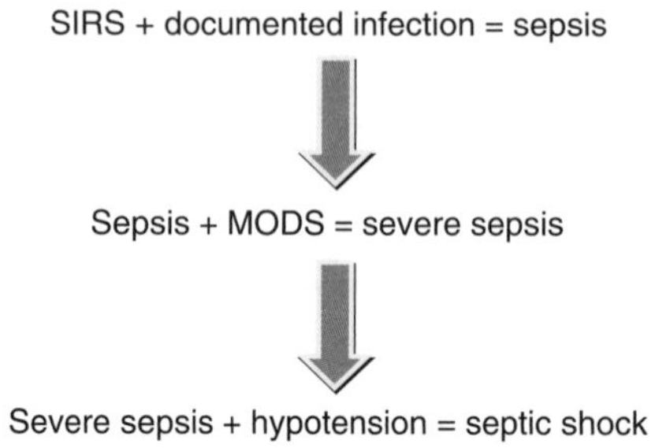

SIRS + documented infection = sepsis

Sepsis + MODS = severe sepsis

Severe sepsis + hypotension = septic shock

Figure 11.1 Overview of the sepsis continuum

Source: Adapted from Galvagno (2003: 205).

stages of sepsis (Table 11.1). However, in the UK, reflective of NICE (2007) guidelines on the care of the acutely ill patient, derangements in the physiology of Fiona should be given initial consideration in both community and hospital settings.

Check point

Sepsis is cunning and moves fast. *Beware of sepsis – be aware of sepsis* (Harper 2011).

Table 11.1 The four main stages of sepsis

Stage	Indications
Stage 1 – SIRS	As the name suggests this is a systemic inflammation resulting from any major insult to the body, e.g. trauma caused from surgery such as LSCS or perineal wound, in which two or more of the vital signs outlined by Garrod et al. (2011) are present + elevated WBC count leading to leukocytosis, leucopenia and raised plasma C-reactive protein > 2 SD above normal values. Clutton-Brock (2011) states that SIRS is confirmed if the WBC is < 4 × 10^9 cells/L or > 12× 10^9 cells/L in non-pregnant women.
	Early recognition and rapid response to the treatment of sepsis at this initial stage will prevent severe sepsis/septic shock developing.

CMACE (2010) highlights the importance of midwives and doctors providing women with health education information about the potential risk of sepsis and its prevention, especially if exposed to young children, family members or general members of the public suffering from sore throat/upper respiratory tract infection. Community-acquired beta-haemolytic *Streptococcus* and infections from group A *Streptococcus pyogenes* were found to play a significant part in the increased number of maternal deaths in the 2006–2008 confidential enquiries into maternal deaths triennial report (Harper 2011).

Stage 2 – Sepsis	Sepsis is identified by the presence of two signs and symptoms outlined above in stage 1, along with suspected or diagnosed infection. The exact aetiology of the infection is not always identified. Thus in order to stave off MODS, there should be no delay in treatment once SIRS is suspected.

Midwives, whether working in the community or hospital setting, should not delay in liaising and referring the woman to the obstetric team at the local maternity consultant-led unit. Early hospitalization means appropriate broad spectrum antibiotic therapy can then be implemented while awaiting result of blood cultures. Proper measures will then be taken to closely monitor vital signs in order to detect signs of organ dysfunction or failure. Any delay in treatment will slow the treatment of sepsis. Harper (2011) states that initial blood culture might be negative, placing emphasis on the need to repeat these blood tests.

Stage 3 – Severe Sepsis	Severe sepsis occurs when a woman who meets the sepsis criteria detailed above develops features suggestive of organ dysfunction e.g. brain, heart, liver, lung, and kidneys.

This stage is confirmed if the woman develops one of the clinical features of organ dysfunction.

It is best to consider the effects of severe sepsis in a systematic way as outlined below:

- Insult to the brain will manifest as neurological changes affecting the woman's mental state and level of consciousness. Cerebral alterations in the form of ischaemia, micro-abscesses, micro-thrombi or haemorrhage may lead to some signs of encephalopathy/alteration in mental state e.g. agitation, confusion, restlessness and possibly coma. Assessment of mental status to determine degree of arousal and responsiveness can be assessed using the *AVPU* method of assessment (see Cases 2 and 10).
- The pathophysiological changes in the CVS may result in a drop in systolic BP (< 90 mmHG), MAP < 65 mmHG, a fall in baseline BP > 30–40 mmHG. Mitchell and Whitehouse (2010) state that CVS changes are most critical. These combined with anuria and acute renal failure, are not uncommon and very testing indeed. However, haemodynamic stability can be achieved if the woman recovers and organ function returns to normal.
- Haematological alterations: reduced platelet count by up to 50% in a matter of days, acutely abnormal prothrombin time or PTT in the absence of any thromboprophylaxis. This may trigger the onset of DIC (Case 5).
- Hepatic/liver changes (hyperbilirubinaemia) – the pathophysiology of severe sepsis may signal an abnormal alteration in serum bilirubin levels > 4 mg/dL or 70 mmol/L and alkaline phosphatase level > 250 units per litre.
- Respiratory changes: Respiratory rate > 24 breaths per minute.

(*Continued overleaf*)

Table 11.1 Continued

Stage	Indications
	• Renal disruptions: oliguria/anuria, risk of fluid overload and electrolyte imbalance may occur + ↑ creatinine level of 0.5 mg/dL.
	• Metabolic acidosis with serum lactate levels > 4 mmol/L as identified by the SSC/sepsis bundles (Dellinger et al 2008).

Once severe sepsis is recognized aggressive treatment in a high dependency/critical care area where there is highly trained and skilled staff in the management of life-threatening illnesses is crucial for the woman's survival. Aided by CVP line, the modified MEOWS and SBAR tool, systems for assessing levels of consciousness such as the AVPU, and ABCDE assessment tools outlined in previous cases should be employed to assess, monitor, evaluate, record and communicate findings relating to vital signs within the interprofessional team. The woman will need oxygen therapy if her oxygen saturation levels fall + catheterization with hourly urine measurements calculated at 0.5 mL/kg/ hour documented on the fluid balance/ MEOWS chart. The anaesthetic team will guide much of the resuscitative and maintenance interventions implemented. This structured approach is crucial to the woman's survival.

Stage 4 – Septic shock   Of all the four stages of sepsis, septic shock is the most critical, having the highest mortality rate. It is defined as severe sepsis with marked hypotension with systolic BP < 90 mmHg + the individual's condition fails to respond to fluid resuscitation, indicative of marked organ dysfunction/failure.

This stage is extremely challenging to manage and the chance of survival is very slim. The aim of treatment should be prevention. Women who develop septic shock will need assisted ventilation and care in an intensive care unit informed by local and national guidelines such as sepsis *resuscitation* and *management* bundles (Dellinger et al. 2008).

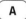 **2**   **How would you account for the epidemiology of sepsis?**

A   Despite improvements in maternity care resulting in a significant decline in maternal morbidity and mortality over the course of several decades (Lewis and Drife 2004; Lewis 2007; CMACE 2011), sepsis remains a real threat in the childbearing context. As outlined by Fiona's case, sepsis represents a wide spectrum of severity amounting to an urgent critical illness and challenging maternity emergency. Maternal physiological adaptation to pregnancy may mask the early onset of the illness until it reaches a critical stage where management becomes futile (Harper 2011). Not surprisingly, the increased mortality rate linked to sepsis makes it the leading cause of direct maternal deaths in the UK (CMACE 2011), at the time of writing. Although recent evidence signifies an increase in the incidence of sepsis as depicted by the trends in the 2006–2008 triennial report on maternal mortality in the UK (CMACE 2011), it is still an uncommon encounter in contemporary practice. Nonetheless, sepsis, when it does occur is a force to be reckoned with. It is associated with increased morbidity and costs (Linde-Zwirble and Angus 2004); the highest price paid may ultimately result in maternal demise. More generally, but equally troubling, is the estimation by Daniels et al. (2010) in their observational cohort study, that the escalating scale of sepsis in the UK in the wider population is likely to result in approximately 37,000 deaths annually.

3 What are the early warning signs of sepsis?

A The early warning signs of sepsis that should trigger a rapid response are previously discussed in Table 11.1 but are summarized again in Box 11.1 to ensure vigilance in identification when assessing, monitoring, reporting and recording vital signs. Fiona presents with a number of worrying signs and symptoms that were not ignored.

Box 11.1 Early warning signs of sepsis

Extremes of body temperature i.e. hypothermia < 36°C or hyperthermia > 38.3°C accompanied by chills/rigours. There may also be noticeable skin changes such as development of a rash or skin feeling unusually warm/cold and clammy to touch.

Disruption to the CVS leading to tachycardia, hypotension and altered tissue perfusion.

Altered respiration as the woman has difficulty breathing with onset of shallow breaths or hyperventilation. Tachypnoea may manifest as a compensatory mechanism.

Neurological changes affecting the brain leading to lethargy, fatigue, general malaise/weakness at best, and to confusion and subsequently coma at worst, especially if sepsis is not recognized and treated early.

(International Sepsis Forum 2003; Sepsis Alliance 2010; Clutton-Brock 2011; Harper 2011)

---

4 What are the common sources of sepsis during pregnancy?

A These are listed in Box 11.2; it is important to remember that any risk factor for infection will escalate the dangers for a pregnant woman such as Fiona, who is already immuno-compromised as a result of her pregnant state. The midwife should be conversant with factors that impact on cellular and humoral immunity such as co-morbidities or underlying medical disorders, e.g. diabetes mellitus, human immunodeficiency virus, renal disease and surgical wounds, as well as women receiving therapeutic interventions (e.g. corticosteroid therapy). Iatrogenic factors that are associated with nosocomial infection should also be considered, e.g. CVP lines, endotracheal tubes and urinary catheters all disturb mucosal and cutaneous integrity.

Box 11.2 Common sources of sepsis during pregnancy

Pyelonephritis
Chorioamnionitis
Upper respiratory tract infections
Septic abortion
Renal calculi
Pancreatitis
Cholecystitis
Postpartum infections associated with surgical operations, i.e. caesarean section or episiotomy wound/incision and complex perineal trauma such as 3rd or 4th degree tear.

(Sheffield 2004; Guinn et al. 2007)

---

5 **What are the causative organisms commonly associated with sepsis?**

A Infection may be associated with Gram-positive or Gram-negative bacteria, fungi or viruses (Box 11.3). Gram-positive bacteria such as *Streptococcus pneumoniae*, Group A *Streptococcus* (GAS) and *Staphylococcus aureus* are more commonly associated with sepsis than Gram-negative microbes such as *E. coli* and *Klebsiella*. A community-acquired infection such as GAS is particularly pervasive (CMACE 2010).

Box 11.3 Causative organisms associated with sepsis

- Beta-haemolytic *streptococcus*/group A *Streptococcus pyogenes* (GAS)
- *Haemophilus influenzae*
- *Staphylococcus aureus*
- Methicillin-resistant *Staphylococcus aureus* (MRSA)
- *Streptococcus pneumoniae*
- *Morganella morganii*
- *Escherichia coli* (*E. coli*)
- *Pseudomonas aeruginosa*
- *Klebsiella*
- *Clostridium sordelli*
- *Clostridium difficile*
- *Clostridium septicum*

(Harrison et al. 2006)

It is important to note that GAS, a community-acquired infection, has played a significant part in the rise in maternal mortality associated with sepsis. This organism is a particular threat during the winter months and is a common cause of sore throat in young children. The spread of the organism is by direct contact or droplet transmission and approximately 5–30 per cent of the general population are carriers, with GAS being transported on the skin or throat (Harper 2011).

6 **A differential diagnosis should be considered in all critical illness. There may be several explanations for Fiona's illness; what are they?**

A Although severe sepsis is confirmed in Fiona's case, her initial signs and symptoms are relatively non-specific. Though tachycardic and tachypnoeic, she is neither hypothermic nor pyrexial. Therefore, her clinical features could be due to a host of causes. 'Flu-like' symptoms are an indication of infection, whether bacterial or viral in nature or related to another inflammatory process. Nausea and vomiting with abdominal pain could be related to a problem with the GI tract or renal system. For these reasons it is important to rule out other causes (Box 11.4).

Box 11.4 Differential diagnosis

Influenza
Pneumonia
Acute pancreatitis
Acute gastroenteritis
Pyelonephritis or other acute urinary tract infection
Acute appendicitis
Acute cholecystitis.

Underlying co-morbidities will have a profound effect on sepsis, not least because pre-existing medical disorders might be further impacted by the onset of a SIRS process. Such individuals, according to Blomqvist (2011), are associated with a higher mortality rate.

Fiona works as a nursery school teacher. Being pregnant means that she would be susceptible to contracting any upper respiratory tract infections passed on by the young children in her care, making her vulnerable to acquiring sepsis. Laboratory and bedside investigations will assist with confirming the diagnosis.

7 **What is the pathophysiology of sepsis?**

A The pathophysiology of sepsis is complex, conflicting and poorly understood. Some of the changes that disrupt normal physiology are previously discussed in Table 11.1. Popular theories partly explain the course of the illness but are still interpreted as ill-defined and inconsistent in relation to the part played by each individual factor in the sepsis cascade. Consequently, it is suggested that multiple derangements exist in sepsis involving a variety of bodily organs (Daniels 2009; Mitchell and Whitehouse 2010).

The response an individual makes to the onset of sepsis is partly genetic and largely biphasic in nature (Saade 2004; Blomqvist 2011). The marked SIRS overwhelms the immune system causing the release of proteins likened to 'a cytokine storm' (Clutton-Brock 2011: 174). Ultimately this may lead to a destructive cascade, including MODS or organ failure plus untimely death. Hence the need for prompt recognition, timely referral coupled with early and efficacious management (Saade 2004; Remick 2007; Dellinger et al. 2008).

The stages of sepsis, as detailed in Table 11.1, are best presented as a continuum; to do otherwise, Daniels (2009) and Daniels and Nutbeam (2010) suggest, is tantamount to being over-simplistic. The flow diagram outlined in Figure 11.2 provides a basic overview of sepsis.

Sepsis is an enigma. Inflammation is the body's normal default response to infection. Well adults are usually equipped with an arsenal of defence to ward off threats against invading microorganisms. With sepsis, this early physiological response to infection is lost, culminating in a systemic and inappropriate inflammatory reaction which is both of overwhelming proportions and detrimental to the individual's immune system (Hotchkiss and Karl 2003; Russell 2006; Daniels 2009).

The resulting SIRS leads to neutrophils, monocytes, macrophages and platelets binding to endothelial cells. Endothelial cells are chiefly responsible for selective permeability to

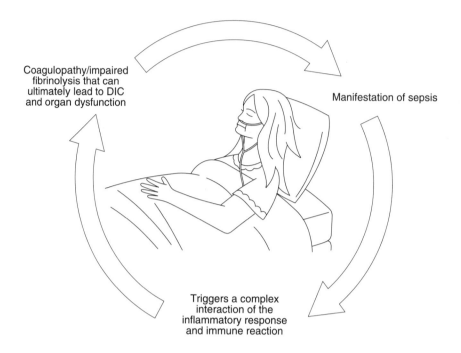

Figure 11.2 Overview of sepsis syndrome

ensure vaso-regulation and act as an anticoagulant interface. Marked phagocytosis occurs, and the combination with leucocytes leads to further release of cytokines and increased vasoconstriction or vasodilatation (Saade 2004).

The pathogenesis of sepsis results in marked capillary permeability or 'leaky' vessels (due to the endothelial damage) and an activated coagulation cascade. These changes lead to mitochondrial disruption in the cells, cell damage and development of micro-thrombi. Cytokines also aid in the stimulation of the liver plus an increase in the production of C-reactive protein (Clutton-Brock 2011).

In summary, sepsis results in altered cardiovascular function due to the development of 'leaky' capillaries leading to reduced blood flow. The presence of any bacterial infection in the blood is known as bacteraemia, becoming septicaemia when the presence of the bacteria in the bloodstream actively multiplies at an alarming rate, escalating to a state that totally debilitates the individual resulting in septic shock (Daniels 2009; Nelson et al. 2009).

8 **What are the main principles of care in the management of sepsis?**

A Expeditious management of Fiona should be premised on the key *resuscitation* and *management* sepsis care bundles as outlined by the Sepsis Alliance (2010), Levy et al. (2010) and Dellinger et al. (2008). Implementation of the Surviving Sepsis Campaign (SSC) recommendations allows the interprofessional team involved in the management of sepsis to standardize their approach to care, following the sequence, timing and goals spelt out by each care bundle. In the first six hours, energy should be focused on goal-directed therapy, where a variety of approaches to management will be necessary to meet Fiona's needs as 'one size does not fit all' (Figure 11.3). Implementation of early goal-directed therapy is associated with a reduction in MODS and mortality (Russell 2006; Guinn et al. 2007; Townsend et al. 2008; Trzeciak et al. 2008).

The Sepsis Alliance (2010) define a 'bundle' as a group of simple, realistic, pragmatic and uniformed approaches to the treatment/management of a given disease. The individual element of each bundle is founded on the best evidence-based practices available. Thus the SSC care bundles are the epitome of the evidence-based principles or recommendations that can be universally instituted and, when implemented together, may result in maximum outcomes better than if implemented individually (Daniels et al. 2010). Individual hospitals can customize the recommendations in the formulation of local clinical guidelines.

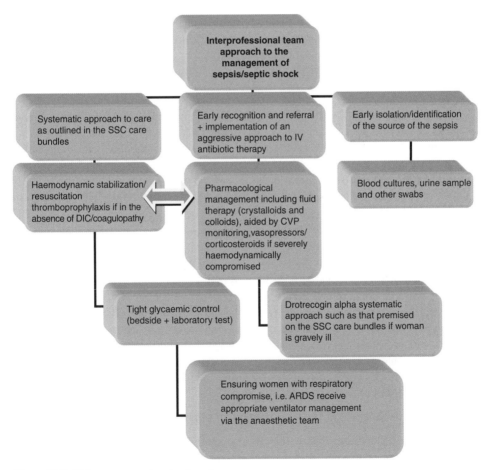

Figure 11.3 Main management goals of sepsis

Early identification/assessment/referral

Early identification/assessment/referral are a crucial part of management in the critically ill to identify the problem. Early identification is paramount as it determines the need for referral, which then triggers speed, extent and urgency of treatment. The challenge, however, as highlighted in the 2006–2008 triennial report on maternal mortality in the UK (CMACE 2011) is that young, healthy pregnant women, such as Fiona, have considerable physiological reserves that may conceal the early warning signs of critical illness, not least sepsis. Assessment plays an important role in decision making as to which element of the sepsis bundles in conjunction with other appropriate interventions will be specifically mobilized to care for Fiona. Careful assessment, monitoring and evaluation of the efficacy of each intervention are necessary to determine the success at each stage.

As stated previously, the ABCDE and AVPU methods of assessment, documented in other cases of the book, are useful in assessing, monitoring, recording and reporting Fiona's vital signs and neurological condition.

The sheer scale and gravity of sepsis must never be underestimated. Nelson et al. (2009) place emphasis on the onset and progression of this critical illness, stating that its subtleties and nuances may be underplayed at the health professional's peril. The onset of sepsis may very well be subtle in its initial stages, but its escalation is known to be rapid and often deadly without due recognition, swift referral and prompt treatment. To highlight the enormity of the problem CMACE (2010: 1) issued an advance briefing to doctors and midwives in the UK with the following warning:

> Sepsis in pregnancy is often insidious in onset but can progress very rapidly. In the postpartum period the risk of serious sepsis should not be overlooked, particularly in the earlier gestations. Early recognition, urgent transfer to hospital and prompt, aggressive treatment is necessary to save lives. Whilst presentation may be atypical, tachypnoea, neutropenia and hypothermia are ominous signs. Diarrhoea is a common symptom of pelvic sepsis and the combination of abdominal and absent fetal heart rate may signify sepsis rather than placental abruption.

Galvagno and Camann (2009) outline the challenge to early recognition of sepsis and management of the critically ill pregnant woman. This is partly because the physiological changes during pregnancy predispose the woman to a number of critical conditions such as VTE episodes, which may complicate the picture and make diagnosis difficult. This highlights the importance of skilful and intelligent management of all women who present with any deviation from normality during pregnancy, labour and the postpartum period.

In summary, the main aim of management is early goal-directed therapy, the majority of which can be achieved via high level care in the maternity unit to stabilize Fiona prior to expediting birth to continue maternal treatment and any subsequent transfer to critical care/ ITU, should the need arise.

9   **What is the midwife's role in the management of sepsis?**

A   The midwife has a significant role to play as a key member of the interprofessional team in the recognition, reporting and management of any critical illness arising in midwifery practice.

The chapter on sepsis by Harper (2011: 85) in the triennial report from CMACE on maternal deaths in the UK (CMACE 2011) emphasizes that midwives and doctors involved in maternity care have a duty to 'be aware of sepsis – beware of sepsis'. This means the midwife must always have a high index of suspicion when caring for any woman such as Fiona, who presents with abdominal pain, sore throat, 'flu-like' symptoms, diarrhoea, vomiting or extremes of body temperature. The midwife also needs to be equipped with an arsenal of skills in her vigilance to recognize early signs of infection during pregnancy, labour or puerperium, e.g. mastitis, offensive vaginal discharge/liquor, lochia, or, at birth, an unexpectedly compromised baby.

The midwife should obtain a full and detailed history, document and refer deviations from normality to the obstetrician (NMC 2004), as well as take appropriate swabs for microbiology investigation from areas such as the genital tract, perineum, ear, throat and skin as per local guidelines. A urine sample should also be obtained and sent for laboratory analysis to isolate possible pathogens responsible for any underlying infection. This can be done at the time of insertion of the urinary catheter to obtain hourly urine measures.

Any pregnant woman postpartum with a LSCS or perineal wound, who cares for young children, is at risk of developing upper respiratory tract infections especially during the winter months, as previously mentioned, due to GAS infection (CMACE 2010). The midwife is best placed to provide health education information about the risk of such infections and the preventative measures to take to avoid cross-infection from hand to mouth. Verbal and written information to convey the message to women, partner and close family members on the dangers of GAS and other microbial infection during pregnancy and the speed by which they can become systemic should be provided (CMACE 2011).

Midwives should ensure care is woman-centred, individualized, dignified, kind, respectful and sensitive to the socio-cultural and psychological needs of both Fiona and her significant others, such as partner and family. Psychosocial support for the relatives to help ameliorate any ensuing stress/anxiety associated with the early goal-directed therapy of the resuscitation and management bundles of the SSC and the technological interventions should not be overlooked.

The signs and symptoms of sepsis are well worth highlighting antenatally in order that women can report early onset of any infection or seek advice, should they have any concerns. Women should be assessed for any signs of urinary tract infections (UTIs), pre-term pre-labour rupture of the membranes (PPROM), and infection of the upper respiratory tract or other sources. Midwives are in repeated contact with childbearing women during the antepartum, labour and postpartum periods and have ample opportunity to detect ensuing infection and initiate a rapid response via referral to the medical team.

The assessment, monitoring and recording of vital signs once sepsis is suspected are a core part of care. Any of the features outlined in Table 11.1 and Figure 11.1 must be reported and acted on promptly. Particular attention should be paid to:

- temperature
- pulse
- blood pressure
- respiration
- hourly urine measurements
- any change to mental/neurological status
- FHR pattern.

Record keeping

All serial values of blood tests/laboratory investigations must be charted in a systematic way. The importance of clear unambiguous documentation when assessing, recording and communicating findings relating to vital signs, cannot be over-emphasized. Instead of stating urine output is average or reduced, or blood sugar (BS) high or low, quantify the findings by specifically stating the amount of urine measured or the exact measurement of the BS. The MEOWS chart should be used to document all vital signs with no omissions. Any exclusion of important findings such as BP, temperature, RR, BS, oxygen saturation levels and urine measurements could be significant, signalling the difference between life and death (Nelson et al. 2009).

Check point

Know the various clinical features of sepsis as the condition does not always result in pyrexia. Women who develop severe sepsis could be hypothermic.

In this case, the onset of sepsis was detected speedily and the swift and intelligent response of the midwife in communicating her suspicions to other key members of the interprofessional team helped save Fiona's life. This is not the case for all women as reported by CMACE (Harper 2011). Sepsis remains a rare occurrence in maternity care in developed countries. Due to its infrequency, it should feature prominently in maternity emergencies skills and drills training for all midwives, doctors and allied health professionals involved in maternity care.

Summary of key points

- Sepsis-related maternal mortality is rare, complex and a significant challenge in contemporary practice. For these reasons it is important to 'be aware of sepsis – beware of sepsis' (Harper 2011).
- Sepsis moves fast and is potentially fatal. Infection does not always result in pyrexia. Women who develop severe sepsis may have a lowered body temperature. Deviation in this vital sign should not be ignored. The mnemonic identified by Garrod et al. (2011) should act as a useful *aide-mémoire*.
- In order to save mothers' lives, prompt recognition/diagnosis, coupled with rapid response and aggressive treatment, are the cornerstones of successful management to arrest the sepsis cascade and prevent rapid progression to septic shock.
- The care/management of pregnant women with septic shock is still evolving.
- Use of the SBAR tool and the MEOWS chart will facilitate timely communication with obstetricians, anaesthetists and other key members of the medical team.
- Hyper-vigilance by midwives in record keeping helps to prevent omissions in documentation of vital signs.

- The midwife has a duty of care to ensure the woman's holistic needs are met. This includes psychosocial support for the woman's partner/relatives to help ameliorate the stress/anxiety associated with medical management and the technological interventions.
- The midwife's professional responsibilities include accurate record keeping and reporting of any deviation or subtle changes in vital signs.
- Good team working and collaboration within the interprofessional team will result in effective care, which will signal the difference between life and death.

REFERENCES

Blomqvist, H. (2011) *Risk Factors*. Available at: https://www.aboutsepsis.com (accessed 12 March 2011).

Centre for Maternal and Child Enquiries (CMACE) (2010) *Saving Mothers' Lives, 2006–2008: CMACE Emergent Theme Briefing #1: Genital Tract Sepsis*. Available at: http://www.cmace.org.uk (accessed 12 January 2011).

Centre for Maternal and Child Enquiries (CMACE) (2011) *Saving Mothers' Lives: Reviewing Maternal Deaths to Make Motherhood Safer: 2006–2008. The Eighth Report on Confidential Enquiries into Maternal Deaths in the United Kingdom*. Ed. G. Lewis. *BJOG: An International British Journal of Obstetrics and Gynaecology*, 118 (Suppl. 1): 1–203.

Clutton-Brock, T. (2011) Critical care, in CMACE *Saving Mothers' Lives: Reviewing Maternal Deaths to Make Motherhood Safer: 2006–2008. The Eighth Report on Confidential Enquiries into Maternal Deaths in the United Kingdom*. Ed. G. Lewis. *BJOG: An International British Journal of Obstetrics and Gynaecology*, 118 (Suppl. 1): 173–80.

Daniels, R. (2009) *Pathophysiology of Sepsis: NHS Evidence – Emergency and Urgent Care, Annual Evidence Update*. Available at: http://www.library.nhs.uk (accessed 12 January 2011).

Daniels, R. and Nutbeam, T. (eds) (2010) The ABC of sepsis, *Journal of Tropical Paediatrics*, 50(4): 287.

Daniels, R., Nutbeam, T., McNamara, G. and Galvin, C. (2010) The sepsis six and the severe sepsis resuscitation bundle: a prospective observational cohort study, *Journal of Emergency Medicine*. Available at: http://emj.bmj.com (accessed 12 January 2011). DOI: 10.1136/emj.2010.095067.

Dellinger, R.P., Levy, M.M., Carlet, J.M., Bion, J., Parker, M.M., Jaeschke, R., Reinhart, K., Angus, D.C., Brun-Buisson, C., Beale, R., Calandra, T., Dhainnaut, J.F., Gerlach, H., Harvey, M., Marini, J.J., Marshall, J., Ranieri, M., Ramsey, G., Sevransky, J., Thompson, B.T., Townsend, S., Vender, J.S., Zimmerman, J.L. and Vincent, J.L. (2008) Surviving Sepsis Campaign: international guidelines for management of severe sepsis and septic shock, *Intensive Care Medicine*, 34(1): 17–60. DOI: 10.1007/s00134-007-0943-2.

Galvagno, S.M. (2003) *Emergency Pathophysiology: Clinical Applications for Pre-Hospital Care*. Jackson: Teton New Media.

Galvagno, S.M. and Camann, W. (2009) Sepsis and acute renal failure in pregnancy. *Anesthesia and Analgesia*, 108(2): 572–5. Available at: http://www.anesthesia-analgesia.org/content/108/2/572.full.pdf (accessed 30 January 2011). DOI: 10.1213/ane.Ob013e3181937b7e.

Garrod, D., Beale, V., Rogers, J. and Miller, A. (2011) Issues for midwives. Conference paper presented at *Saving Mothers' Lives Conference: Reviewing Maternal Deaths to Make Motherhood Safer: 2006–2008. BJOG: An International British Journal of Obstetrics and Gynaecology*, 118 (Suppl. 1): 149–57.

Guinn, D., Abel, D. and Tomlinson, M. (2007) Early goal directed therapy for sepsis during pregnancy, *Obstetrics and Gynecology in Clinics of North America*, 34(3): 459–79. Available at: http://www. obgyn.theclinics.com (accessed 30 January 2011).

Harper, A. (2011) Sepsis, in Centre for Maternal and Child Enquiries (CMACE) *Saving Mothers' Lives: Reviewing Maternal Deaths to Make Motherhood Safer: 2006–2008. The Eighth Report on Confidential Enquiries into Maternal Deaths in the United Kingdom.* Ed. G. Lewis. *BJOG: An International British Journal of Obstetrics and Gynaecology*; 118 (Suppl. 1): 85–96.

Harrison, D.A., Welch, C.A. and Eddleston, J.M. (2006) The epidemiology of severe sepsis in England, Wales and Northern Ireland, 1996 to 2004: secondary analysis of a high quality clinical database, the ICNARC Case Mix Programme Database, *Critical Care*, 10(R42). Available at: http://www.ccforum.com/content/10/2/R42 (accessed 30 January 2011). DOI: 10.1186/cc4854.

Hotchkiss, R.S. and Karl, I.E. (2003) The pathophysiology and treatment of sepsis, *New England Journal of Medicine*, 348(2): 138–50.

International Sepsis Forum (2003) *Promoting a Better Understanding of Sepsis*, 2nd edn. Available at: http://www.sepsisforum.org (accessed 12 January 2011).

Levy, M.M., Dellinger, R.P., Townsend, S.R., Lindle-Zwirble, W.T., Marshall, J.C., Bion, J., Schorr, C., Artigas, A., Ramsey, G., Beale, R., Parker, M.M., Gerlach, H., Reinhart, K., Silva, E., Harvey, M., Regan, S. and Angus, D.C. (2010) The Surviving Sepsis Campaign: results of an international guideline based performance improvement program targeting severe sepsis, *Intensive Care Medicine*, 36(1): 222–31. DOI: 10.1007/s00134-009-1738-3.

Lewis, G. (ed.) (2007) *Saving Mothers' Lives: Reviewing Maternal Deaths to Make Motherhood Safer: 2003–2005. The Seventh Report on Confidential Enquiries into Maternal Deaths in the United Kingdom.* London: CEMACH.

Lewis, G. and Drife, J. (eds) (2004) *Why Mothers Die 2000–2002: The Sixth Report of the Confidential Enquiries into Maternal Deaths in the United Kingdom.* London: RCOG.

Linde-Zwirble, W.T. and Angus, D.C. (2004) Severe sepsis epidemiology: sampling, selection and society, *Critical Care*, 8(4): 222–6.

Mitchell, E. and Whitehouse, T. (2010) The pathophysiology of sepsis, in R. Daniels and T. Nutbeam (eds) *The ABC of Sepsis.* Oxford: Wiley-Blackwell.

National Institute for Health and Clinical Excellence (NICE) (2007) *Acutely Ill Patients in Hospital: Recognition of and Response to Acute Illness in Adults in Hospital.* Clinical Guideline No. 50. London: NICE. Available at: http://www.nice.org.uk (accessed 12 January 2011).

Nelson, D.P., LeMaster, T.H., Plost, G.N. and Zahner, M.L. (2009) Recognising sepsis in the adult patient, *American Journal of Nursing*, 109(3): 40–5.

Nursing and Midwifery Council (2004) *Midwives Rules and Standards.* London: NMC.

Remick, D.G. (2007) Biological perspectives: pathophysiology of sepsis, *American Journal of Pathology*, 170(5). DOI: 10.2353/ajpath.2007.060872.

Russell, J.A. (2006) Management of sepsis, *New England Journal of Medicine*, 355(16): 1699–713.

Saade, G.R. (2004) Maternal sepsis, in M.R. Foley, T. H. Strong and T.J. Garite (eds) *Obstetric Intensive Care Manual.* New York: McGraw-Hill, pp. 113–19.

Sepsis Alliance (2010) *Surviving Sepsis Campaign.* Available at: http://www.sepsisalliance.org (accessed 12 January 2011).

Sheffield, J. (2004) Sepsis and septic shock in pregnancy, *Critical Care Clinics*, 20(4): 651 – 60. Available at: http://www.ncbi.nlm.nih.gov/pubmed/15388194 (accessed 12 January 2011).

Townsend, S.R., Schorr, C., Levy, M.M. and Dellinger, R.P. (2008) Reducing mortality in severe sepsis: the surviving sepsis campaign, *Clinics in Chest Medicine*, 29(4): 721–33.

Trzeciak, S., McCoy, J.V., Dellinger, P., Arnold, R.C., Rizzuto, M., Abate, N.L., Shapiro, N.I., Parrillo, J.E., Hollenburg, S.M. on behalf of the Microcirculatory Alterations in Resuscitation and Shock (MARS) Investigators (2008) Early increases in microcirculatory perfusion protocol-directed resuscitation are associated with reduced multi-organ failure at 24 hours in patients with sepsis, *Intensive Care Medicine*, 34(12): 17–60. DOI: 10.1007/s00134-008-1193-6.

ANNOTATED FURTHER READING

Fourrie, F. (2004) Recombinant human activated protein C in the treatment of severe sepsis: an evidence-based review, *Critical Care Medicine*, 32 (Suppl.): S534–S541.

A useful review of rhAPC or Drotrecogin alfa (activated) in the treatment of severe sepsis.

Robson, W.P. and Daniel, R. (2008) Helping the sepsis six: helping patients to survive sepsis, *British Journal of Nursing*, 17(1): 16–21.

Raises some key points that are transferable to midwifery practice.

Vaughan, D., Robinson, N., Lucas, N. and Arulkumaran, S. (2010) *Handbook of Obstetric High Dependency Care*. Chichester: Wiley-Blackwell.

Provides a useful overview of the context of high dependency care.

USEFUL WEBSITES

http://www.aagbi.org	The Association of Anaesthetists of Great Britain and Ireland
https://www.aboutsepsis.com	About Sepsis (this website is aimed at health care professionals, who need to register online in order to use the site)
http://www.advanceinsepsis.com	Advances in Sepsis
http://www.alert-course.com	ALERT system of assessment
http://www.esicm.org	European Society of Intensive Care Medicine
http://www.nice.org.uk	National Institute for Health and Clinical Excellence
http://www.npeu.ox.ac.uk	National Perinatal Epidemiology Unit (from 1 April 2011 NPEU takes over the role of the former CMACE)
http://www.rcog.org.uk	Royal College of Obstetricians and Gynaecologists
http://wwwsccm.org	Society of Critical Care Medicine
http://www.sepsisalliance.org	Sepsis Alliance
http://www.sepsisforum.org	International Sepsis Forum
http://www.sisna.org	Surgical Infection Society
http://www.survivingsepsis.org	Surviving Sepsis Campaign (use this link to access the surviving sepsis care bundles for resuscitation and management)

Cardiac arrest

Sam Bharmal and Maureen D. Raynor

Pre-requisites for the chapter: the reader should have an understanding of:

- Physiology of the cardiovascular and respiratory system and maternal physiological adaptation to these changes.
- How circulatory arrest is diagnosed.
- Causes of cardiac arrest in pregnancy.
- Types and causes of shock.
- Current advanced life support guidelines.
- The role of defibrillation.
- Physiological changes of pregnancy that contribute to rapid deterioration.
- Modifications required for maternal cardiopulmonary resuscitation.
- The role of perimortem delivery of the fetus.
- Drugs/medicines used in resuscitation.
- Post-resuscitation care.

Pre-reading self-assessment

1 What is the relationship between venous return, cardiac output, and blood pressure?
2 How may cardiac arrest be prevented in a hospital setting?
3 What are the immediate resuscitative measures required when cardio-respiratory arrest is suspected?
4 Describe the goal of basic life support and the challenges pregnancy presents to this.
5 Compare causes of cardiac arrest to those of respiratory arrest in adults.

Recommended prior reading

Department of Health (DH) (2009) *Competencies for Recognising and Responding to Acutely Ill Patients in Hospital*. London: DH. Available at: http://www.dh.gov.uk/en/ Publicationsandstatistics/Publications/PublicationsPolicyAndGuidance/DH_096989

De Swiet, M., Williamson, C. and Lewis, G. (2011) Other indirect deaths, in Centre for Maternal and Child Enquiries (CMACE) *Saving Mothers' Lives: Reviewing Maternal Deaths to Make Motherhood Safer: 2006-2008. The Eighth Report of the Confidential Enquiries into Maternal Deaths in the United Kingdom (UK)*, ed. G. Lewis. *BJOG*,118 (Suppl. 1): 119–31.

(Continued overleaf)

National Confidential Enquiry into Patient Outcome and Death (2005) *An Acute Problem*. London: NCEPOD. Available at: http://www.ncepod.org.uk/2005aap.htm

National Institute for Health and Clinical Excellence (NICE) (2007) *Acutely Ill Patients in Hospitals: Recognition of and Response to Acute Illness in Adults in Hospital*. Clinical Guideline No. 50. Available at: http://www.nice.org.uk (accessed 10 May 2011)

National Patient Safety Agency (2007a) *Safer Care for the Acutely Ill Patient: Learning from Serious Incidents*. London: NPSA. Available at: http://www.npsa.nhs.uk/nrls/alerts-and-directives/directives-guidance/acutely-ill-patient/

National Patient Safety Agency (2007b) *Recognising and Responding Appropriately to Early Signs of Deterioration in Hospitalised Patients*. Available at: http://www.npsa.nhs.uk/nrls/alerts-and-directives/directives-guidance/acutely-ill-patient/deterioration-in-hospitalised-patients/

CASE STUDY

Amy is brought in by ambulance to the emergency department (ED). She is 37 weeks pregnant and has been involved in a road traffic accident/collision. She was a front-seat passenger, wearing her seatbelt. The car was hit from the passenger side while travelling at 30 miles per hour, spun around, and collided with a lamp post.

Amy is accompanied by her husband who is not injured but is extremely anxious. She is wearing a hard collar and has been put on a spinal board. When she arrives, she is able to give a full account of the accident and looks shaken but well. She complains of some chest pain, especially on the left side, and severe pain in her left thigh. Her BP is 130/85 mmHg, pulse 90 bpm, saturation 97 per cent on air, RR is 16 breaths per minute. Her left leg is obviously deformed mid-thigh.

Examination reveals tenderness in her lower abdomen and some bruising over the left upper chest in keeping with a seatbelt injury. Amy confirms feeling fetal movement. A midwife and portable fetal monitoring device are requested. Amy has two wide-bore cannulae inserted; blood samples are obtained and sent to the laboratory for FBC, Gp & S, U & Es and glucose.

A chest X-ray (CXR) is suggestive of three fractured ribs on the left, and an XR of Amy's thigh confirms a fractured femur. Cervical spine XR looks normal. It is not possible to have a clear assessment of Amy's cervical spine clinically and the emergency department registrar requests and organizes a CT scan of her neck. When she is leaving ED for the scan, Amy becomes very anxious. Her heart rate is 110 bpm and her RR is 20 breaths/min. Her BP remains 130/85 mmHg.

Thirty minutes later, a cardiac arrest team is called to the CT scan department where Amy has been taken.

1 **Describe the key features of trauma assessment of a pregnant woman and list the factors that affect the resuscitation of a pregnant woman who is in cardiac arrest.**

A Trauma is an important cause of morbidity and mortality in the pregnant woman as outlined in the case study. The highest proportion of trauma in pregnant women occurs in the third trimester of pregnancy, with road traffic accident being the most common cause (Lewis 2007).

It is evident that abdominal injuries are on the increase and it should be remembered that these may be from both accidental and non-accidental causes as reported by Lewis (2007, 2011), writing on behalf of CEMACH and CMACE respectively. During early pregnancy, the uterus is contained within the pelvis, which confers it some protection. Later, it lies anterior to abdominal viscera and itself acts as protection to blunt any penetrating trauma. While uterine muscle is elastic, the placenta is fixed, and may easily be sheared off the uterine wall by deceleration injuries. Incorrectly placed seatbelts may cause placental abruption and uterine rupture, as well as damage to other abdominal organs (bowel and omentum, liver, spleen, stomach). Even relatively minor injury can cause placental abruption which is fatal to the fetus, and sufficient to cause severe morbidity to the mother. Factors such as these may not be immediately apparent to non-obstetricians dealing with pregnant women in the emergency department, and it is therefore imperative that multidisciplinary involvement is sought early.

Principles of assessment and treatment are exactly the same as those of a non-pregnant woman. It is important, however, to avoid aorto-caval compression by TILTING the woman in a left-lateral position (Figure 12.1), using a wedge if necessary to aid venous return (Hull and Bennett 2007; Campbell and Sanson 2009).

Pregnant women have a greater tolerance to blood loss but the fetus does not. By the third trimester, plasma volume has increased by approximately 50 per cent, and up to half of young women with significant abdominal haemorrhage will have minimal or no signs on initial assessment, as outlined by Weintraub et al. (2006) and the MOET manual (Grady et al. 2007). However, compensatory mechanisms include reduction of placental blood flow to preserve maternal circulation, and fetal compromise may be an early indicator of hypovolaemia.

Where available, the presence of a multidisciplinary trauma team provides immediate specialist input and many hands. It is important to include a senior obstetrician, midwife and paediatrician. A good history should include the factors identified by the acronym MIST as detailed in Box 12.1.

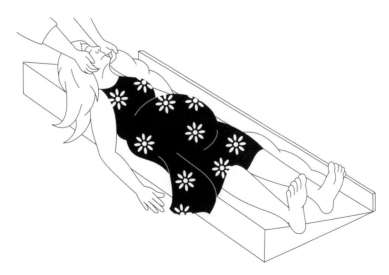

Figure 12.1 The wedged lateral tilt position
Note left lateral tilt to avoid aorto-caval compression. Remember to avoid head tilt and chin lift in favour of jaw thrust if cervical spine injury suspected.

Box 12.1 A good history should account for the acronym MIST

M	**M**echanism of injury
I	**I**njuries already identified
S	**S**ymptoms and signs
T	**T**reatment already received

The above considerations during the process of history taking will provide invaluable information and guide further investigation. Details of the pregnancy should be sought, along with past medical history, medication and allergies (Grady et al. 2007).

The primary survey consists of assessment and management of life-threatening conditions as they are identified. Basic monitoring (pulse oximetry, ECG, non-invasive blood pressure, respiratory rate, end tidal carbon dioxide in an intubated individual) should be applied while this is taking place.

Employing a systematic approach ensures that nothing is missed. There should also be ongoing appraisal as constant re-evaluation is the key to early detection of problems.

Check point

A systematic approach should be used in the assessment of any severely ill or unconscious pregnant woman.

It is best to consider the process of assessment as being two-fold:

1 *the primary survey*: this should employ the ABCDE method of assessment (see Figure 12.2), as identified by the ALERT Course Development Group (Smith et al. 2002) (see Case 2).
2 *the secondary survey*: this is a top-to-toe, back and front examination of the woman that should be carried out once the primary survey has been completed and any immediate threats to life treated. Its purpose is to identify any other injuries sustained, especially ones that may themselves become life-threatening.

The interprofessional team members attending the woman should consider:

• Rectal and vaginal examination.
• ECG and review of CXR may reveal cardiac or lung contusion. CT scan may reveal injury to the diaphragm, mediastinum or spine, or chest pathology not visible on CXR.

The Confidential Enquiry into Maternal Deaths in the UK for the triennium, 2006–2008 (CMACE 2011), reports 17 deaths from road traffic accidents (up from 8 in the previous triennium) in women who were either pregnant or within 6 weeks of birth. Two were

[A = AIRWAY with cervical spine protection]
- Clear and open the airway (avoid head tilt, chin lift in favour of jaw thrust if cervical spine injury suspected).
- Compromise is more likely if reduced level of consciousness.
- Remember risk of aspiration – early intubation may be indicated.

[B = BREATHING]
- Give high flow oxygen (15 litre/min. through a non-rebreathable mask).
- Ventilatory assistance as required, especially if suspected underlying brain injury.
- Prevent secondary brain injury by avoiding hypoxia and hypercarbia.
- Consider presence of rib fractures, flail chest, pneumothorax, haemothorax, lung contusion.
- Decompress tension pneumothorax (doctor will insert large-bore cannula in second intercostal space, mid-clavicular line).
- Doctor will place chest drain as indicated (essential after needle decompression of chest).
- Remember that the diaphragm is elevated during pregnancy, risking damage to liver, spleen or stomach if the drain is placed too low. The fifth intercostal space, anterior to the mid-axillary line is recommended as outlined by MOET manual (Grady et al. 2007).

[C = CIRCULATION]
- Lateral TILT if not already done (see Figure 12.1).
- Place 2 large-bore cannulae.
- Take blood for grouping or cross-matching, and Kleihauer test (even if Rhesus-positive, can give an idea of degree of feto-maternal transfusion). Remember need for anti-D in Rh -ve mother.
- Aggressive replacement of fluid.
- Remember availability of O -ve blood (in accordance with local guidelines).
- Warm fluid where possible to avoid worsening any coagulopathy.
- Remember causes of concealed haemorrhage; **"blood on the floor and four more" (five in pregnancy)** :
  Placental abruption/uterine rupture
  Haemothorax
  Abdominal/retroperitoneal bleeding
  Pelvic fracture, damage to venous plexuses
  Long bone fractures (over 1000 mL for a femur alone).
- Exclude tension pneumothorax and cardiac tamponade.
- Consider cardiac contusion if arrhythmias or shock.
- FAST scan of abdomen:
  Early detection of abdominal free fluid
  Presence of fetal heart noting rate/rhythm and any abnormalities.
- Insert urinary catheter for hourly measurements.

(Continued overleaf)

THE INTERPROFESSIONAL TEAM MAY NEED TO DELIVER FETUS EVEN IF DEAD TO
AID MATERNAL RESUSCITATION AND ALLOW ACCESS FOR HAEMORRHAGE
CONTROL.

[D = DISABILITY]
- AVPU and Glasgow Coma Scale (see Cases 1 and 10).
- Consider airway protection if = 8, or deterioration of 2 points.
- Check pupil size and reactivity (head injury).
- Check glucose.
- Consider causes of lowered level of consciousness.
- Hypoxia and hypercarbia secondary to compromised airway or breathing:
  Poor cerebral perfusion secondary to hypotension or cardiac arrest
  Postictal state due to eclamptic or epileptic fit
  Intracranial pathology:
      bleeding (subdural, extradural, subarachnoid)
      thrombosis
      tumour
      infection (meningitis, encephalitis).
  Drugs, alcohol or poisons (carbon monoxide if burns).

[E = EXPOSURE/ENVIRONMENTAL CONTROL]
- Visual inspection looking for current and old injuries (e.g. non-accidental), evidence of infection, calf swelling, abdominal distension etc.
- Keep the woman warm.

FETAL ASSESSMENT
Assessment of fetal heart is an integral part of the care. However, it should be remembered that the best way to resuscitate the fetus is by resuscitating the mother.

Figure 12.2 The ABCDE method of assessment.

pedestrians. In only one of the remaining 15 cases was the woman known not to be wearing a seatbelt. Four women underwent perimortem caesarean section in the ED. None of the babies survived. These deaths are classed as 'Coincidental' by CMACE (Lewis 2011).

2   **Define shock, with particular reference to hypovolaemic shock.**

A   Shock occurs when there is inadequate oxygen supply to organs, and inadequate waste product removal from organs. It is very important to appreciate that this condition is diagnosed by detailed clinical evaluation of a pregnant woman or non-pregnant individual, and is not definable by a set of vital sign observations. Evidence of shock may be very subtle to detect initially, and a high index of suspicion and continued vigilance are needed.

The activation of physiological compensatory mechanisms in fit women can mask the severity of the underlying disturbance until the situation is far advanced; cardiac arrest may then rapidly ensue. Furthermore, the normal physiological changes occurring during pregnancy can lead to a false sense of security.

The causes of shock can be classified as hypovolaemic, septic, neurogenic, cardiogenic and anaphylactic as detailed in Box 12.2. These conditions can co-exist to varying degrees.

Box 12.2 Classification and causes of shock

- *Hypovolaemic shock*: This is the most likely kind of shock to be encountered in pregnancy and results from loss of circulating blood volume due to maternal haemorrhage. It will be discussed in more detail below.
- *Septic shock*: This occurs in response to infection from organisms, is extremely common in the hospital setting and is further discussed in Case 11. It has been recognized as the leading cause of maternal death in the latest CMACE (Lewis 2011) report, prompting a number of key recommendations.
- *Neurogenic shock*: This occurs as a result of acute injury to the spinal cord resulting in vasodilatation, manifest by hypotension and warm peripheries. Injuries occurring at or above the high thoracic level can interrupt sympathetic innervation to the heart, leading to a bradycardia. Treatment involves judicious fluid replacement, vasopressors, and management of bradycardia. There is little data on spinal shock in pregnancy.
- *Cardiogenic shock*: This occurs as a result of myocardial dysfunction, and management is in conjunction with a cardiologist and intensive care physician. Ionotropes may well be required.
- *Anaphylactic shock*: This is an abnormal immunological response to an allergen, which the woman may not be aware of, or to which she may even have been uneventfully exposed previously. It is thankfully rare. The main physiological changes include vasodilatation and an increase in vascular permeability, resulting in a loss of circulating blood volume. This is discussed in Case 10.

(Grady et al. 2007)

Hypovolaemic shock in pregnancy can be due to a number of causes. Some are visually obvious (blood on the floor). Others have to be actively sought (abruptio placentae, blood pooling in an atonic uterus or the vagina, genital tract trauma, uterine rupture, abdominal bleeding post-surgery, trauma causing bleeding into the chest, abdomen, retroperitoneal space, pelvis or long bones). Common signs of hypovolaemia are outlined in Figure 12.3.

Anxiety is an early symptom, progressing to confusion, aggression and eventually loss of consciousness as cerebral perfusion deteriorates. Hypotension is usually a late sign, when compensatory mechanisms (tachycardia and vasoconstriction) are no longer sufficient to maintain venous return.

Early and aggressive volume replacement is the only way to improve venous return and cardiac output, and to restore adequate organ perfusion.

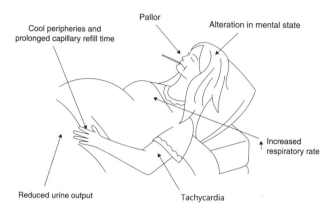

Figure 12.3 Signs of hypovolaemia

In the non-pregnant adult, the blood volume is approximately 70 mL/kg or 5000 mL in a 70 kg individual (Grady et al. 2007). In pregnancy, an increase in red cell mass and plasma volume results in a blood volume of 100 mL/kg, an increase of nearly 40 per cent. A pregnant woman can lose up to 35 per cent (1000–1500 mL) of her circulating volume before even mounting a tachycardia. In addition, blood can be diverted from the fetoplacental unit. An early sign of maternal hypovolaemia may be signs of fetal compromise; assessment of the fetus may provide valuable clues to the status of the mother. A high index of suspicion for bleeding must be maintained in these women as expected signs and symptoms associated with hypovolaemia may not be present until very late, in some cases too late.

When in the supine position in later pregnancy, the gravid uterus can cause compression of the abdominal aorta and inferior vena cava. The resulting reduction in venous return can decrease cardiac output by a third, significantly worsening any hypotension due to hypovolaemia. In order to prevent this, the uterus must be displaced, either by tilting the woman, or by manually lifting it to the left.

When classifying shock, a common *aide-mémoire*, according to Grady (2007) is to think of it in four stages as detailed in Table 12.1. Any cause of shock, if left untreated, can lead to cardiac arrest. When deterioration does occur, it is precipitous and catastrophic.

Writing on behalf of CMACE in the triennial report for 2006–2008, Hulbert (2011) identifies 27 recordable maternal deaths in the ED or shortly after the women were transferred to another critical care area. Most of these women had suffered a cardiac arrest prior to arrival with the minority actually arresting in the ED. Cardiopulmonary resuscitation (CPR) was performed in all the reported cases. Ten women were successfully resuscitated and transferred to other critical care areas. Resuscitation was discontinued for the remaining 17 women while they were still in the ED. The overall conclusion is that resuscitation guidelines were efficiently implemented. The findings also convey the well-recognized but disturbing fact that outcomes from pre-hospital arrests are universally poor (Schiff and Holt 2005; Chames and Pearlman 2008; Campbell and Sanson 2009).

Table 12.1 Classifications of circulating volume in non-pregnant women

Class	Loss of circulatory volume (%)	Amount in a 70 kg adult (mL)	Clinical features and management
1	0–15	< 750	Minimal features of tachycardia are the only abnormal sign in healthy adults due to compensatory response of the sympathetic pathway of the autonomic nervous system that plays a key role in BP control via the diversion of blood via the GI tract (splenic capsule constriction). Hyper-vigilance needed to observe for early signs of deterioration, bearing in mind that there may be steady occult bleeding internally (Table 12.3).
11	15–30	750–1500	Significant changes in clinical features include ↑ pulse, ↑ RR and ↑ diastolic BP to compensate for volume loss. Crystalloids are the first choice as fluid replacement therapy.
111	30–40	1500–2000	Noticeably symptomatic with a rapid pulse rate, ↑ RR and on assessment using the AVPU scale changes in mental status may be obvious, e.g. anxiety, restlessness and thirst. Grady (2007) states that it is only at this stage that the systolic BP will be affected (postural hypotension). Peripheral vasoconstriction is no longer effective in compensating for the increased loss in circulatory blood volume. Cool peripheries and prolonged capillary refill time are usually present. Fluid replacement therapy at this stage should consider use of colloids (blood transfusion, Gelofusine) when necessary. Crystalloids may not be effective on their own.
1V	> 40	> 2000	Serious and life-threatening stage with marked tachycardia, ↑ RR and air hunger. Breathing may be shallow and laboured with ↓ BP. Urine output is reduced. Mental status will be altered with reduced oxygen saturation levels. Loss of consciousness is likely to result if there is a loss of circulating volume > 50 per cent. This stage requires aggressive resuscitation including fluid replacement therapy in the form of blood replacement products and possibly surgical intervention. Death is a real possibility without early resuscitative measures.

Source: Adapted from Grady (2007: 99).

A perimortem caesarean section was performed on all 17 women who died in the E D. The reported outcome for those neonates is as follows: 1 live birth, 5 early neonatal deaths and 11 stillbirths. These pregnancies were between 20 and 39 weeks. The outcome was extremely grave for the neonates born by perimortem caesarean section performed at 28 gestational weeks or less: none survived. Not surprisingly, the survival rates were more favourable with increased gestational age. A reported 47 per cent of the neonates who were born by perimortem caesarean section at ≥ 36 weeks gestation survived. However, all but one followed a collapse while the mother was already hospitalized.

Perimortem caesarean section is part of the resuscitative procedure that should be considered in any woman who experiences a cardiac arrest in the last 20 weeks of pregnancy (Whitty 2002; Hulbert 2007; Dijkman et al. 2010). This intervention is necessary to ensure that effective maternal C PR can be achieved. Hulbert (2007) and Katz et al. (1986) highlight that the procedure must be performed within 5 minutes of the arrest where there is no initial response to advanced C PR in the tilted position. Table 12.2 outlines the parameters the multidisciplinary team would consider prior to perimortem caesarean section.

Table 12.2 Perimortem caesarean section

Benefits

Immediate relief of aorto-caval compression, increasing venous return.
Allows continuation of C PR in supine position.
Reduction of maternal oxygen consumption.
Facilitates ventilation.
70 per cent chance of neonatal survival if delivered within 5 minutes (no neurological sequelae, but dependent on gestation) (Katz et al. 1986, 2005; Shields and Fausett 2010).

Timing

Should begin within 4 minutes of the onset of C PR.
Birth of baby should be within 5 minutes of onset of C PR.
Applicable to pregnancy beyond 20 weeks.
DO NOT stop CPR during procedure.

Conduct

As speed is of the essence, no need to transfer to operating theatre providing basic equipment is available.
Surgical approach depends on preference and skill of operator.
No evidence that lower segment C S any better or worse than classical.
In theory, only need scalpel and forceps. Most larger E Ds carry obstetric trays.
Airway should be protected by intubation at earliest opportunity as risk of aspiration is high.
Facility for neonatal resuscitation is desirable and neonatal team essential.

Post-birth

If resuscitation successful, transfer to theatre to complete surgery.
Give anaesthesia/analgesia.
Continue treating cause of arrest (four 'Hs' and four 'Ts' – these are explained in Box 12.4).

3 **What are the possible causes of Amy's cardiac arrest?**

A Cardiac arrest in pregnancy is very rare (Price et al. 2008; Campbell and Sanson 2009). On arrival, it was clear that Amy had been involved in a significant collision. The mechanism of injury (passenger-side impact sufficient to spin the car, deceleration when the car hit the lamp post, significant intrusion into passenger compartment) and her advanced stage of pregnancy should have ensured her transfer to a trauma centre and triggered a trauma team alert (Gray et al. 1997; Sharma 2005) with separate calls to the obstetric, midwifery and neonatal teams.

Her pre-hospital care involved immobilization of her cervical spine in a hard collar, and she had been placed on a spinal board for protection of the rest of her spine. She had been administered oxygen and IV access had been secured. On arrival, she was talking and lucid, suggesting a clear airway, adequate breathing and a blood pressure sufficient to ensure cerebral perfusion.

Her significant injuries were a fractured femur and fractured ribs on the left. These alone could account for a 2000 mL blood loss. Grady (2007) in the MOET manual, identifies the different injuries that may contribute to significant blood loss and may result in shock, especially if there are multiple injuries (see Table 12.3).

Injuries that should have been specifically sought and excluded are:

- pneumothorax, flail chest, pulmonary contusion (from rib fractures);
- haemothorax (rib fractures);
- intra-abdominal bleeding from a ruptured or punctured spleen (lower rib fractures, blunt trauma);
- other intra-abdominal injury;
- placental abruption or uterine rupture (shearing injury, blunt trauma);
- fractured pelvis.

Any one of the above factors may have contributed to severe hypovolaemia. Unless the whole spinal board was tilted, aorto-caval compression would have significantly exacerbated Amy's condition.

As with otherwise fit young adults, and especially due to pregnancy, Amy's physiological

Table 12.3 Blood loss from different injuries

Type of injury	Blood volume lost (litres)
Closed fracture	1.5
Fracture of the pelvis	3.0
Fractured ribs (individual rib)	0.15
One blood-filled hemithorax	2.0
A closed tibial fracture	0.5
An open wound the size of an adult hand	0.5
A clot the size of an adult fist	0.5

Source: Adapted from Grady (2007: 101).

reserve and compensatory mechanisms prevented her from showing many of the classic signs of blood loss. It is important that members of the multidisciplinary team involved in the care of pregnant women admitted to the E D have knowledge of the physiological parameters of pregnancy. This will enable them to recognize early deterioration in women's condition during pregnancy and identify critical illness, a recurrent theme in successive triennial reports (Lewis 2007, 2011).

More subtle signs and clinical suspicion should have alerted clinicians to the risk of occult blood loss. Think 'blood on the floor and four (five in pregnancy) more', as previously outlined.

Amy's mild tachycardia, rise in respiratory rate, and increasing anxiety should prompt further examination and early fluid resuscitation. A repeat Hb might have shown a drop from her initial result, although often not. An arterial blood gas interpreted within pregnancy ranges may have given clues to poor perfusion by showing an abnormally high lactate level (suggesting poor tissue perfusion) and a compensatory respiratory alkalosis. Hb from this sample might again have confirmed a drop from previous values. A 'normal' blood pressure was maintained until significant blood loss had occurred.

Before sending a woman such as Amy to a remote site such as the CT scanner, it is imperative to ensure that cardiovascular and respiratory stability are maintained. Once again, lying in the supine position in the scanner will have significantly impaired venous return. Regular monitoring may have shown a rising pulse. Verbal contact would have confirmed a decrease in conscious level but this is often difficult during such an examination.

Other causes of arrest that should be considered are detailed in Box 12.3.

Box 12.3 Other causes of cardiac arrest

- Amniotic fluid embolism.
- Seizures due to head injury, hypoxia, hypercarbia or eclampsia.
- Tension pneumothorax.
- Cardiac tamponade.
- Arrhythmias secondary to cardiac contusion.
- Aortic dissection/disruption.
- Massive pulmonary embolus.

---

4 **Describe basic and advanced life support in a pregnant woman.**

A Amy should be placed on her back with left lateral tilt, as depicted in Figure 12.1. This can be on a wedge, or with the rescuers beneath her right hip. Effective C P R is incredibly difficult in this position (Morris and Stacey 2003) and the required depth of compression of *at least* a third of chest diameter is unlikely to be achievable. The procedure for C P R should follow the revised guidelines issued by R C U K (2010) as illustrated by the algorithm in Figure 12.4.

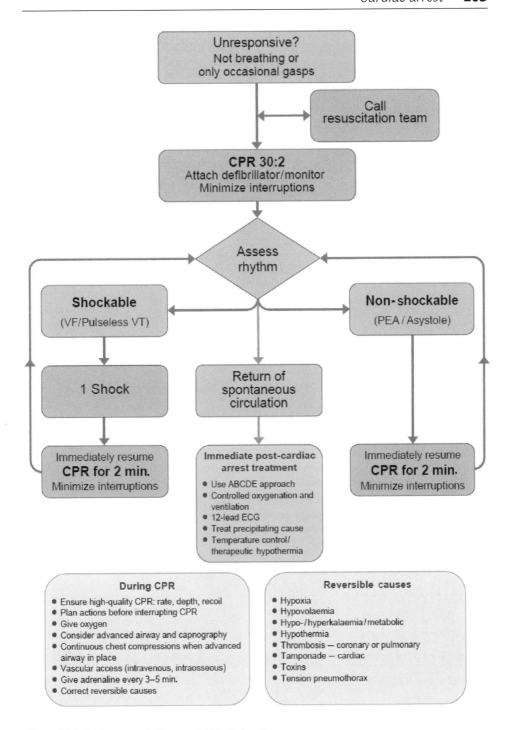

Figure 12.4 Adult advanced life support (ALS) algorithm

Source: Resuscitation Council UK (2010) Adult Advanced Life Support. In: *2010 Resuscitation guidelines* (chapter 7: 60). London: RCUK www.resus.org.uk. Accessed 27 April 2011. Reproduced with kind permission. All rights reserved.

Check points

- Advanced life support is identical in the pregnant and non-pregnant individual.
- All physiological values should be interpreted in the light of changes due to pregnancy (e.g. arterial blood gases, urea and creatinine, fibrinogen levels).
- Use of a MEOWS system (see Case 1), with appropriate tracking and triggering is invaluable in the potential prevention of cardiac arrest.

---

5 **Compare the causes of shockable versus non-shockable rhythms.**

A There are two ECG rhythms that should be instantly recognizable as requiring electrical cardioversion (shockable). These are ventricular fibrillation and pulseless ventricular tachycardia.

Ventricular fibrillation (VF) is characterized by uncoordinated electrical activity and no recognizable QRS complexes (Figure 12.5). There is no cardiac output and CPR should be started immediately. A shock should be administered as quickly as possible, but good quality cardiac compressions should be carried on while preparation for this is occurring.

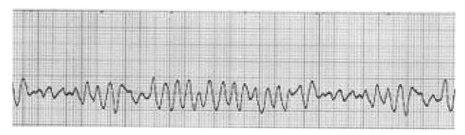

Figure 12.5 Ventricular fibrillation

Ventricular tachycardia can be pulseless or associated with an output. It shows a broad QRS complex and fast but regular rate (Figure 12.6). If it is associated with a pulse, a shock is not immediately indicated providing the woman is conscious, with an acceptable blood pressure and no signs of compromise. If there is no cardiac output, treatment is the same as for VF.

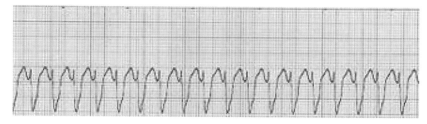

Figure 12.6 Ventricular tachycardia

There are similarly two non-shockable rhythms. The first is pulseless electrical activity (Figure 12.7), which is associated with massive haemorrhage and pulmonary embolus. To all intents and purposes, it looks identical to normal sinus rhythm, but is not associated with an output. CPR should be continued while reversible causes are sought and corrected.

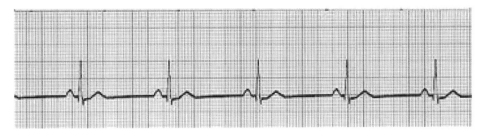

Figure 12.7 Pulseless electrical activity

The second non-shockable rhythm is asystole (Figure 12.8), the complete absence of electrical activity.

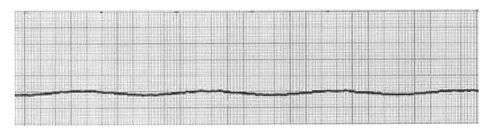

Figure 12.8 Asystole

Check point

It should be remembered that straight lines rarely exist in nature, and an electronic flat line suggests disconnection or monitoring failure.

---

6 **List and discuss the reversible causes of arrest.**

A Reversible causes of arrest applicable to pregnancy are outlined in Box 12.4 based on RCUK (2010) guidelines. Whenever cardiac arrest occurs in a pregnant woman, the possible aetiology or precipitating factors for which specific treatment exists must be identified. For ease of recall these factors are divided into two groups of four, based upon their initial letter, either H or T as outlined in Box 12.4.

Box 12.4 Reversible causes of arrest

The Four 'Hs'

1 *Hypoxia*: To reduce the risk of hypoxia, it is best to ensure effective ventilation of the lungs with 100 per cent oxygen via high concentration mask. There should be ongoing evaluation to confirm adequate chest rise as well as bilateral breath sounds.

(Continued overleaf)

A skilled member of the interprofessional team, more commonly the anaesthetist, should make a careful assessment to determine the correct placement of the tracheal tube.

2 *Hypovolaemia*: Careful ECG monitoring will reveal early abnormalities in cardiac rhythm, e.g. pulseless electrical activity resulting from hypovolaemia is usually attributable to severe haemorrhage. Such bleeding may be directly related to the trauma, ruptured aortic aneurysm or bleeding from damaged internal organs or gastrointestinal tract. Homeostasis can be achieved by early fluid replacement therapy and urgent corrective surgery to arrest the bleeding.

3 *Hyperkalaemia, hypokalaemia, hypocalcaemia,* acidaemia, and other metabolic disorders: These are identified by appropriate biochemical tests as well as careful screening of the woman's medical records to detect any relevant history. An ECG might provide useful information. Intravenous calcium gluconate is the treatment of choice in cases of magnesium sulphate toxicity. Care should be exercised in the treatment of any woman receiving magnesium sulphate in severe pre-eclampsia. The need for calcium chloride is indicated in the presence of hyperkalaemia, hypocalcaemia, and calcium channel-blocking drug overdose.

4 *Hypothermia*: This is a real possibility in any drowning incident and should be screened for using a low-reading thermometer. It is also important to remember that hypothermia can be a feature of sepsis (Case 11).

The Four 'Ts'

1 *Tension pneumothorax*: A tension pneumothorax is always a risk and must be ruled out by a member of the medical team as it may be the primary cause of pulseless electrical activity. It might result from medical iatrogenesis such as attempts to insert a central venous catheter.

2 *Tamponade*: Cardiac tamponade is a medical emergency which occurs when fluid such as blood or gas accumulates in the pericardial space. This leads to reduced ventricular filling and pericardial effusion with the unwanted sequelae of haemodynamic compromise. It must be recognized and treated speedily in order to prevent fatality. Yet paradoxically it is challenging to diagnose as the actual urgency of cardiac arrest obscures its features. However, RCUK (2010) states that ensuing cardiac arrest following penetrating chest trauma is usually suggestive of tamponade. This warrants hyper-vigilance by the multidisciplinary team.

3 *Toxic substances*: The use of toxic substances can precipitate cardiac arrest. Laboratory tests will aid diagnosis when a specific history is not discernible. Appropriate antidotes where available must be mobilized or guidance sought from one of the national toxicology units that provide information for health professionals such as Toxbase: www.toxbase.co.uk or www.spib.scot.nhs.uk.

4 *Thromboembolism* (pulmonary embolus/coronary thrombosis): CMACE (Lewis 2011) highlights VTE as being the third commonest cause of maternal mortality for the triennium 2006–2008 in the UK. Cardiac arrest is always a risk when a pregnant woman develops VTE (see Case 4). The implementation of routine thromboprophylaxis post-LSCS has seen a steady decrease in maternal deaths from

VTE. Such preventative measures should be considered when cardiac arrest occurs during pregnancy, not least because of the physiological increase in clotting factors during pregnancy.

(RCUK 2010; Soar et al. 2010)

7 **Outline the key principles of immediate post-resuscitation care.**

A Meticulous post-resuscitation care is vital to optimize Amy's chances of a good recovery and should be thought of as a continuum of resuscitation. The main principle of care should be aimed at achieving the return of spontaneous circulation (ROSC), ensuring stabilization and normal cerebral function through vigilance at re-evaluation of ABCDE (Shapiro 2006; Price et al. 2008; King 2009). Good oxygenation with close monitoring of fluid replacement therapy will ensure adequate tissue perfusion, cardiac function and maintenance of normal parameters of all vital signs. This is necessary before Amy is transferred to a high dependency/critical care area. Thromboprophylaxis will be required to prevent VTE. There should be clear and accurate documentation; all observations should be recorded on the MEOWS chart. In order not to compromise recovery, Amy's pain should be well managed by the anaesthetic team. Effective teamwork within the multidisciplinary team is essential to ensure seamless and robust communication. The baby's well-being will be dependent on any insult experienced as a result of Amy's injuries coupled with the timing/need for perimortem caesarean section (El-Kady 2007). A thorough assessment should be performed by the paediatric team.

Psychosocial aspects of care should not be overlooked, including spiritual needs. It is important in terms of supporting the partner/family members and keeping them informed of developments or the breaking of any bad news. The midwife should ensure she fulfils her statutory obligations in relation to documentation and immediate care of the mother and baby (NMC 2004).

Check point

Although the physiological alterations of pregnancy present a major challenge to all body systems, cardiac arrest in young, healthy, pregnant women is rare. Due to its rarity, it should be a regular feature in multiprofessional 'skills and drills' training.

CASE REVIEW

Post-surgery, Amy was transferred to ICU and her baby son was transferred to NICU for specialist care. He was born with an APGAR of 5 at 1 minute, 7 at 5 minutes and 7 at 10 minutes.

Summary of key points

- Trauma such as a road traffic accident can culminate in cardiac emergencies/ cardiac arrest or untimely death without prompt and appropriate response.
- Cardiac arrest is a rarity in pregnancy; it is paramount to determine the aetiology whether related to pregnancy or the non-pregnant state.
- Cardiac arrest poses a set of complex challenges to the life of mother and fetus.
- Knowledge of maternal physiology as well as the modifications needed in pregnancy including the alleviation of aorto-caval compression by the gravid uterus, are essential for optimal outcomes.
- Swift response to the early onset of critical illness requires knowledgeable and skilled health professionals able to recognize the early warning signs in pregnancy.
- ROSC is a pivotal step in the resuscitation chain.
- Clinical urgency is paramount to ensure immediate resuscitation of the mother to maximize the chances of a good outcome for mother and baby.
- Fetal compromise is an early warning sign of deterioration in maternal well-being; assessment of FHR is important.
- Rapid perimortem caesarean section when indicated is necessary to save the life of mother and baby.

REFERENCES

Campbell, T.A. and Sanson, T.G. (2009) Cardiac arrest and pregnancy, *Journal of Emergency, Trauma and Shock*, 2(1): 34–42.

Centre for Maternal and Child Enquiries (2011) *Saving Mothers' Lives: Reviewing Maternal Deaths to Make Motherhood Safer: 2006–2008. The Eighth Report of the Confidential Enquiries into Maternal Deaths in the United Kingdom*, ed. G. Lewis. *BJOG: An International British Journal of Obstetrics and Gynaecology*, 118 (Suppl. 1): 1–203.

Chames, M.C. and Pearlman, M.D. (2008) Trauma during pregnancy: outcomes and clinical management, *Clinical Obstetrics and Gynaecology*, 51(2): 398–408.

Dijkman, A., Huisman, C.M.A., Smit, M., Schutte, J.M., Zwart, J.J., van Roosmalen, J.J. and Oepkes, D. (2010) Cardiac arrest in pregnancy: increasing use of perimortem caesarean section due to emergency skills training? *BJOG: An International British Journal of Obstetrics and Gynaecology*, 117(3): 282–7.

El-Kady, D. (2007) Perinatal outcomes of traumatic injuries during pregnancy, *Clinical Obstetrics and Gynaecology*, 51(3): 582–91.

Grady, K. (2007) Shock, in K. Grady, C. Howell and C. Cox (eds) *Managing Obstetric Emergencies and Trauma: The MOET Course*, 2nd edn. London: RCOG.

Grady, K., Howell, C. and Cox, C. (eds) (2007) *Managing Obstetric Emergencies and Trauma: The MOET Course*, 2nd edn. London: RCOG .

Gray, A., Goyber, E.C., Goodacre, S.W. and Johnson, G.S. (1997) Trauma triage: a comparison of CRAMS and TRTs in a UL population, *Injury*, 28(2): 97–101.

Hulbert, D. (2007) Emergency medicine, in G. Lewis (ed.) *The Confidential Enquiry into Maternal and Child Health (CEMACH). Saving Mothers' Lives: Reviewing Maternal Deaths to Make Motherhood Safer: 2003–2005. The Seventh Report on Confidential Enquiries into Maternal Deaths in the United Kingdom*. London: CEMACH, pp. 230–7.

Hulbert, D. (2011) Emergency medicine, in C MAC E *Saving Mothers' Lives: Reviewing Maternal Deaths to Make Motherhood Safer: 2006–2008. The Eighth Report of the Confidential Enquiries into Maternal Deaths in the United Kingdom*, ed. G. Lewis. *BJOG: An International British Journal of Obstetrics and Gynaecology*, 118 (Suppl. 1):167–72.

Hull, S. and Bennett, S. (2007) The pregnant trauma patient: assessment and anaesthetic management, *International Anesthesiology Clinics*, 45(3) 1–18.

Katz, V.L., Balderston, K. and DeFreest, M. (2005) Perimortem caesarean delivery: were our assumptions correct? *American Journal of Obstetrics and Gynecology*, 192 (6): 1916–20 (p. 1921 discussion).

Katz, V.L., Dotters, D.J. and Droegemueller, W. (1986) Perimortem caesarean delivery, *Obstetrics and Gynecology*, 68(4): 571–6.

King, B. (2009) Post-resuscitation care, in P. Moule and J.W. Albarran (eds) *Practical Resuscitation for Healthcare Professionals*, 2nd edn. Chichester: Wiley-Blackwell, pp. 184–94.

Lewis, G. (ed.) (2007) *The Confidential Enquiry into Maternal and Child Health (CEMACH). Saving Mothers' Lives: Reviewing Maternal Deaths to Make Motherhood Safer: 2003–2005. The Seventh Report on Confidential Enquiries into Maternal Deaths in the United Kingdom*. London: CEMACH.

Lewis, G. (2011) Deaths apparently unrelated to pregnancy from Coincidental and Late causes including domestic abuse, in C MAC E *Saving Mothers' Lives: Reviewing Maternal Deaths to Make Motherhood Safer: 2006–2008. The Eighth Report of the Confidential Enquiries into Maternal Deaths in the United Kingdom*, ed. G. Lewis. *BJOG: An International British Journal of Obstetrics and Gynaecology*, 118 (Suppl. 1): 146–51.

Morris, S. and Stacey, M. (2003) Resuscitation in pregnancy, *British Medical Journal*, 327(7426): 1277–9.

Nursing and Midwifery Council (N MC) (2004) *Midwives Rules and Standards*. London: N MC.

Price, L.C., Slack, A. and Nelson-Piercy, C. (2008) Aims of obstetric critical care management, *Best Practice and Research Clinical Obstetrics and Gynaecology*, 22(5): 775–99.

Resuscitation Council (U K) (2010) *2010 Resuscitation Guidelines*. London: RCU K.

Schiff, M.A. and Holt, V.L. (2005) Pregnancy outcomes following hospitalization for motor vehicle crashes in Washington State from 1989–2001, *American Journal of Epidemiology*, 162(2): 197.

Shapiro, J. (2006) Critical care of the obstetric patient, *Journal of Intensive Care Medicine*, 21(5): 278–86.

Sharma, B.R. (2005) Development of pre-hospital trauma-care system: an overview, *Injury*, 36(5): 579–87.

Shields, A. and Fausett, M.B. (2010) Cardiopulmonary resuscitation in pregnancy, in M.A. Belfort, G.R. Saade, M.R. Foley, J.P. Phelan and G.A. Dildy (eds) *Critical Care Obstetrics*, 5th edn. Chichester: Wiley-Blackwell, pp. 93–107.

Smith, S.B., Osgood, V.M. and Crane, S. (2002) A LERT T M: a multiprofessional training course in the care of the acutely ill adult patient, *Resuscitation*, 52(3): 281–6.

Soar, G.D., Perkins, G., Abbas, G., Alfonzo, A., Barelli, A., Bierens, J.J., Brugger, H., Deakin, C.D., Dunning, J., Georgiou, M., Handley, A.J., Lockey, D.J., Paal, P., Sandroni, C., Thies, K.C., Zideman, D.A. and Nolan, J.P. (2010) European Resuscitation Council Guidelines for Resuscitation 2010. Section 8. Cardiac arrest in special circumstances: electrolyte abnormalities, poisoning, drowning, accidental hypothermia, hyperthermia, asthma, anaphylaxis, cardiac surgery, trauma, pregnancy, electrocution, *Resuscitation*, 81(10): 1400–33.

Weintraub, A.Y., Leron, E. and Mazor, M. (2006) The pathophysiology of trauma in pregnancy: a review, *Journal of Maternal, Fetal and Neonatal Medicine*, 19(10): 601–5.

Whitty, J. (2002) Maternal cardiac arrest in pregnancy, *Clinical Obstetrics and Gynaecology*, 45(2): 377–92.

ANNOTATED FURTHER READING

Parrillo, J.E. and Dellinger, P. (eds) (2008) *Critical Care Medicine: Principles of Diagnosis and Management in the Adult*, 3rd edn. London: Mosby, Chapter 82.

Provides an informative chapter on critical illness during pregnancy.

Simpson, H. (2006) Respiratory Assessment, *British Journal of Nursing*, 15(9): 484–8.

Provides helpful tips on respiratory assessment.

Torgersen, C. and Curran, C. (2006) A systematic approach to the physiologic adaptations of pregnancy, *Critical Care Nursing Quarterly*, 29(1): 2–19.

A useful review of maternal adjustment to the physiological demands of pregnancy.

Waterhouse, C. (2005) The Glasgow Coma Scale and other neurological observations, *Nursing Standard*, 19(33): 56–64.

A helpful guide.

USEFUL WEBSITES

http://www.aagbi.org	The Association of Anaesthetists of Great Britain and Ireland
http://www.alert-course.com	ALERT system of assessment
http://www.alsg.org	Advanced life support group
http://www.bcs.com	British Cardiovascular Society
http://www.dh.gov.uk	UK Department of Health
http://www.gmcriticalcare skillsinstitute.org.uk	Greater Manchester Critical Care Skills Institute
http://www.ncepod.org.uk	National Confidential Enquiry into Patient Outcome and Death
http://www.nice.org.uk	National Institute for Health and Clinical Excellence
http://www.npeu.ox.ac.uk	National Perinatal Epidemiology Unit
http://www.rcoa.ac.uk	The Royal College of Anaesthetists
http://www.rcog.org.uk	Royal College of Obstetricians and Gynaecologists (RCOG)
http://www.resus.org.uk	Resuscitation Council UK
http://www.sign.ac.uk	Scottish Intercollegiate Group Network
http://www.trauma.org	Website that provides useful resources, e.g. articles and interactive scenarios on trauma

Diabetic coma
Andrew Simm and Maureen D. Raynor

Pre-requisites for the chapter: the reader should have an understanding of:

- Physiological process of carbohydrate/glucose metabolism.
- Physiological function of pancreatic endocrine hormones insulin and glucagon.
- Hormonal changes and functions during pregnancy, especially human placental lactogen.
- Definitions, diagnosis, classification and management of diabetes mellitus during pregnancy (pre-conception, antepartum, intrapartum and postpartum periods).
- Resuscitation – basic and advanced life support of adult and neonate.
- Relevant pharmacology for effective glycaemic control, e.g. types of insulin and oral hypoglycaemic agents.
- Value of the Modified Early Obstetric Warning Score System (MEOWS) and SBAR (Situation, Background, Assessment and Recommendation) tool of reporting/communication.
- Ways of maximizing effective communication and interprofessional team working.
- Public health role/responsibilities of the midwife in caring for the pregnant woman with diabetes mellitus.

Pre-reading self-assessment

Define the following terms and state their significance:

1 glycogenolysis
2 gluconeogenesis
3 hypoglycaemia
4 hyperglycaemia
5 polydipsia
6 glycosuria
7 ketonuria
8 ketonaemia
9 acidaemia
10 neuroglycopenia

(Continued overleaf)

Recommended prior reading

Confidential Enquiry into Maternal and Child Health (2007) *Diabetes in Pregnancy: Are We Providing the Best Care? Findings of a National Enquiry, England, Wales and Northern Ireland*. Available at: www.cmace.org.uk (accessed 22 August 2010).

Department of Health (DH) (2010) *Six Years On: Delivering the Diabetes National Service Framework*. Available at: www.dh.gov.uk

De Swiet, M., Williamson, C. and Lewis, G. (2011) Other indirect deaths, in Centre for Maternal and Child Enquiries (CMACE) *Saving Mothers' Lives: Reviewing Maternal Deaths to Make Motherhood Safer: 2006–2008. The Eighth Report of the Confidential Enquiries into Maternal Deaths in the United Kingdom (UK)*, ed. G. Lewis. BJOG, 118 (Suppl. 1): 119–31.

National Institute for Health and Clinical Excellence (NICE) (2007) *Acutely Ill Patients in Hospitals: Recognition of and Response to Acute Illness in Adults in Hospital*. Clinical Guideline No. 50. Available at: www.nice.org.uk (accessed 10 May 2011)

CASE STUDY

Sophie, a 23-year-old primigravid woman, is admitted to the antenatal ward at 32 weeks gestation with nausea and some vomiting. Detailed assessment reveals that Sophie has had type 1 diabetes for 11 years. Her booking weight was 64 kg and her body mass index was recorded as 22 in the maternity records.

Her partner, Harry, reports that last night Sophie thought she was getting 'flu-like' symptoms and she complained of feeling shivery and achy. She had some back pain. He went to work in the morning as planned after Sophie reassured him that she would be fine. However, he returned from work at lunch time to find Sophie lying on the settee complaining of feeling unwell, experiencing dull abdominal pain and back pain, a general loss of appetite, nausea and occasional vomiting.

Sophie had not undertaken any blood glucose readings since the day before. An intravenous infusion of crystalloids was already in progress, which the paramedics had sited prior to transfer. Their record of Sophie's vital signs at the time of the initial assessment and during the transfer period revealed signs of haemodynamic decompensation: BP 88/60 mmHg (booking BP 128/72 mmHg), P 110 bpm, T 35°C and RR 26 breaths per min. On admission, following a full assessment by the midwife and obstetrician, a MEOWS chart was commenced and a self-retaining urinary catheter for hourly urine drainage and urinalysis inserted. Urinalysis revealed ketones +++, glucose +++, nitrites and protein +.

1 **What are the possible explanations for Sophie's condition?**

A Sophie's symptoms are relatively non-specific, and could be attributed to a number of problems. 'Flu-like' symptoms are suggestive of a viral or bacterial infection, but could be attributable to some other inflammatory process. Abdominal and back pains are suggestive of an intra-abdominal source, and it is important to try and establish a clearer history as to the nature of the pain experienced, e.g. colicky or constant, any radiation of the pain, and any associated gastro-intestinal or urinary symptoms. It is also important to consider pregnancy-specific diseases which can be variable in presentation, e.g. pre-eclampsia.

Symptoms must be considered in the context of Sophie's medical history and her pregnancy. The initial observations are indicative of diabetic ketoacidosis (DKA), and her symptoms of abdominal pain, nausea and vomiting would be consistent with this. This can be precipitated by infection, but the pregnancy itself can be sufficient, especially if compliance with therapy is not optimal. Nonetheless, investigations into potential underlying causes should be undertaken as outlined in Box 13.3.

Box 13.1 lists the differential diagnoses that should be considered when assessing Sophie on admission to hospital.

Box 13.1 Differential diagnoses

Urinary tract infection/pyelonephritis
Acute appendicitis
Acute cholecystitis
Acute pancreatitis
Acute gastroenteritis
Peptic ulceration
Pneumonia
Influenza
Diabetic ketoacidosis
Pre-eclampsia

In this instance, the nitrites in the urine are suggestive of an underlying urinary tract infection that may be the precipitant of the DKA.

2 **The reason for Sophie being so unwell appears to be 'diabetic ketoacidosis'. With reference to relevant pathophysiology, how can you explain the pathogenesis of this hyperglycaemic emergency?**

A Best practice guidelines from the Joint British Diabetes Society's Inpatient Care Group (Diabetic UK 2010) on the management of DKA in adults emphasize the gravity of the condition by highlighting the significant morbidity and mortality associated with it. They describe the pathophysiology as a complex disordered metabolic state characterized by the biochemical triad detailed in Figure 13.1.

DKA results from absolute or relative insulin deficiency accompanied by an increase in counter-regulatory hormones (i.e. glucagon, growth hormone, the stress hormones cortisol and the catecholamines, and free fatty acids).

Insulin is needed to facilitate the entry of glucose into the cells to be utilized as energy by the body, and as a result it brings about a lowering of blood glucose levels. The glucose is used by cells to produce energy. With insulin deficiency, blood glucose cannot enter cells for energy consumption. The counter-regulatory hormones enhance gluconeogenesis and glycogenolysis resulting in marked hyperglycaemia (Diabetic UK 2010), but without insulin the glucose remains unable to enter the cells. Thus an alternative source of energy must be found. The body mobilizes its fat stores (lipolysis) to provide essential energy for sustaining vital organs and maintaining life. The process of oxidation converts fatty acids to acetyl-CoA which is then used to produce energy. However, during high rates of fatty acid oxidation, some of the acetyl-CoA is converted to ketone bodies. Their production exceeds the capacity of the brain, heart

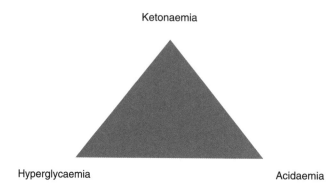

Figure 13.1 Biochemical triad of DKA (Diabetes UK 2010)

and skeletal muscle to use them for energy. As they are relatively strong acids, acidification of the blood occurs, one consequence of which is impairing the ability of haemoglobin to bind to oxygen.

Hyperventilation occurs in an attempt to overcome the metabolic acidosis by blowing off more carbon dioxide (respiratory alkalosis). The high blood glucose levels spill over into the urine and produce an osmotic diuresis. Consequently there is marked glycosuria, polyuria and dehydration, the latter often exacerbated by vomiting. Electrolytes become depleted. The key features are outlined in Box 13.2.

Box 13.2 Biochemical indices of DKA

- Ketonaemia: 3 mmol/L and over

or

- Significant ketonuria (> 2+ on standard urinalysis)
- Blood glucose > 11 mmol/L or known diabetes mellitus
- Bicarbonate (HCO_3^-) below 15 mmol/L and/or venous pH < 7.3

Adapted from Diabetes UK (2010: 5)

The hyperglycaemia, acidosis, electrolyte disturbances and dehydration all present a threat to the well-being of both the mother and her baby.

3   **Why does DKA pose a significant threat to the well-being of both Sophie and her developing fetus?**

A   The incidence of DKA in pregnancy is relatively low, and is quoted between 1 and 3 per cent. Fetal mortality is variably quoted at between 9 and 35 per cent, and maternal mortality between 4 and 15 per cent (Kamalakannan et al. 2003). There are several reasons why ketoacidosis may be more likely in pregnancy, not least the insulin resistance that develops as pregnancy progresses, and the relative state of accelerated starvation. Bicarbonate levels (the buffer of hydrogen ions) are already slightly lower in pregnancy, resulting in the potential for more rapid development of ketoacidosis, and at lower glucose levels. Fortunately the intensive surveillance of women with diabetes in pregnancy, aiming for tight glycaemic control to reduce the risks, keeps the incidence of ketoacidosis low. Particular groups at risk are those with poor glycaemic control who are not compliant with treatment, and women threatening pre-term labour who require steroids to aid maturity of the fetal lungs (steroids oppose insulin action and promote gluconeogenesis).

Check point

Intercurrent illness can also predispose to DKA, as this case highlights.

Once the ketoacidosis has developed, the mother becomes progressively dehydrated with attendant electrolyte disturbances. These can exacerbate the vomiting. Acidosis is dangerous to cells, and oxygen delivery is impaired.

There may be various effects on the fetus, but the relative contribution to fetal risk from each is still not fully known. Dehydration may impair uteroplacental blood flow, and electrolyte disturbance may be manifest in both mother and fetus. The maternal acidosis may make oxygen delivery to the fetus more difficult, at a time when fetal hyperinsulinaemia (a response to the high glucose levels crossing the placenta) is already increasing metabolic demand. Acidosis may also develop in the fetus. Any combination of these poses a threat to the well-being of the fetus, and tests of fetal well-being may show abnormalities.

4   **What are the main investigations that should be undertaken following Sophie's admission to hospital?**

A   Table 13.1 lists the principal investigations that should be undertaken following Sophie's admission, the reasoning behind the investigations, and the results obtained.

Traditionally acidosis has been determined by sampling arterial blood, but in most instances this is no longer considered necessary; venous sampling is technically much easier. Much of the testing can be done on bedside meters (blood glucose and ketones, if available), and blood gas analysers (venous pH, bicarbonate and electrolytes) with the advantage that results are available rapidly, given there is no waiting for the laboratory to process the sample. These results both confirm the diagnosis and guide management. Nonetheless, abnormal results should usually be verified on a sample sent to the laboratory.

The midstream urine sample and blood cultures are taken as there is suspicion of urinary tract infection. In someone who is this unwell, there may be more widespread infection with bacteraemia, thus blood cultures are advisable despite the temperature not being elevated. In fact, a low temperature, as in this case, can be found in association with sepsis (see Case 11), as demonstrated by the findings illuminated in the 2006–2008 triennial report from CMACE (2011) on maternal mortality in the UK.

Maternal well-being is of prime importance, and when the mother is extremely unwell, fetal well-being should not take priority. In this case it would be worthwhile establishing fetal well-being by way of a CTG once treatment of the mother has been instituted. If abnormalities are present on the CTG, these are often secondary to the underlying ketoacidosis. Correction of this may result in improvement of the CTG.

Table 13.1 Principal investigations, reasoning and results of investigations

Investigation	Reason	Results
Capillary blood glucose	Quick bedside test to establish presence of hyperglycaemia	18.0 mmol/L
Venous plasma glucose	To confirm accuracy of capillary glucose	18.6 mmol/L
Blood urea and electrolytes	Dehydration may be reflected in elevated urea and creatinine levels (normal levels usually lower in pregnancy). Electrolyte disturbances are common	Na^+ 133 mmol/L K^+ 4.7 mmol/L Urea 5.1 mmol/L Creatinine 88 micromol/L
Venous bicarbonate	To evaluate degree of acidosis	10 mmol/L
Venous pH	To evaluate degree of acidosis	pH 7.24
Blood ketones (if available)	To establish presence of ketonaemia	4 mmol/L
Full blood count	White cell count elevated in infection	Hb 13.8 g/dL WCC 23 × 10⁹/L Platelets 287 × 10⁹/L
Midstream urine culture	To establish whether urinary tract infection present and, if so, determine antibiotic sensitivities	*E. coli* in significant numbers
Blood culture	To establish whether there is bacteraemia when sepsis is suspected	Negative
Cardiotocograph	To establish fetal well-being	Normal

5   **What is the initial management of Sophie?**

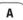 Management should be undertaken by a multidisciplinary team that includes senior obstetricians and midwives, but must also involve a diabetes specialist team (Diabetes UK 2010; SIGN 2010). This should take place in a unit with facilities for high level care or equivalent area offering level 2 critical care (Intensive Care Society 2009). Management will be guided by the results of investigations, but the main principles of treatment are:

- appropriate fluid replacement;
- insulin administration;
- treatment of any precipitating cause.

Fluid replacement needs to be aggressive, using crystalloids, i.e. normal saline or Hartmann's solution. This restores circulatory volume, clears ketones, and can be used to correct electrolyte imbalance (potassium supplementation should be guided by blood levels that should be checked at regular intervals). Insulin therapy given via an intravenous infusion reduces blood glucose levels and suppresses ketogenesis. Once the blood glucose falls below a certain level, intravenous dextrose should be run alongside the insulin infusion. Fluid replacement with normal saline or Hartmann's solution should be additional to this.

In Sophie's case, intravenous antibiotics should be administered while awaiting the urine culture result, as urinary tract infection is considered likely. Intravenous therapy should be used until the vomiting has resolved. The midwife should maintain a strict fluid balance chart and in conjunction with the obstetric team, ensure that Sophie's fluids and electrolytes are monitored closely and recorded accurately and contemporaneously.

6   **What are the implications of pre-existing diabetes in pregnancy?**

A   Diabetes mellitus is the most common pre-existing medical disorder complicating pregnancy in the UK. Approximately 1:250 pregnant women have pre-existing diabetes (NICE 2008; Diabetic UK 2010; SIGN 2010). This can be type 1 or type 2 diabetes, both are associated with increased perinatal mortality. The implications of diabetes in pregnancy can be looked at in different ways, either looking at the effects of diabetes on the pregnancy and vice versa, or potential effects on mother and fetus. Boxes 13.3 and 13.4 outline the principal effects of diabetes on the pregnancy coupled with the impact of pregnancy on the diabetic state, as reflected in the NICE (2008) guideline for diabetes in pregnancy, the CEMACH (2005) report on pregnancy with type 1 and type 2 diabetes, and the SIGN (2010) management of diabetes guidelines.

Box 13.3 Risks of diabetes in pregnancy

- Miscarriage.
- Congenital malformation.
- Fetal macrosomia.
- Intra-uterine growth restriction (IUGR)/pre-eclampsia, especially in women with vascular complications of diabetes, e.g. nephropathy.
- Stillbirth.
- Pre-term delivery (spontaneous and iatrogenic).
- Induction of labour.
- Caesarean section.
- Birth trauma (to mother and fetus).
- Transient neonatal morbidity (e.g. hypoglycaemia).
- Neonatal death.
- Obesity and/or diabetes developing later in the baby's life.

Box 13.4 Effects of pregnancy on diabetes

- Changing glucose levels resulting in more difficult control.
- Risk of diabetic ketoacidosis.
- Risk of hypoglycaemia owing to tight control in pregnancy.
- Worsening of underlying vascular complications, e.g. nephropathy, retinopathy.

As stated previously, the risks of diabetes in pregnancy mean that management of these women should be conducted by a multidisciplinary team comprising a diabetes physician, a specialist nurse in diabetes, a specialist midwife, a dietician and an obstetrician. Frequent review is necessary to regularly evaluate the blood sugar profiles and adjust therapy accordingly. The use of ultrasound scan is an integral part of care as a detailed anomaly scan is important in looking for cardiac and neural tube defects that are more frequent in diabetes. Fetal growth velocity is reviewed by monthly scans in the third trimester; birth should occur by 40 weeks to minimize the risk of late stillbirth (Temple et al. 2002; Penney et al. 2003; Macintosh et al. 2006).

7 **Define the terms 'hyperglycaemia' and 'hypoglycaemia'. What blood glucose targets for women with diabetes are recommended in pregnancy, and how are these achieved?**

A *Hyperglycaemia* is the term used for expressing high blood sugar, the exact value of which is variably defined in the literature (usually between 8 and 15 mmol/L). Chronic hyperglycaemia is the defining feature of diabetes mellitus. Acute hyperglycaemia can occur outside of diabetes, precipitants including stress, e.g. associated with myocardial infarction, or medications including steroids. It is important to note that in managing DKA, the focus has changed from concentrating on the hyperglycaemia to looking at the ketonaemia, given that this is the fundamental abnormality.

Hypoglycaemia is a state of having lower than normal blood glucose. From a practical perspective, any blood glucose less than 4 mmol/L should be treated in someone with diabetes requiring hospital admission. This should not be confused with levels in adults without diabetes, where normal glucose levels are 3.5–7.0 mmol/L.

Challenges to good glycaemic control can manifest in the first, second and third trimesters of pregnancy due to insulin resistance, culminating in an elevated insulin secretion. This is a well-recognized phenomenon known to occur to stave off an abnormal rise in glucose, free fatty acids and amino acids. These alterations in pregnancy, coupled with the onset of nausea and vomiting for some women, mean this is a particularly testing time. The hormones of pregnancy, especially the main culprit human placental lactogen (HPL), which has a similar effect to growth hormone, contribute to the insulin resistance, freeing up glucose in favour of the fetus. However, the effects of HPL also increase free fatty acids – a source of energy for the mother and fetus during periods of body starvation.

It is important to note that hypoglycaemia may present in a non-specific way as outlined in Box 13.5.

Box 13.5 Signs and symptoms of hypoglycaemia

- Palpitations
- Nausea
- Sweating, skin clammy and cool to touch
- Hunger
- Tremulousness/jitteriness/poor co-ordination (jerky or shaky movements)
- Malaise or headache

- Odd or atypical behaviour such as resistive behaviour or unexpected aggression
- Speech difficulty, e.g. slurring of words
- Drowsiness or confusion.

The above clinical features are thought to be attributable to an autonomic response brought about by the sympatho-adrenal system. When the brain is starved of the glucose supply needed to sustain cerebral function, features of neuroglycopenia develop, leading to disruption of cognitive performance.

Whatever the type of diabetes, national guidelines advocate tight glycaemic control during pregnancy (NICE 2008; Diabetic UK 2010; SIGN 2010). Women should be advised to check fasting and 1-hour postprandial glucose levels after every meal during pregnancy. They should also test before retiring to bed. The target ranges for glucose in pregnancy are a fasting level between 3.5 and 5.9 mmol/L and 1-hour post-prandial glucose below 7.8 mmol/L (NICE 2008). The glucose level before retiring to bed should usually be between 6 and 7 mmol/L. These targets are achieved through a combination of dietary adjustment with or without additional therapy with insulin or oral hypoglycaemic agents.

8 **What is the management of symptomatic hypoglycaemia?**

A The guideline *Hospital Management of Hypoglycaemia in Adults with Diabetes Mellitus* (Stannistreet et al. 2010) outlines the management of adults with hypoglycaemia according to the severity of their symptoms. Although applicable to the whole adult population with diabetes, the principles are applicable to pregnant women with diabetes requiring treatment.

In women who are conscious, orientated and able to swallow, 1–20 g of quick-acting carbohydrate should be given. This might include:

- 150–200 mL of pure fruit juice
- 90–120 mL of original Lucozade®
- 5–7 Dextrosol® tablets.

If the capillary blood glucose measurement remains below 4 mmol/L after 10–15 minutes, administration of one of the above can be repeated. Hypoglycaemia resistant to these measures may require glucagon or intravenous dextrose. Once the glucose is above 4 mmol/L and the woman has recovered, a long-acting carbohydrate should be given, for example, two biscuits or a slice of bread/toast. Normal insulin, if due to be administered, should not be omitted (Stannistreet et al. 2010).

If the woman is conscious but unco-operative, and can swallow, 1.5–2 tubes of GlucoGel® can be squeezed into the mouth between the teeth and gums.

If unconscious, immediate medical assistance should be sought. Intravenous dextrose or glucagon IM are required. The ABCDE principles of assessment as outlined in Cases 1, 11 and 12 should be adhered to. Stannistreet et al. (2010) stress that attention should be paid to the following:

- **A** – airway management – establishing, securing and maintaining an adequate flow of oxygen.
- **B** – breathing – good oxygenation is important to ventilation of the lungs and sustaining breathing.
- **C** – circulation – ensuring adequate circulatory blood volume like the other first-line resuscitative measures is also critical to both maternal and fetal well-being.
- **D** – disability – assessment of the degree of any underlying diasability (including neurological assessment and blood glucose monitoring) is vital.
- **E** – exposure – allowance should also be made for this aspect, including assessment and recording of core body temperature on the MEOWS chart coupled with a complete review of other records and an overall thorough examination of Sophie.

Check point

When assessing state of consciousness using the AVPU scale as detailed in previous cases, the midwife must be aware of the importance of reporting *P* and *U* levels to the maternity emergency team.

ONGOING CARE

Hypoglycaemia is an ever-looming threat in the early months of pregnancy. Three maternal deaths from hypoglycaemia are documented in the CMACE report for the triennium 2006–2008 (De Swiet et al. 2011). The deaths of these women highlight the tightrope negotiated by women who present with type 1 diabetes mellitus during pregnancy, which is complicated by other co-morbidities such as infection. Not surprisingly, hypoglycaemia and DKA are perhaps the most feared complications of diabetes mellitus during pregnancy. Good follow-up education is important for ongoing compliance. Pregnancy is a time when women are highly motivated to improve their health to ensure optimal health and a good outcome for their babies. Every opportunity should be taken to capitalize on women's thirst for knowledge during the antepartum period, given the repeated contact with the interprofessional team during this time (Lewis and Drife 2004; Lewis 2007).

Women should be informed about the benefits of treating early onset of any ensuing infection, a common precipitating factor of DKA previously outlined. Educational information that illuminates the gains of good glycaemic control is more likely to result in positive outcomes being associated with reduced perinatal morbidity and mortality, including neonatal respiratory distress syndrome and hypoglycaemia (Temple et al. 2002; Penney et al. 2003; Macintosh et al. 2006).

Having a clear understanding of the prevention, pathogenesis, contributory factors, clinical features and first-line management of diabetic coma is essential. This will ensure the midwife and other key members of the interprofessional team are adequately prepared to recognize early such critical conditions. This will enable optimal outcomes for mother and baby. Being prepared is being forearmed.

Summary of key points

- DKA is a rare complication during pregnancy but an ever-present threat, therefore prevention is always fundamentally better than cure.
- Both hypoglycaemia and DKA are unwelcome and challenging complications of diabetes that may result in an emergency.
- Pre-conception education and counselling are highly recommended for all women of childbearing years with diabetes mellitus.
- The focus of managing diabetic DKA should be directed at correcting ketonaemia, the crux of the problem.
- Hypoglycaemia is a real risk during pregnancy, especially the first trimester. Achieving optimal glycaemic control while safeguarding the well-being of the pregnant woman and her developing fetus remains a challenge as borne out in the report by CMACE (2011).
- Having a clear understanding of the prevention, pathogenesis, contributory factors, clinical features and first-line management of hypoglycaemia and DKA is crucial.

REFERENCES

CMACE (2011) *Saving Mothers' Lives: Reviewing Maternal Deaths to Make Motherhood Safer: 2006–2008. The Eighth Report of the Confidential Enquiries into Maternal Deaths in the United Kingdom*. Ed. G. Lewis. *BJOG: An International British Journal of Obstetrics and Gynaecology*, 118 (Suppl. 1): 1–203.

Confidential Enquiries into Maternal and Child Health (2005) *Pregnancy in Women with Type 1 and Type 2 Diabetes: England, Wales and Northern Ireland*. London: CEMACH.

Confidential Enquiries into Maternal and Child Health (2007) *Diabetes in Pregnancy: Are We Providing the Best Care? Findings of a National Enquiry: England, Wales and Northern Ireland*. London: CEMACH.

Department of Health (DH) (2010) *Six Years On: Delivering the Diabetes National Service Framework*. Available at: http://www.dh.gov.uk

De Swiet, M., Williamson, C. and Lewis, G. (2011) Other indirect deaths, in Centre for Maternal and Child Enquiries (CMACE) *Saving Mothers' Lives: Reviewing Maternal Deaths to Make Motherhood Safer: 2006–2008. The Eighth Report of the Confidential Enquiries into Maternal Deaths in the United Kingdom (UK)*, ed. G. Lewis. *BJOG*, 118 (Suppl. 1): 119–31.

Diabetes UK (2010) *Report of the Joint British Diabetes Societies Inpatient Care Group: Management of Ketoacidosis in Adults*. Available at: http://www.diabetes.nhs.uk (accessed 22 August 2010).

Intensive Care Society (2009) *Levels of Critical Care for Adult Patients: Standards and Guidelines*. London: Intensive Care Society. Available at: http://www.ics.ac.uk (accessed 1 April 2011).

Kamalakannan, D., Baskar, V., Darton, D. and Abdu, T. (2003) Diabetic ketoacidosis in pregnancy, *Postgraduate Medical Journal*, 79(934): 454–7. Available at: http://www.ncbi.nlm.nih.gov/pmc/articles/PMC1742779/ (accessed 25 March 2011). DOI: 10.1136/pmj.79.934.454.

Lewis, G. (ed.) (2007) *The Confidential Enquiry into Maternal and Child Health (CEMACH). Saving Mothers' Lives: Reviewing Maternal Deaths to Make Motherhood Safer: 2003–2005. The Seventh Report on Confidential Enquiries into Maternal Deaths in the United Kingdom*. London: CEMACH.

Lewis, G. and Drife, J. (eds) (2004) *Why Mothers Die: 2000–2002: The Sixth Report of the Confidential Enquiries into Maternal Deaths in the United Kingdom*. Available at: http://www.cmace.org.uk (accessed 10 April 2011).

Macintosh, M.C.M., Fleming, K.M., Bailey, J.A., Doyle, P., Modder, J., Acolet, D., Golightly, S. and Miller, A. (2006) Perinatal mortality and congenital anomalies in babies of women with type 1 and 2 diabetes in England, Wales and Northern Ireland: population based study, *BMJ*, 333(7560): 177. Available at: http://www.bmj.com (accessed 1 April 2011). DOI: 10.1136/bmj.38856.692986.AE.

National Institute for Health and Clinical Excellence (NICE) (2007) *Acutely Ill Patients in Hospitals: Recognition of and Response to Acute Illness in Adults in Hospital*. Clinical Guideline No. 50. Available at: http://www.nice.org.uk (accessed 22 August 2010).

National Institute for Health and Clinical Excellence (NICE) (2008) *Diabetes in Pregnancy: Management of Diabetes from Pre-Conception to Postnatal Period*. Clinical Guideline No. 63. Available at: http://www.nice.org.uk. (accessed 22 August 2010).

Penney, G.C., Mair, G. and Pearson, D.W.M. (2003) Outcomes of pregnancies in women with type 1 diabetes in Scotland: a national population study, *British Journal of Obstetrics and Gynaecology*, 110(3): 315–18.

Scottish Intercollegiate Guidelines Network (2010) *Management of Diabetes: A National Clinical Guideline No. 116*. Available at: http://www.sign.ac.uk (accessed 22 August 2010).

Stannistreet, D., Walden, E., Jones, C. and Graveling, A. (2010) *The Hospital Management of Hypoglycaemia in Adults with Diabetes Mellitus (On Behalf of the Joint British Diabetes Society and Diabetes UK)*. Available at: http://www.diabetes.nhs.uk (accessed 1 April 2011).

Temple, R., Aldridge, V., Greenwood, R., Heyburn, P., Sampson, M. and Stanley, K. (2002) Association between outcome of pregnancy and glycaemic control in early pregnancy in type 1 diabetes: population based study, *BMJ*, 325(7375): 1275. Available at: http://www.bmj.com (accessed 1 April 2011). DOI: 10.1136/bmj.325.7375.1275.

ANNOTATED FURTHER READING

Confidential Enquiries into Maternal and Child Health (2007) *Diabetes in Pregnancy: Caring for the Baby after Birth: Findings of a National Enquiry. England, Wales and Northern Ireland*. London: CEMACH.

Provides useful guidelines on the care of the neonate born to a mother with diabetes mellitus.

Frier, B.M. and Fisher, M. (eds) (2007) *Hypoglycaemia in Clinical Diabetes*, 2nd edn. Chichester: Wiley.

Has an informative chapter on risks of diabetes mellitus for the mother, fetus and neonate.

King, J.C. (2006) Maternal obesity, metabolism, and pregnancy outcome, *Annual Review of Nutrition*, 26: 271–91. DOI: 10.1146/annurev.nutr.24.012003.132249.

Highlights the challenges posed by obesity to carbohydrats metabolism and the risk of developing diabetes mellitus.

Lavender, T., Platt, M.J., Tsekiri, E.K., Casson, I., Byrom, S., Baker, L. and Walkinshaw, S. (2009) Women's perceptions of being pregnant and having pregestational diabetes, *Midwifery*. Full text DOI:10.1016/j.midw.2009.01.003.

A useful article.

Ramussen, B., O'Connell, B., Dunning, P. and Cox, H. (2007) Young women with type 1 diabetes: management of turning points and transitions, *Quality Health Research*, 17(3): 300–10.

A useful insight into diabetes as a major transitional crisis, coupled with the psychological processes/coping strategies employed by women with diabetes mellitus.

USEFUL WEBSITES

http://www.aagbi.org	The Association of Anaesthetists of Great Britain and Ireland
http://www.alert-course.com	A L E R T system of assessment
http://www.dh.gov.uk	U K Department of Health
http://www.diabetes.nhs.uk	N H S Diabetes
http://www.diabetes.org.uk	Diabetes U K
http://www.ncepod.org.uk/2005aap.htm	National Confidential Enquiry into Patient Outcome and Death
http://www.nice.org.uk	National Institute for Health and Clinical Excellence
http://www.npeu.ox.ac.uk/mbrrace-uk	National Perinatal Epidemiology Unit
http://www.npsa.nhs.uk	National Patient Safety Agency
http://www.rcog.org.uk	Royal College of Obstetricians and Gynaecologists
http://www.sign.ac.uk	Scottish Intercollegiate Guidelines Network

CASE STUDY 14
Shoulder dystocia
Susan Brydon and Maureen D. Raynor

Pre-requisites for the chapter: the reader should have an understanding of:

- The anatomy and physiology of the pelvic variants, including their diameters.
- The physiological mechanisms during the second stage of labour which are necessary for a normal birth.
- Optimal birth positions.
- The midwife's role and responsibilities during normal and complicated birth.
- The midwife's role and responsibilities within the interprofessional team.
- Local National Health Service (NHS) Trust clinical governance/risk management procedures relating to the reporting of critical incidents and Clinical Negligence Scheme for Trusts (CNST) requirements.
- Current national and local recommendations for the management of shoulder dystocia.
- Types of brachial plexus birth injury.
- The medico-legal imperative of record keeping.

Pre-reading self-assessment

1 What internal rotation will the fetus undergo during passage through the birth canal in order to realize a normal birth?
2 What is the definition of macrosomia?
3 What is the current understanding of the mechanism for shoulder dystocia?
4 What is meant by the term 'maternal propulsive forces'?
5 What physiological changes occur during the adoption of the McRoberts' manoeuvre?
6 Differentiate between Erb's palsy and Klumpke's palsy.

Recommended prior reading

Department of Health (DH) (1998) *Confidential Enquiry into Stillbirths and Deaths in Infancy (CESDI): Fifth Annual Report.* London: Maternal and Child Health Research Consortium.
Department of Health (DH) (1999) *Confidential Enquiry into Stillbirths and Deaths in Infancy: Sixth Annual Report.* London: Maternal and Child Health Research Consortium. Current local clinical guideline on the management of shoulder dystocia.

CASE STUDY

Anna is a 29 year old who is admitted at 40 weeks and 5 days of pregnancy to her local M L U in spontaneous labour. It is her second pregnancy; the first had resulted in a spontaneous birth with no complications. She is accompanied by her husband George. On arrival in the unit, the previous history, the reason for admission and maternal and fetal well-being are assessed and normal observations of maternal T PR, B P and urinalysis are confirmed. There is no evidence of any adverse history that could affect the labour or progress of the birth. The previous baby weighed 3.2 kg and was born in good condition with Apgar scores of 10 at 1 and 5 minutes respectively.

Findings on abdominal examination are longitudinal lie, cephalic presentation, R O L position, 2/5ths engaged, and S P F H measures 37 cm. There is no indication for E F M; therefore structured I A is performed using a Pinard stethoscope for one full minute in accordance with the N I C E (2007) guideline. The F H is within the normal range at 146 bpm with no abnormalities detected during auscultation. The contraction pattern and Anna's general demeanour indicate that labour is established and advancing. Therefore, the midwife decides that a V E is unnecessary at this stage.

Because Anna appears to be in established labour, the midwife continues to monitor the F H intermittently at 15-minute intervals during the first stage of labour, with all recordings within the normal range. Anna is coping well with labour; 45 minutes after admission she reports that she is experiencing rectal pressure. Five minutes later a strong urge to push is experienced and the contractions are expulsive. The baby's head is born 15 minutes later and the midwife notices that the head is tightly pressed against the perineum. There is evidence of some restitution before the next contraction. With the subsequent contraction the midwife applies routine traction in order to guide the baby out of the birth canal but there is no advance of the shoulders.

1   **What is the pathophysiology and likely cause of the delay in the birth of the baby's shoulders?**

A   The likeliest cause of the delay in the birth of the baby's shoulders is failure of the bisacromial diameter to rotate into the widest diameter of the pelvic outlet, the anteroposterior diameter, causing the anterior shoulder to become trapped behind or above the symphysis pubis. This results in anterior shoulder dystocia, a serious maternity emergency associated with a high risk of perinatal morbidity/mortality and maternal complications (Draycott et al. 2005).

On reviewing the evidence, there are a number of theories about the pathophysiology of shoulder dystocia. Sandmire and DeMott (2008) provide a simple explanation, stating that in births complicated by shoulder dystocia, the shoulders are attempting to enter the pelvic inlet in the short anteroposterior diameter and this can result in persistent obstruction leading to the diagnosis of shoulder dystocia after the head is born. Moreover, the fetal head will continue its descent down the birth canal while the stuck shoulder remains stationary, resulting in the stretching of the neck and brachial plexus.

Piper and McDonald (1994) agree and add a further theory, stating that in some cases the shoulders of a macrosomic fetus may enter the pelvis in the normal oblique diameter of the pelvis and become impacted as they attempt to rotate to the anteroposterior diameter of the outlet. This theory suggests that the obstruction in some cases is not at the inlet but occurs within the pelvis due to the presence of large fetal shoulders and body.

Gherman's (2002) explanation of the pathophysiology starts quite plausibly, stating that shoulder dystocia is the result of a recognized inconsistency between the bisacromial diameter (fetal shoulders) and the pelvic inlet. However, curiously, his clarification of the problem further suggests that failure of the shoulders to engage in the widest diameter of the pelvis can be additionally sub-categorized into:

1 *High form of shoulder dystocia:* non-engagement of both shoulders.
2 *Mid-form of shoulder dystocia*: non-rotation of the bisacromial diameter in the mid-cavity of the pelvis. Slight degree of restitution is notable and the characteristic 'turtle sign' is absent.
3 *Low form of shoulder dystocia*: non-engagement of one shoulder only, which commonly is the anterior shoulder.

This explanation is unhelpful as it implies grading of the shoulder dystocia, which is not the practice in the UK. At best, it is confusing and, at worst, it is anatomically unreliable as it appears to suggest that the fetal head can be born when both shoulders are retained above the pelvic inlet. This view is repeated in the literature (Benedetti and Gabbe 1978; Piper and McDonald 1994) and popular midwifery textbooks. As the distance from the sacral promontory to the vaginal outlet is 12–13 cm, it is implausible to consider that the fetal head could be born if the posterior shoulder was still above the sacral promontory. In cases of posterior shoulder impaction, where the posterior shoulder is impacted at the level of the sacral promontory, the impaction will have to be overcome by maternal propulsive forces or internal rotation in order for the head to be born.

It is worth noting that in the 'low form of shoulder dystocia', where there is non-engagement of one shoulder, the anterior, the distance between the vaginal outlet and the inlet of the pelvis is at least 5 cm. This is still a considerable distance and it is unreasonable to consider that the brachial plexus would not be stretched if the head was born and the anterior shoulder remained impacted above the symphysis pubis. Understanding of the anatomy and the forces exerted during normal birth has led to challenges to the dominant theory about the causation of obstetric brachial plexus palsy injury (OBPPI), as it is now argued that such injuries can be caused during the process of the birth rather than by any action of the midwife/doctor (Gonik et al. 2000; Gherman et al. 2006; Sandmire and DeMott 2008, 2009).

Check points

- A failure of the shoulders to deliver with the next uterine contraction after the birth of the head should be identified as shoulder dystocia.
- Regardless of the suspected cause, traction should only be used in conjunction with a specific manoeuvre until there is evidence that the shoulders have been freed from the bony pelvis. Such evidence includes significant forward movement of the baby or visualization of the shoulder(s) at the vaginal outlet.
- Shoulder dystocia is largely unpreventable and unpredictable, therefore midwives and obstetricians should be aware of the possibility of shoulder dystocia with all vaginal births, regardless of risk indicators.

2   **What other explanations could there be for the failure of the shoulders to deliver?**

A   Delay in the birth of the shoulders can occur if the posterior shoulder is transiently obstructed at the pelvic brim on the promontory of the sacrum and the fetus continues to descend under the influence of maternal propulsive forces (Sandmire and DeMott 2009). By the time the head is born, the transient obstruction will have resolved but delay in the birth can occur, resulting in a diagnosis of shoulder dystocia.

OTHER CAUSES OF TRANSIENT DELAY IN THE BIRTH OF THE SHOULDERS

There are a number of passive physiological movements the fetus makes during its journey through the birth canal in the second stage of labour. During this process there are a number of physiological explanations for the transient delay in the birth of the fetal shoulders as highlighted in Box 14.1.

Box 14.1 Reasons for transient delay in the birth of the fetal shoulders during the second stage of labour:

Nuchal cord   In rare cases the cord is wrapped tightly around the fetal neck, shortening the cord and preventing descent of the shoulders.

Body dystocia   This is where the size of the fetus inhibits normal progress through the birth canal despite the shoulders being free of the bony pelvis, e.g. large abdominal-thoracic ratio.

Compound presentation   A phenomenon that occurs when the hand and arm are alongside the fetal head/shoulders; this can prevent descent of the shoulders and birth of the body. Removal of the hand from the birth canal by gentle traction will usually resolve this problem.

If the baby is born with an Erb's palsy, it is important to identify whether the affected shoulder was anterior or posterior at the time of the birth. This is because damage to the posterior shoulder plexus is not attributable to the actions of the attending midwife or doctor (Stirrat and Taylor 2002).

In order to differentiate between anterior and posterior shoulder dystocia, it is important that the position of the fetus is recorded following each abdominal palpation and/or VE prior to the birth and that the direction in which the baby's head is facing after restitution is described. The former may be considered more reliable as it provides an independent assessment of fetal position before the emergency arose.

3 **What is the incidence of shoulder dystocia?**

A The incidence of shoulder dystocia is variously described in the literature, with quoted rates as low as 0.6 per cent and as high as 2–2.4 per cent (Draycott et al. 2005, 2008). This variation in incidence may be related to under- or over-reporting. Some clinicians will report shoulder dystocia if specific manoeuvres are required in order to free the baby, and this is the diagnostic test recommended in most of the current literature. This can distort the true incidence, however, as some clinicians will use one of the recognized manoeuvres prophylactically, usually McRoberts', when there is a suspicion, rather than a definite diagnosis of shoulder dystocia. Consequently, this may result in some vaginal births being classified as complicated by shoulder dystocia when in fact the birth has proceeded without complication. In addition, some cases of shoulder dystocia are incorrectly described as simply 'difficulty with the shoulders', which may lead to the shoulder dystocia being unreported (Mahran et al. 2008).

Whether the incidence of shoulder dystocia is increasing is not possible to accurately determine, although more recent studies have shown a small increase (Mackenzie et al. 2007; Draycott et al. 2008) despite the considerable rise in the CS rate and consequent reduction in the vaginal birth rate. The explanation for the increase is unclear but may be related to enhanced awareness and identification or factors as yet not quantified.

4 **What are the commonly cited antenatal and intrapartum risk indicators for shoulder dystocia?**

A A number of risk associated factors have been identified with the phenomenon of shoulder dystocia. These are outlined in Box 14.2 for both the antenatal and intrapartum periods and should be seen as having a poor predictive rather than definitive value, primarily because they are commonly encountered in normal pregnancy and provide little in the way of predicting shoulder dystocia.

Box 14.2

Associated antenatal risk factors for shoulder dystocia (Nocon et al. 1993; Nocon and Weisbrod 1995; Draycott et al. 2005)

Previous shoulder dystocia;

Maternal diabetes;

Maternal obesity (BMI > 30);

Fetal macrosomia (estimated fetal weight > 4.5 kg);

Post-dates pregnancy.

Associated intrapartum risk indicators for shoulder dystocia (Gupta et al. 2010; Nesbitt et al. 1998)

Augmented or induced labour;

Prolonged first stage;

Prolonged second stage;

(Continued overleaf)

Instrumental birth, e.g. mid-cavity forceps;

'Turtling' sign – head retracts tightly against the mother's perineum, causing the baby's cheeks to bulge.

Slow advance of the baby's head/difficulty in freeing the face and chin from the vagina.

Check point

Again it should be noted that all of the associated risk indicators are commonly encountered during labour and birth and are not sufficiently predictive to assist in the decision-making process.

---

5 **Can shoulder dystocia be prevented?**

A Studies have demonstrated that many of the frequently quoted risk indicators are not associated with an increased risk of shoulder dystocia and that only 25 per cent of shoulder dystocia cases had at least one significant risk factor. When considered another way, three-quarters of all shoulder dystocia occurred in the absence of any risk indicator. According to Lewis et al. (1998) and Gherman (2002), the positive predictive value of antenatal risk factors for shoulder dystocia is less than 2 per cent individually, 3 per cent when combined.

Induction of labour in an attempt to prevent shoulder dystocia will not achieve its aim, even in cases where the fetus is suspected to be macrosomic (birth weight suspected to be > 4.5 kg) (Irion and Boulvain 2004). There is some evidence that induction of labour for suspected macrosomia in women with diabetes may reduce the incidence of shoulder dystocia and macrosomia but there is no evidence of a reduction in maternal or neonatal morbidity (Irion and Boulvain 2004).

Shoulder dystocia can only be prevented by elective caesarean section but this is not recommended as a method of reducing potential perinatal morbidity, even in cases of suspected macrosomia, in the absence of diabetes, as the method of assessing fetal weight is subject to considerable error and most large babies are born without shoulder dystocia (Naef and Martin 1995).

The evidence shows that in cases of suspected macrosomia, performing an elective LSCS in an attempt to prevent shoulder dystocia will significantly increase the CS rate and add millions of pounds to the health care budget, but will not improve maternal or fetal outcome. Another important aspect to consider is that such a policy would subject large numbers of women to unnecessary surgery and expose them to the increased risks associated with such delivery, without any recordable benefit. CS should be considered for women with diabetes (see Case 13) and suspected fetal macrosomia or if the estimated fetal weight is greater than 4.5 kg without diabetes (Draycott et al. 2005).

It is clear that efforts to reduce the numbers of shoulder dystocia cases and any resulting OBPPI have to date been unsuccessful (Mackenzie et al. 2007; Sandmire and DeMott 2008) and that induction of labour or birth by CS are not feasible options. Adherence to these options would appear therefore to be grounded in defensive practice intended to protect the clinician.

There is good evidence to indicate that OBPPI may have occurred well before the midwife or the doctor attempts to assist the birth of the baby (Gherman 2002; Gherman et al. 2006). This is important to consider from a medico-legal perspective in an increasingly litigious NHS. It is also worth bearing in mind that the rise in CS globally and better education of midwives and doctors through regular skills and drills training (Crofts et al. 2006, 2007, 2008a, 2008b) have not resulted in a reduction in OBPPI. Moreover, studies have shown that the number of LSCS would increase by over 2000 to prevent a single permanent injury following shoulder dystocia (Rouse and Owen 1999).

Despite the relationship between excessive fetal size and shoulder dystocia, the majority of babies will birth without complication and estimation of fetal size is therefore not a good predictor of shoulder dystocia. The problem here is that clinical fetal weight estimation is unreliable, with at least a 10 per cent margin for error for actual birth weight and a sensitivity of just 60 per cent for macrosomia (over 4.5kgs) (Rouse and Owen 1999).

It can be concluded that many of the risk indicators described in the literature have a poor positive predictive value and do not play a useful part in the predication of shoulder dystocia (Gherman 2002). In the absence of effective predictive indicators, it is not possible to prevent most cases of shoulder dystocia.

6 **What is the first-line management of shoulder dystocia?**

A As stated earlier, shoulder dystocia is a serious maternal emergency that is both rare and largely unpredictable. Antenatal risk factors provide an imprecise assessment of the likely occurrence of the problem during labour, thus its presentation in the majority of cases is unexpected. Shoulder dystocia has grave implications for the physical, psychological well-being of the mother (Athukorala et al. 2006) as well as for fetal and neonatal morbidity/ mortality. In the UK, midwives are the lead professionals in attendance in the majority of vaginal births and will play a key role in the management of shoulder dystocia. All midwives working as pivotal members of the interprofessional team should have a mental plan of action, one that reflects a systematic approach to management, gives direction in a crisis, and converts terror to a reasoned response.

All practitioners involved in intrapartum care should be ready with a defined, pre-determined and clearly structured algorithm or clinical guideline of what to do when faced with the challenge of shoulder dystocia. Historical Confidential Enquiry into Stillbirths and Deaths in Infancy reports (DH 1998, 1999) support this axiom, recommending that all maternity units must have a 'drill' for action when shoulder dystocia occurs, and this 'drill' should be frequently practised to maintain skills and competence as highlighted by the SaFE randomized controlled study team (Crofts et al. 2006). Nonetheless, it should be remembered that care plans, clinical guidelines and 'fire-drills' are only adjuncts to effective care. They cannot and should not substitute for good clinical judgement (Nocon 2000).

Given that Anna is birthing her baby in a MLU, the midwife should consider simple external manoeuvres first such as 'all fours' position or Gaskin manoeuvre (Bruner et al. 1998) (Figure 14.1a) or McRoberts' technique (Figure 14.1b) accompanied by suprapubic pressure (Figure 14.1c) before trying any of the internal manoeuvres (Figures 14.1d and 14.1e). These figures outline the external and internal manoeuvres that are internationally recognized and recommended for the management of shoulder dystocia.

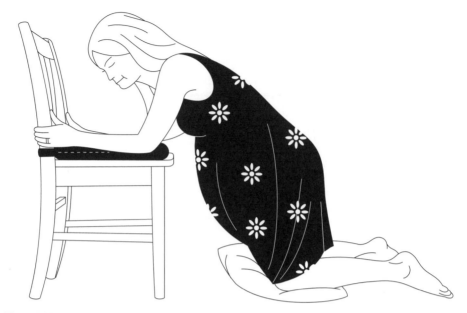

Figure 14.1a All fours i.e. kneeling position or the Gaskin manoeuvre

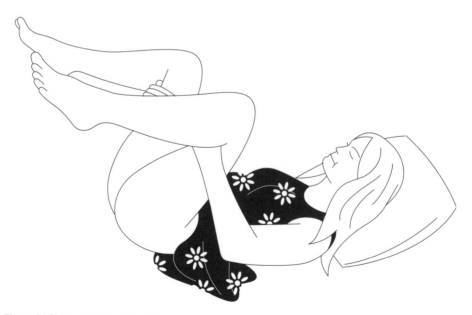

Figure 14.1b The McRoberts' technique

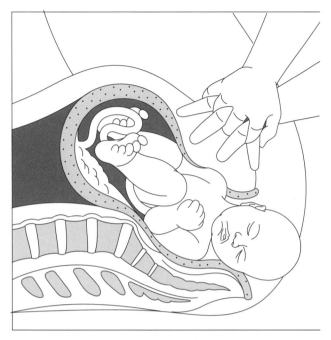

Figure 14.1c Hand position to affect suprapubic pressure. The hand is clasped similar to that used when performing adult cardiac massage during CPR. It is important to position the hands over the suprapubic area where the back is located.

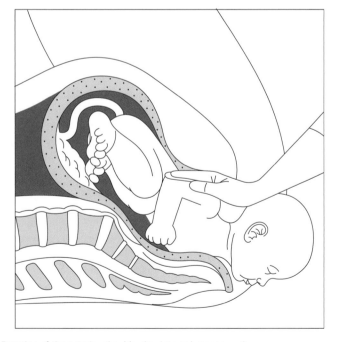

Figure 14.1d Rotation of the anterior shoulder (an internal manoeuvre)

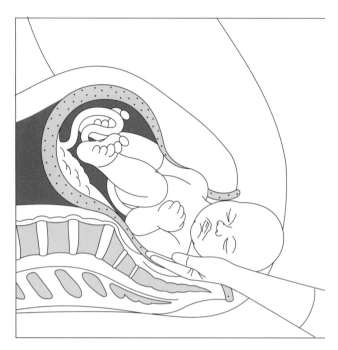

Figure 14.1e Gaining access to the pelvis where the space is usually greatest, i.e. the hollow of the sacrum, and removing the posterior arm.

7 **What is the second-line management of shoulder dystocia?**

A Second-line management of shoulder dystocia includes evaluating the need for episiotomy, internal manoeuvres and a further change in maternal position.

It is important to consider that an episiotomy will not relieve the bony obstruction and that, in most cases, the shoulder dystocia will be overcome using the McRoberts' manoeuvre and suprapubic pressure alone (Gherman et al. 1998). It should usually be considered at the point at which internal manoeuvres are required. In many cases access to the vagina can be gained without the need for an episiotomy and therefore this intervention may not be necessary and is not mandatory (Gurewitsch et al. 2004; Draycott et al. 2005).

8 **Which actions are to be avoided in the management of shoulder dystocia?**

A *Do not* attempt to prevent shoulder dystocia by laying the woman flat(ter) during a vaginal birth or by adopting prophylactic McRoberts'. There is no evidence that prophylactic McRoberts' is effective in preventing traction force (Poggi et al. 2004), shoulder dystocia or neonatal injury. Laying the woman flat without hyperflexing the legs can reduce the angle of the pelvis at the outlet and decrease the available anterior space as it causes a downward displacement of the symphysis pubis by 1–1.5 cm (Borell and Fernstrom 1957). When the mother is lying in a supine position, the movement of the sacrum and coccyx are restricted (McGeown 2001). When the legs are hyperflexed as part of McRoberts' technique (Figure 14.1b), the coccyx will lift off the bed, allowing more room posteriorly, and in addition there will be a flattening of the sacrum and a significant increase in the angle of inclination between the top of the symphysis and the top of the sacral promontory as a result of a marked cephalad rotation of the symphysis pubis (Gherman et al. 2000).

Any attempt to adopt the McRoberts' position when there are too few staff to assist with holding the legs in position will make the accoucher vulnerable to criticism if the baby is subsequently born with an OBPPI. McRoberts' technique is a recommended first-line management of shoulder dystocia and can only be applied if the legs are effectively hyper-flexed and the mother is laid flat (Draycott et al. 2005) and for this to be achieved, assistance will usually be required.

The adoption of prophylactic McRoberts' technique can cause problems when auditing the incidence and management of shoulder dystocia and, probably more importantly, subject women to an undignified and uncomfortable position without justification.

Do not hesitate to identify shoulder dystocia and to call for assistance. Attempting to free the shoulders by making a further attempt to pull on the head when resistance has been encountered can increase the obstruction at the pelvic outlet and may increase the risk of OBPPI if the anterior shoulder has not rotated into the pelvic outlet.

Once shoulder dystocia has been diagnosed, do not attempt further traction until recog-nized manoeuvres are in place. An instinctive human reaction to any difficulty is to try harder. With shoulder dystocia, this can translate into the application of increasingly forceful traction as the accoucher attempts to overcome the obstruction and complete the birth. Any traction that is applied in an effort to pull the shoulder free from the bony pelvis could increase the pressure on the brachial plexus, which will already be stretched within the pelvis (Sandmire and DeMott 2008), thus risking OBPPI (Baskett and Allen 1995). Although there is evidence to show that the incidence of OBPPI has remained unchanged despite the introduction of skills and drills training and the emphasis on avoidance of strong traction (Crofts et al. 2006; Mackenzie et al. 2007; Sandmire and DeMott 2008), it is counterintuitive to consider that the application of such traction could not increase the pressure on an already stretched brachial plexus and so it should always be avoided.

Do not encourage the mother to push, as this will not resolve the shoulder dystocia and may result in further impaction of the shoulder (Gonik et al. 2003). Pushing should only be encouraged when the shoulders are free of the bony pelvis and the birth is proceeding.

Do not attempt to grade the amount of traction that is applied during a birth complicated by shoulder dystocia. All traction should be comparable with the traction used to guide the baby from the vagina during a normal uncomplicated birth and should be ceased immediately if there is any evidence of resistance. Any traction that can be graded as stronger than guiding traction is inconsistent with reasonable practice and should not be used.

Do not leave the scribe to decide what actions are being taken and when. Tell the scribe what is happening as this will avoid misunderstandings and discrepancies in the notes.

Do not use fundal pressure; this can further increase the impaction of the shoulders and cause neonatal/maternal injury resulting in short- or long-term morbidity (DH 1998).

9 **How would you account for the maternal and fetal/neonatal morbidity associated with shoulder dystocia?**

A For the mother: shoulder dystocia carries a high burden of risk for both psychological and physical trauma (Athukorala et al. 2006), due to:

1 *PPH*: This presents the greatest danger to the mother following shoulder dystocia, with a reported incidence at 11 per cent (Gherman et al. 1997). The haemorrhage rate is

associated with uterine atony resulting from the delay in the birth but can also result from trauma to the cervix, vagina or rectum.

2   *Trauma*: Perineal trauma, including third and fourth degree tears, have been reported following shoulder dystocia.

3   *Psychological impact*: Although it is not possible to quantify, there seems little doubt that the added maternal anxiety arising from a traumatic birth, personal injury and the grief associated with neonatal injury or loss is a source of maternal morbidity (Piper and McDonald 1994).

For the fetus/neonate:

1   *Asphyxia*: Neonatal asphyxia complicates 5.7–9.7 per cent of shoulder dystocia cases (DH 1998).

2   *OBPPI*: This is associated with shoulder dystocia and the quoted rates of incidence vary. OBPPI as a complication of vaginal birth is a rare event, occurring in 0.9 per cent of all births (Perlow et al. 1996) and there is some evidence that the rate is increasing (Mollberg et al. 2005) or remaining constant over time (Gurewitsch et al. 2006; Mackenzie et al. 2007). There is little evidence to suggest a fall in the rate, although one trial has described this (Draycott et al. 2008). Why the rate of OBPPI has not fallen has so far not been explained satisfactorily. In a large retrospective analysis of births between 1954–1959 and 1987–1991, the OBPPI rate was 0.10 per cent, despite the fact that the LSCS rate rose from 5 per cent to 20 per cent over the same period (Graham et al. 1997).

  Transient OBPPI is more common than permanent and will usually resolve within 6 months of the birth. Permanent OBPPI is rare, occurring in 2 per 10,000 births (Sandmire and DeMott 2008).

3   *Fractures*: Fractures of the clavicle and humerus have been identified following shoulder dystocia and usually heal well without long-term complications. Again there is variation in the rates quoted in the literature and overall fracture rates of 5.1 per cent have been quoted (Baskett and Allen 1995). In another study, clavicular fracture rates as high as 9.5 per cent and humeral fracture rates of 4.2 per cent have been quoted (Gherman et al. 1998).

10 **Documentation is important in all cases of shoulder dystocia. From a medico-legal perspective, how would you justify this statement?**

A Accurate, legible, timely and concise record keeping in all cases of shoulder dystocia is paramount, not least from a medico-legal, risk management and clinical governance perspective. Indeed, it could be argued that in an increasingly litigious society, the best defence in any litigation case involving shoulder dystocia or any other maternity emergency is the considered and intelligent decision-making actions taken and documented during the course of management. All NHS Trusts in the UK are required to have a robust system of record keeping and communication, a requirement of CNST Standard 4, set by the NHSLA (2011).

  After managing the shoulder dystocia in Anna's case, the interprofessional team should strive to learn lessons from the critical incident through a thorough review. Reflection and discussion on what happened via appraisal of the documentation will help the team identify any gaps in knowledge and practice, and more generally, help pinpoint any other key issues for further improvement. Shoulder dystocia may also trigger a medico-legal investigation especially if the outcome for the neonate is poor. It is good practice to allocate a scribe once shoulder dystocia is diagnosed and help arrives in the form of the maternity emergency team. A proforma such as the one devised by the RCOG (Draycott et al. 2005) and detailed in Appendix 14.1 helps to provide structure, standardization and a systematic approach to documentation, to ensure no salient aspect of record keeping is omitted.

Getting together soon after managing the critical incident to review the records helps the team to employ a consistent and joined-up approach to documenting step by step the sequence of events that unfolded. All entries must be made *as contemporaneously as reasonably possible*, signed with no omissions. This will avoid discrepancies in documentation between what the allocated scribe writes, entries made by the midwife, obstetrician, student, paediatrician/neonatologist and other members of the interprofessional team. The team should also document any recommendation(s) that could be useful for the planning of future births as well as for medico-legal reasons (DH 1998, 1999; Draycott et al. 2005). The details of the documentation should account for all the areas outlined in Table 14.1.

Table 14.1 Record-keeping checklist

	What to document – do write	
Timings:	Position of the fetal head/back during labour e.g. ROA/LOA. Birth of the baby's head coupled with the recognition of the problem + which shoulder emerged first, i.e. anterior or posterior.	✓
	Time interval between birth of the head and body.	✓
	Help summoned; arrival of the team and their designation. Details of exact timings of the corrective manoeuvre(s) employed, which should include:	✓
	☛ Who did what?	✓
	☛ At what time?	✓
	☛ For how long?	✓
Description of the corrective manoeuvres employed	☛ Position change?	✓
	☛ McRoberts' manoeuvre by whom and who held which leg.	✓
	☛ Which aspect of the maternal abdomen was the fetal back palpated/located + position of the fetal shoulders/arms.	✓
	☛ When was suprapubic pressure employed, from which side and by whom + was it applied from behind/the back of the fetal anterior shoulder?	✓
	☛ Sequence/order/timing of any internal manoeuvres employed and who effected the intervention(s).	✓
	☛ Was it necessary to perform an episiotomy? If yes, or no, is the rationale clearly stated?	✓
An estimate of the traction forces that were exerted	Evidence provided by Crofts et al. (2006, 2007, 2008a, 2008b) highlights the importance of being very aware of the damage that can be caused by excess traction.	
	☛ Was any initial force used to free the shoulders before dystocia was recognized? Use measurable terms such as 'normal' as this reflects the norm or non-forced traction that would be used at any vaginal birth.	✓

(Continued overleaf)

Table 14.1 Continued

	What to document – do write	
Details of any injuries to mother and baby	☞ Is fetal outcome clearly stated including Apgars, resuscitative measures, and results of the analysis of paired cord blood samples?	✓
	☞ Details of any fetal weight estimation antenatally and how does it compare to the actual birth weight?	✓
	☞ Details of thorough neonatal examination performed by a neonatologist/paediatrician immediately after birth to detect birth injuries, e.g. OBPPI. If evidence of Erb's palsy it is vital to state the position of the affected shoulder at the time of birth, i.e. anterior or posterior.	✓
	☞ Is there evidence of maternal analgesia during the management process?	✓
	☞ Details of meticulous inspection of the woman's genital tract, identification, classification and early repair of any genital tract trauma (including who performed the repair, timing, location, post-repair analgesia and health education advice).	✓
	☞ EBL (including postpartum haemorrhage).	✓
	☞ Evidence of any bladder trauma, catheterization and after care.	✓
Measures to limit psychological sequelae should be explicit, the records should account for details of the psychosocial support provided for the woman and her birth companion during and after the crisis (DH 1998, 1999).		
	What not to document – do not write	
Avoid ambiguous statements	☞ Subjective entries, e.g. 'moderate shoulder dystocia'.	X
	☞ 'Tight fit', when what is meant is baby's head advances slowly with difficulty freeing the face from the vagina with evidence of 'turtling sign'.	X
	☞ 'Difficulty with shoulders corrected by strong traction' (Mahran et al. 2008), when what is meant is shoulder dystocia corrected by one of the recognized manoeuvres, which must be stated.	X
	☞ 'Fundal pressure' employed when what is really meant is suprapubic pressure.	X
	☞ 'Extended perineal laceration which has been repaired', when what is actually meant is a 3a, 3b, 3c or 4th degree tear that fits with the classification of NICE (2007).	X
Avoid unnecessary morbidity: do not use fundal pressure or increasingly forceful traction on the fetal head. These actions are associated with OBPPI (Crofts et al. 2007; Draycott et al. 2008).		

COMMUNICATION

Poor communication is perhaps the single most common reason for complaints in the NHS and maternity care in general (NHSLA 2011). White et al. (2005) identify communication problems are attributable to 1:7 legal claims in the maternity sector. Reasons for adverse outcomes in shoulder dystocia are complex and multifaceted and have been linked to diverse factors, not only communication difficulties. However, poor teamwork coupled with poor interpersonal relationships within the interprofessional team may culminate in poor outcomes (Smith and Dixon 2007). Like all women, effective communication will be essential to Anna's satisfaction with care (Barker et al. 2005; White et al. 2005; Draycott and Crofts 2006; Redshaw and Heikkila 2010).

Check point

Effective communication and thorough documentation help in risk management, quality assurance, and the sharpening of interprofessional relationships and interpersonal skills, especially in cases of shoulder dystocia (Draycott 2006; Crofts 2008b).

CASE REVIEW

The birth of Anna's baby girl, Adele, was complete with the removal of the posterior arm by the attending midwife. Baby Adele emerged pale and floppy needing advanced CPR by the neonatal team. She was later transferred to the NICU with a suspected fractured clavicle. Anna had a 2nd degree perineal laceration that was promptly repaired and an EBL of 600 mL.

Summary of key points

- Shoulder dystocia is largely a rare, unpreventable and unpredictable maternity emergency.
- Shoulder dystocia imposes a high risk of injury to mother and baby of both a psychological and physical nature (Athukorala et al. 2006).
- The rarity of shoulder dystocia demands preparedness to manage it well at all vaginal births. As shoulder dystocia is a rare and largely unpredictable event, all staff should be regularly trained to recognize and manage it in accordance with national and local guidelines.
- Shoulder dystocia requires prompt recognition plus intelligent, skilful and timely management, which includes execution of the well-recognized and rehearsed manoeuvres, as these can be life-saving.
- All labour suites should have a clear evidence-based and up-to-date guideline on the management of shoulder dystocia (DH 1998, 1999; NHSLA 2011).
- Experienced members of the interprofessional team should be notified whenever shoulder dystocia is anticipated/recognized during a vaginal birth.
- OBPPI is often the result of intrinsic factors unrelated to the actual facilitation of the vaginal birth.
- Clear, accurate, contemporaneous, systematic, concise and consistent documentation is perhaps the single best defence in any medico-legal case involving shoulder dystocia.

Appendix 14.1 Shoulder dystocia proforma to assist with systematic documentation

SHOULDER DYSTOCIA

Date ....

Delivery of head   Spontaneous ☐   Instrumental ☐

Registrar called   Yes ☐   No ☐   Time Registrar called............. Arrived...................................

Senior midwife called   Yes ☐   No ☐   Time .... Arrived ....

Paediatrician called   Yes ☐   No ☐   Time .... Arrived ....

PROCEDURE USED TO ASSIST DELIVERY OF THE SHOULDERS

	Tick	Order	Time	Performed by (print name)
McRoberts' manoeuvre	☐	☐	....	....
Suprapubic pressure and routine traction*	☐	☐	....	....
Evaluation for episiotomy (reason if not performed)	☐	☐	....	....
Episiotomy	☐	☐	....	....
Delivery of posterior arm	☐	☐	....	....
Wood screw manoeuvre	☐	☐	....	....
Mother on all fours/other	☐	☐	....	....

Time of delivery of head ....   **Time of delivery of body** ....

At Delivery: Head facing mother's Left ☐   **Head facing mother's right** ☐

FETAL CONDITION

Weight ....kg   **Apgar**   1 minute ☐   5 minutes ☐   10 minutes ☐

Cord pH: Arterial .... Venous..............
Paediatric assessment at delivery..
....
....

* Routine traction refers to the traction required for delivery of the shoulders in a normal vaginal delivery
  where there is no difficulty with the shoulders.

Signed.. Print name...

REFERENCES

Athukorala, C., Middleton, P. and Crowther, C.A. (2006) Intrapartum interventions for preventing shoulder dystocia, *Cochrane Database of Systematic Reviews*. Issue 4. Art. No.: CD005543. DOI: 10.1002/14651858.CD005543.pub2.

Barker, S.R., Choi, P.Y.L. and Henshaw, C.A. (2005) 'I felt as though I'd been in jail': women's experiences of maternity care during labour, delivery and the immediate postpartum, *Feminism Psychology*, 15(3): 315–42.

Baskett, T.F. and Allen, A.C. (1995) Perinatal implications of shoulder dystocia, *Obstetrics and Gynecology*, 86(1): 14–17.

Benedetti, T.J. and Gabbe, S.G. (1978) Shoulder dystocia: a complication of fetal macrosomia and prolonged second stage of labour with midpelvic delivery, *Obstetrics and Gynecology*, 52(5): 526–9.

Borrell, U. and Fernstrom, I. (1957) A pelvimetric method for the assessment of pelvic mouldability. *Acta Radiol*, 47: 365–70, cited in R.B. Gherman, J.Tramont, P. Muffley, T. Goodwin, and M. Murphy (2000) Analysis of McRoberts' manoever by X-ray pelvimetry, *Obstetrics and Gynecology*, 95(1): 43–7.

Boulvain, M., Stan, C.M. and Irion, O. (2001) Elective delivery in diabetic pregnant women, *Cochrane Database of Systematic Reviews*; Issue 2. Art. No.: CD001997. DOI: 10.1002/14651858. CD001997.

Bruner, J.P., Drummond, S., Meenan, A.L. and Gaskin, I.M. (1998) All-fours maneuver for reducing shoulder dystocia during labor, *Journal of Reproductive Medicine*, 43(5): 439–43.

Crofts, J.F., Bartlett, C., Ellis, D., Fox, R. and Draycott, T.J. (2008a) Documentation of simulated shoulder dystocia: accurate and complete? *BJOG: An International Journal of Obstetrics and Gynaecology*, 115(10): 1303–8.

Crofts, J.F., Bartlett, C., Ellis, D., Hunt, L.P., Fox, R. and Draycott, T.J. (2006) Training for shoulder dystocia: a trial of simulation using low-fidelity and high-fidelity mannequins, *Obstetrics and Gynecology*, 108(6): 1477–85.

Crofts, J.F., Ellis, D., Draycott, T.J., Winter, C., Hunt, L.P. and Akande, V.A. (2007) Change in knowledge of midwives and obstetricians following obstetric emergency training – a randomised controlled trial of local hospital, simulation centre and team work training, *BJOG: An International Journal of Obstetrics and Gynaecology*, 114(12): 1534–41.

Crofts, J.F., Fox, R., Ellis, D., Winter, C., Hinshaw, K. and Draycott, T.J. (2008b) Observations from 450 shoulder dystocia simulations: lessons for skills training, *Obstetrics and Gynecology*, 112(4): 906–12.

Department of Health (DH) (1998) *Confidential Enquiry into Stillbirths and Deaths in Infancy: Fifth Annual Report*. London: Maternal and Child Health Research Consortium

Department of Health (DH) (1999) *Confidential Enquiry into Stillbirths and Deaths in Infancy: Sixth Annual Report*. London: Maternal and Child Health Research Consortium.

Draycott, T.J. and Crofts, J.F. (2006) Structured team training in obstetrics and its impact on outcome, *Fetal and Medicine Review*, 17(3): 229–37.

Draycott, T.J., Ash, J.P., Wilson, L.V., Yard, E., Sibana, T. and Whitelaw, A. (2008) Improving neonatal outcome through practical shoulder dystocia training, *Obstetrics and Gynaecology*, 112(1): 14–20.

Draycott, T.J., Fox, R. and Montague, I.A. (2005) *Shoulder Dystocia*. Green Top Guideline No. 42. London: RCOG. Available at: http://www.rcog.org.uk (accessed 10 April 2011).

Gherman, R.B. (2002) Shoulder dystocia: an evidence-based evaluation of the obstetric nightmare, *Clinical Obstetrics and Gynecology*, 45(2): 345–62.

Gherman, R.B., Chauhan, S., Ouzounian, J.G., Lerner, H., Gonik, B. and Goodwin, T.M. (2006) Shoulder dystocia: the unpreventable obstetric emergency with empiric management guidelines, *American Journal of Obstetrics and Gynecology*, 195(3): 657–72.

Gherman, R.B., Goodwin, T.M., Souter, I., Neumann, K., Ouzounian, J.G. and Paul, R.H. (1997) The McRoberts maneuver for the alleviation of shoulder dystocia: how successful is it? *American Journal of Obstetrics and Gynecology*, 176(3):656–61.

Gherman, R.B., Ouzounian, J.G. and Goodwin, T.M. (1998) Obstetric maneuvres for shoulder dystocia and associated fetal morbidity, *American Journal of Obstetric and Gynecology*, 178(6): 1126–30.

Gherman, R.B., Tramont, J., Muffley, P., Goodwin, T. and Murphy, M. (2000) Analysis of McRoberts' manoever by X-ray pelvimetry, *Obstetrics and Gynecology*, 95(1): 43–7.

Gonik, B., Walker, A. and Grimm, M. (2000) Mathematic modelling of forces associated with shoulder dystocia: a comparison of endogenous and exogenous sources, *American Journal of Obstetric and Gynecology*, 182(3): 689–91.

Gonik, B., Zhang, N. and Grimm, M.J. (2003) Defining forces that are associated with shoulder dystocia: the use of a mathematic dynamic computer model, *American Journal of Obstetric and Gynecology*, 188(4): 1068–72.

Graham, E.M., Forouzan, I. and Morgan, M. (1997) A retrospective analysis of Erb's Palsy cases and their relation to birth weight and trauma at delivery, *The Journal of Maternal-fetal Medicine*, 6(1): 1–5.

Gupta, M., Hockley, C., Quigley, M.A., Yeh, P., and Impey, L. (2010) Antenatal and intrapartum prediction of shoulder dystocia, *European Journal of Obstetrics and Gynecology and Reproductive Biology*, 151(2): 134–9.

Gurewitsch, E.D., Donithan, H., Stallings, S., Moore, P.L., Agarwal, S., Allen, L.M and Allen, R.H. (2004) Episiotomy versus fetal manipulation maneuvers in managing severe shoulder dystocia: a comparison of outcomes, *American Journal of Obstetrics and Gynecology*, 191(3): 911–16.

Gurewitsch, E.D., Johnson, E., Hamzehzadeh, S. and Allen, R.H. (2006) Risk factors for brachial plexus injury with and without shoulder dystocia, *American Journal of Obstetrics and Gynecology*, 2(194): 486–92.

Irion, O. and Boulvain, M. (2004) Induction of labour for suspected fetal macrosomia, *Cochrane Database of Systematic Reviews*; Issue 2. Art. No.: CD000938. DOI: 10.1002/14651858. CD000938.

Lewis, D.F., Edwards, M.S., Asrat, T., Adair, C.D., Brooks, G. and London, S. (1998) Can shoulder dystocia be predicted? Preconceptual and prenatal factors, *Journal of Reproductive Medicine*, 43(8): 654–8.

Mackenzie, I.Z., Shah, M., Lean, K., Dutton, S., Newdick, H. and Tucker, D.E. (2007) Management of shoulder dystocia: trends in incidence and maternal morbidity, *Obstetrics and Gynecology*, 110(5): 1059–68.

Mahran, M.A., Sayed, A.T. and Imoh-Ita, F. (2008) Avoiding over-diagnosis of shoulder dystocia, *Journal of Obstetrics and Gynaecology*, 28(2): 173–6.

McGeown, P. (2001) Practice recommendations for obstetric emergencies, *British Journal of Midwifery*, 9(2): 71–4.

Mollberg, M., Hagberg, H., Bager, B., Hakan, L. and Ladfors, L. (2005) High birth weight and shoulder dystocia: the strongest risk factors for Obstetric Plexus Palsy in a Swedish population based study, *Acta Obstetricia et Gynecoligica Scandinavica*, 84(7): 654–9.

Naef, R.W. and Martin, J.N. (1995) Emergent management of shoulder dystocia, *Obstetrics and Gynecology Clinics of North America*, 22(2): 247–9.

National Health Service Litigation Authority (2011) *Clinical Negligence Scheme for Trusts: Maternity Clinical Risk Management Standards*, Version 1 2011/12. Available at: http://www.nhsla.com (accessed 20 April 2011).

National Institute for Health and Clinical Excellence (2007) *Intrapartum Care: Care of Healthy Women and Their Babies During Childbirth*. Clinical Guideline No. 55: London: NICE.

Nesbitt, T.S., Gilbert, W.M. and Herrchen, B. (1998) Shoulder dystocia and associated risk factors with macrosomic infants born in California, *American Journal of Obstetrics Gynecology*, 179(2): 476–80.

Nocon, J. (2000) Shoulder dystocia and macrosomia, in L.H. Kean, P.N. Baker and D.I. Edelstone (eds) *Best Practice in Labor Ward Management*, 1st edn. Edinburgh: WB Saunders, pp. 167–86.

Nocon, J.J. and Weisbrod, L. (1995) Shoulder dystocia, in J.P. O'Grady, M.L. Gimovsky and C.J. McIlhargie (eds) *Operative Obstetrics*. Baltimore, MD: Williams and Wilkins, pp. 339–53.

Nocon, J.J., McKenzie, D.K., Thomas, L.J. and Hansell, R.S. (1993) Shoulder dystocia: an analysis of risks and obstetric maneuvers, *American Journal of Obstetrics and Gynecology*, 168(6 Pt 1): 1732–9.

Perlow, J.H., Wigton, T., Hart, J., Strassner, H.T., Nageotte, M.P. and Wolk, B.M. (1996) Birth trauma: a five year review of incidence and associated perinatal factor, *Journal of Reproductive Medicine*, 41(10): 754–60.

Piper, M. and McDonald, P. (1994) Management of anticipated and actual shoulder dystocia: interpreting the literature, *Journal of Nurse-Midwifery*, 39(2) (Suppl. 1): S91–S105.

Poggi, S.H., Allen, R.H., Patel, C.R., Ghidini, A., Pezzullo, J.C. and Spong, C.Y. (2004) Randomized trial of McRoberts' versus lithotomy positioning to decrease the force that is applied to the fetus during delivery, *American Journal of Obstetrics and Gynecology*, 191(3): 874–8.

Redshaw, M. and Heikkila, K. (2010) *Delivered with Care: A National Survey of Women's Experience of Maternity Care 2010*. Available at: http://www.npeu.ox.ac.uk/maternitysurveys (accessed 20 April 2011).

Rouse, D.J. and Owen, J. (1999) Prophylactic caesarean delivery for fetal macrosomia diagnosed by means of ultrasonography: a Faustian bargain? *American Journal of Obstetrics and Gynecology*, 181(2): 332–8.

Sandmire, H.F. and DeMott, R.K. (2008) Newborn brachial plexus palsy, *Journal of Obstetrics and Gynaecology*, 28(6): 567–72.

Sandmire, H.F. and DeMott, R.K. (2009) Controversies surrounding the causes of brachial plexus injury, *International Journal of Gynecology and Obstetrics*, 104(1): 9–13.

Smith, A. and Dixon, A. (2007) *The Safety of Maternity Services in England*. London: King's Fund.

Stirrat, G. and Taylor, R. (2002) Mechanisms of obstetric brachial plexus palsy: a critical analysis, *Clinical Risks*, 8(6): 218–22.

White, A.A., Pitchert, J.W., Bledsoe, S.H., Irwin, C. and Entman, S.S. (2005) Cause and effect analysis of closed claims in obstetrics and gynaecology, *Obstetrics and Gynecology*, 105(5–part 1): 1031–8.

ANNOTATED FURTHER READING

Breeze, A.C.G. and Lees, C.C. (2004) Managing shoulder dystocia, *The Lancet*, 364(9452): 2160–1.

A useful review of the management of shoulder dystocia.

Gurewitsch, E.D., Kim, E.J., Yang, J.H., Outland, K.E., McDonald, M.K. and Allen, R.H. (2005) Comparing McRoberts' and Rubin's maneuvers for initial management of shoulder dystocia: an objective evaluation, *American Journal of Obstetrics and Gynecology*, 192: 153–60.

An evaluative piece on the value of some corrective manoeuvres employed in the management of shoulder dystocia.

Hope, P., Breslin, S., Lamont, L., Lucas, A., Martin, D., Moore, I., Pearson, J., Saunders, D. and Settatree, R. (1998) Fatal shoulder dystocia: a review of 56 cases reported to the Confidential Enquiry into Stillbirths and Deaths in Infancy, *BJOG: An International Journal of Obstetrics and Gynaecology*, 105: 1256–61. DOI: 10.1111/j.1471-0528.1998.tb10003.x.

An informative read for learning lessons from poor outcomes.

King's Fund (2008) *Safe Births: Everybody's Business. Independent Inquiry into the Safety of Maternity Services in England.* London: King's Fund. Available at: http://www.kingsfund.org.uk (accessed 20 April 2011).

An insightful report that addresses the importance of balancing risks and safety in maternity care through effective team working, leadership and training.

USEFUL WEBSITES

http://www.erbspalsy.ie/	Erb's Palsy Association of Ireland
http://www.erbspalsygroup.co.uk/	Erb's Palsy Group, UK
http://www.kingsfund.org.uk	King's Fund
http://www.nhsla.com	National Health Service Litigation Authority
http://www.npeu.ox.ac.uk	National Perinatal Epidemiology Unit
http://www.rcm.org.uk	Royal College of Midwives
http://www.rcog.org.uk	Royal College of Obstetricians and Gynaecologists

Index

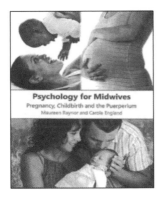

PSYCHOLOGY FOR MIDWIVES

Maureen Raynor and Carole England

9780335234332 (Paperback)
2010

eBook also available

"Psychology for Midwives is an excellent aid in grasping the key concepts of psychology in a focused way, clearly demonstrating how the key concepts can be used within modern day midwifery practice settings. This is an easy to use, informative guide, with up to date sources of evidence."
Kimberley Skinner, Student Midwife, Anglia Ruskin University, UK

Key features:

- Addresses many core concepts and principles of psychology
- Provides simple explanations for why psychological care matters in midwifery practice
- Contains reflective questions, activities, illustrations, tables, summary boxes and a glossary help readers navigate the book

www.openup.co.uk

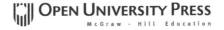

OPEN UNIVERSITY PRESS
McGraw - Hill Education

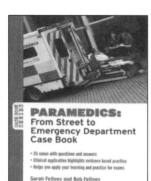
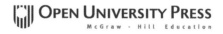

NURSING THE ACUTELY ILL ADULT CASE BOOK

Karen Page and Aidin McKinney

9780335243099 (Paperback)
October 2012

eBook also available

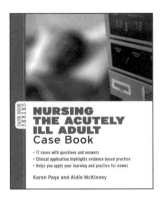

This book takes a unique case study approach to teaching and learning. It comprises of a number of case scenarios which focus on the care of the acutely ill adult. This text will help students integrate their knowledge of pathophysiology, pharmacology and nursing care so they can apply it in professional practice.

Key features:

- 20 realistic case scenarios including asthma, strokes, liver failure and burns which link theory to practice
- Assists students to integrate their understanding of pathophysiology, pharmacology and nursing skills
- Packed with Q&A's, further resources, and learning tools in order to track and further learning

www.openup.co.uk

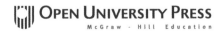

MENTAL HEALTH NURSING CASE BOOK

Nick Wrycraft

9780335242955 (Paperback)
September 2012

eBook also available

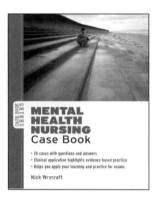

Part of the case book series, this unique book contains a wide range of mental health diagnoses from common problems such as anxiety or depression through to severe and enduring conditions such as schizophrenia. The practical cases link theory to practice and their grounding in reality will really help bring the subject to life.

Key features:

- Cases are organised into sections by life stage from childhood through to old age
- Considers the biological, psychological, social and physical aspects of each scenario featured
- Takes a positive, person centred approach focusing on recovery outcomes

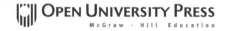

www.openup.co.uk

OPEN UNIVERSITY PRESS
McGraw - Hill Education